HPV: A Handbook to Infections with Human Papillomavirus

HPV: A Handbook to Infections with Human Papillomavirus

Edited by Luna Jefferson

hayle medical

New York

Hayle Medical,
750 Third Avenue, 9th Floor,
New York, NY 10017, USA

Visit us on the World Wide Web at:
www.haylemedical.com

ISBN: 978-1-63241-879-1

Cataloging-in-Publication Data

HPV : a handbook to infections with human papillomavirus / edited by Luna Jefferson.
p. cm.
Includes bibliographical references and index.
ISBN 978-1-63241-879-1
1. Papillomaviruses. 2. Papillomavirus diseases. 3. Virus diseases. I. Jefferson, Luna.
RC168.P15 H68 2020
616.911--dc23

Table of Contents

Preface

I am honored to present to you this unique book which encompasses the most up-to-date data in the field. I was extremely pleased to get this opportunity of editing the work of experts from across the globe. I have also written papers in this field and researched the various aspects revolving around the progress of the discipline. I have tried to unify my knowledge along with that of stalwarts from every corner of the world, to produce a text which not only benefits the readers but also facilitates the growth of the field.

Human papillomavirus infection is an infection caused by the human papillomavirus (HPV). HPV infection is the most prevalent sexually transmitted infection. Most HPV infections cause little to no symptoms and resolve spontaneously. An HPV infection may persist and result in warts or precancerous lesions, which can later cause cancer of the cervix, penis, vulva, vagina, anus, mouth or throat. Some of the risk factors associated with persistent HPV infections are sexual intercourse with multiple partners, poor immune function, early age of first sexual intercourse and smoking. HPV vaccines are effective in the prevention of most common infections. HPV infections can be prevented through sexual abstinence and use of condoms. The immune system clears HPV naturally within a period of two years for the majority of the cases, but it is debated whether the virus gets completely eliminated from the body or reduced to undetectable levels. This book provides comprehensive insights into human papillomavirus. It aims to shed light on the clinical aspects of human papillomavirus infections and the recent researches in this domain. Coherent flow of topics, student-friendly language and extensive use of examples make this book an invaluable source of knowledge.

Finally, I would like to thank all the contributing authors for their valuable time and contributions. This book would not have been possible without their efforts. I would also like to thank my friends and family for their constant support.

Editor

1

The Diagnostic of Cervical Carcinoma: From Theory to Practice

J. Rajčáni, K. Kajo, O. el Hassoun, M. Adamkov and M. Benčat

Abstract

Humanpapillomaviruses(HPV)arenakedparticlescomposedof72subunits,eachformed by 2 structural proteins designated L1 and L2 (L = late). HPV does not grow outside of squamous epithelium cells, in which it infects the suprabasal prickle cell layer. The viral double-stranded DNA (vDNA) has about 8 kilobase pairs (kbp) and also encodes several non-structural polypeptides, designated E1–E7 (E = early). At least 3 early oncoproteins (E5, E6, and E7) induce host cell proliferation, driving them into permanent division. During long-term latency, the circularized HPV DNA may get integrated into the host cell DNA molecule. The circular HPV DNA is then interrupted, usually within the E2 open reading frame (ORF), which then cannot exert its regulatory (feedback) effect on the early gene expression. The increased expression of E6/E7 proteins seriously affects the regulation of host cell division mainly via dysregulation of the functions of p53 and Rp proteins. HPV infects the female genital tract representing the main cause of cervical dysplasia and subsequent squamous cell carcinoma (SCa). The HPV isolates exist mainly in the form of amplified DNAs; based on the similarity and/or variations (dissimilarity) of their L1 capsid polypeptide sequence, 96 human genotypes were included into five genera of the *Papillomaviridae* family. The clinically most important genotypes that cause lesions at mucosal membranes and/or on the skin, belong mainly to the Alphapapillomavirus genus. The genotypes, associated with severe dysplastic changes and/or cervical cancer, were designated as high risk (HR-HPV). The prevalence of the integrated HPV DNA sequence over the episomal molecules appears in a proportion smears-graded LSIL (low-gradesquamousintraepitheliallesion).Lateron,carriercellsrevealingtheintegrated HPVgenomeexpressiontheoncoproteins(E6/E7)clearlyprevailespeciallyinHSIL(high-grade squamous intraepithelial lesion) smears and in the cervical cancer itself. What is crucialforthemoderndiagnosticofcervicaldysplasia,isthep16/INK4A(inhibitorkinase) polypeptide, which itself represents a form of cell defense against the viral oncogenic proteins. The p16 antigen shows a continuous parabasal staining in the CIN I lesion. If dysplastic cells occupy at least one half (or two thirds) of squamous epithelium, the designation CIN II/HSIL is correct, and at the stage of CIN III/HSIL, dysplastic cells replace the entire squamous epithelium. Another frequently used immunohistochemical marker of intraepithelial cervical dysplasia so far is the Ki-67 antigen, which occurs in the nuclei of proliferating and/or repeatedly dividing (immortalized) cells. Women revealing p16-positive ASCUS (atypical smear cells of unknown significance) as well as those showing LSIL (low-grade cytological changes) should be examined for the presence of the HPV DNA. The detection of HPV DNA alone, that is, in the absence of cytological screening, has a relatively lower prediction value, though the HR HPV positive DNA test in the absence of morphological alterations may in part predict the possible progression into malignancy. Nevertheless, only the combined cytological as well as molecular follow-up (cervical smear examined for cytology as well as for HPV DNA) is regarded for the most reliable diagnostic approach.

Keywords: Human papillomavirus, Cervical intraepithelial neoplasia (CIN), Cervical dysplasia, Squamous cell carcinoma, p16/INK4A Polypeptide, Ki-67 polypeptide, Laboratory diagnostic, PA smears, Squamous intraepithelial lesion (SIL), Liquid-based cytology (lbc), Cervical biopsy, Histology, HPV DNA testing

1. Introduction

Virus infection had been for a long time anticipated in the pathogenesis of cervical cancer. The suspected role of herpes simplex virus 2 (HSV 2) early protein as suggested by Aurelian et al. [1] was not confirmed, since several carefully designed prospective and/or serological studies following the significance of elevated anti-HSV 2 antibody levels did not confirm any association. Although certain isolated DNA fragments coming from the HSV genome may transform the tissue culture cells of rodent origin, their relevance in the induction of human cervical carcinoma has not met any further approval [2, 3]. Contemporarily, the human papillomavirus (HPV) has been accepted to represent the most probable infectious agent in respect of cervical cancer [4]. During the last decades, a great bulk of convincing data has accumulated in favor of the latter assumption, which has become widely accepted. Thus, based on substantial clinical and biological evidence, strong relationship exists between HPV infection and the development of cervical cancer. Nevertheless, in line with a few but independent observations, a hypothesis has repeatedly emerged saying that HSV 2 co-infection might represent an accelerating cofactor for cervical carcinoma formation [5]. Novel reports from Brazil and/or some other comparative studies on the given issue, which had been performed simultaneously among Indonesian and Swedish population, confirmed the possible role of HSV 2 in the former but not the in the latter geographical area [6].

Our paper reconciles the role of latent HPV infection (mainly based on the detection of corresponding DNA sequences and/or their fragments) in the stratified squamous epithelium cells of oral, vaginal, and/or anal mucosa (especially at their transition sites to cylindrical epithelium, such as uterine cervix) and/or in the keratinized squamous skin epithelium cells. Regarding to the role of the HPV genome in the pathogenesis of cervical cancer, we shall point at the importance of a complex diagnostic approach overcoming the possible barriers between scientific disciplines such as virology, pathology, and molecular biology on one hand and explain the need of the rapid application of novel achievements in diagnostic pathology, biochemistry, cytology as well as in the clinical practice. Despite of the difficulties of any interdisciplinary approach, the introduction of molecular virology (such the HPV DNA test) and immunohistochemical procedures (p16 and Ki-67 antigen detection) into diagnostic pathology and/or cytology when done in close cooperation with gynecologists has led to a dramatic decrease of the frequency of cervical cancer in several European countries, Slovakia not excluding. Reporting the frequency of positive cervical smears was registered in the terms of the conventional Papanicolaou (PA) test, which is still most suitable for large-scale screening. **Table 1** summarizes six annual reports of one of several Alpha medical Company Ltd Diagnostic Centres, which were destined for domestic insurance companies. The categories of classification of cervical dysplasia in given statistics do not correspond to the Bethesda classification system [7, 8]. According to the latter, atypical squamous cells of unknown significance (ASCUS) should be distinguished from non-neoplastic reactive changes of cervical squamous epithelium cells using the criteria summarized in **Table 2**. The squamous intraepithelial lesion (SIL) can be recognized by the presence of dysplastic cells, which show either mild (low grade) or more severe (high grade) alterations (**Table 3**). The original cytological nomenclature used to describe the appearance of cells in conventional PA smears before the introduction of Bethesda classification system has been repeatedly compared by several authors [9, 10] with the recently adopted definitions. Based on these data, we proved the individual categories of the so-called MKCH classification system (Slovak abbreviation for the expression International Classification of Diseases). To achieve an upmost precise interpretation, we used terms essentially resembling to the CIN (cervical intraepithelial lesion) classification, namely a similar three-degree scale (I—low, II—medium, and III—high). Evaluating in detail each protocol from the archives of the Pathology Diagnostic Centre of Alpha medical Company in Martin coming from a single-year period, that is, the year 2015 (compare **Table 4**), we found that the medium-grade cervical dysplasia category from the MKCH statistics in fact encompassed as many as 64% of smears-graded LSIL, while the proportion smears scored HSIL in the same category was approximately 6%. Noteworthy, another 6% fall into the group of patients with negative smears and the rest protocols revealed the diagnosis of ASCUS and/or ASC-H (in 24%). It should be mentioned that out of 516 samples of the given MKCH category, 110 had been repeatedly tested patients (these women were re-examined within 4–6 months intervals, i.e., at least twice during the same year). Thus, the MKCH category "medium-grade cervical dysplasia" consisted of 516 smears coming from 457 women. In the group of repeatedly examined patients, 10% underwent spontaneous healing during the relatively short 1-year follow-up period (data not shown). The repeatedly negative smears came mainly from patients, which were at first examination scored ASCUS. Unfortunately, their HPV DNA status is not always determined, even though in this group ("medium-grade cervical dysplasia") during the year 2015, altogether 162 of smears were tested HPV DNA, from which 74 were positive (a proportion of 39.5%), while 13 were HPV type 16 positive and 6 were HPV type 18 positive. While only 32% of screened patients were examined by cytology as well as for HPV, many HPV tests were made in the absence of cytology and/or *vice versa* (compare paragraphs 4 and 5, see also **Table 12**).

Diagnosis	Patient number		Per cent	Modified[4]
	Positive	Total examined		
Low-grade cervical dysplasia*,1	3070**	206,317	1.5%	3943 (1.9%)
Medium-grade cervical dysplasia[2]	1456		0.7%	Cancelled
High-grade cervical dysplasia[3]	263		0.13%	466 (0.23%)
ASCUS (includes also ASC-H, from low and medium dysplasias)[1,2]				230 (0.13%)
Carcinoma *in situ*	36		0.02%	No change
Cervical (spinocellular) carcinoma	16***		0.007%	No change

[1]Corresponds to LSIL (88%) and/or ASCUS (12%).[2]Corresponds to LSIL (60%), ASC-H/ASCUS (18%) and/or to HSIL (10%).[3]Corresponds to HSIL.[4]Modified according to above mentioned[1,2,3], remarks (see text for details).*Designation of given statistical categories according to author´s translation (from Slovak).**Positive smears after excluding the negative ones or those referred to as reactive changes.***Including 5 cases showing invasive growth into distant into (surrounding) tissues.#From report of Pathology Diagnostic Centre, Alpha medical Company Ltd, Martin (Slovakia) for domestic authorities (with permission).

Table 1. Frequency of cervical dysplasia and/or cervical cancer by screening of cytological smears from 1 January 2010 to 31 December 2015#.

Atypical cells of unknown significance (ASCUS)	Reactive changes due to inflammation
Size of nuclei increased significantly (three times)	Slightly enlarged nuclei (up most two times)
Cells revealing doubled nuclei may be present	
Moderately dense chromatin staining	Slight hyperchromatic staining only
The fine granular chromatin is dispersed throughout nucleus	
Nuclei may be slightly elliptic, but regularly are nearly round shaped	
The nuclear/cytoplasm ratio (N/C) in moderately increased	
	Atrophic or shrink nuclei
	The cytoplasm may be vacuolated
	Polymorphonuclear leukocytes are present
	Bacteria may be present
Koilocytes (proving HPV) can be recognized	
Hyperchomatosis, dense chromatin granules.	
The nuclear membrane has irregular appearance	
A faint perinuclear ring may be visible	

* Based on the data from corresponding manuals [11, 12].

Table 2. Definition of ASCUS versus reactive changes in cervical smears*.

LSIL	HSIL
Nuclei relatively enlarged (over three times)	Nuclei increased in size, shrink cytoplasm
	Dysplastic cells frequent, smaller in size
	The small dysplastic squamous cells form larger aggregates
The N/C ratio increased not only due to larger nuclei but also by loss of cytoplasm	
The size of nuclei varies, multiple nuclei* (larger polykaryocytes)**	
Evident hyperchromatosis, dark nuclei	
Chromatin shows irregular distribution	
Relatively fine nuclear granules	Coarse grainy chromatin
Occasionally irregular nuclear membrane	Undulate nuclear membrane
Nucleoli may be visible	Nucleoli are not seen
	The cytoplasm may show keratin granules

* Based on data from corresponding manuals [11, 12].

Table 3. Definition of low-grade versus high-grade squamous intraepitelial lesion (SIL)*.

Diagnosis	Patient number		Per cent
	Positive	Total examined	
Low-grade squamous intraepithelial lesion*	1324	37,414	3.54%
High-grade squamous intraepithelial lesion**	151		0.4%
Atypical cells of unknown significance***	231		0.621%
Carcinoma *in situ*	3		0.04%
Cervical carcinoma (SCa)[1]	2		0.005%

* LSIL ** HSIL *** ASCUS.
[1] Squamous cell carcinomas.

Table 4. The frequency of cervical dysplasia and/or cervical cancer by screening of cytological smears from 1 January 2015 to 31 December 2015.

Alternatively, we analyzed a proportion of still available original protocols from a limited number of women (300 at random chosen patients were re-evaluated out of 1425, i.e., 20.6%), in order to assess the estimate number of LSIL and HSIL cases in result of cancelling the undesired category of "medium-grade dysplasia". Despite of some doubts concerning the precision of such calculations, we could demonstrate the decreased incidence as well as a significantly lower morbidity for cervical carcinoma within the last 6-years period. Regarding to the frequency of 7.5 positive smears out of 100,000 samples enrolled, and comparing this number with the overall morbidity rate of 15.4/100,000 as reported for Slovakia in 1999 [13], the estimated decrease of cervical carcinoma cases should be much higher than 50%. Namely, the former number reflects the relative proportion of positive samples out of the total enrolled, while the latter represents the frequency of disease in whole women population (either in the fertile and/or post-fertile age). The estimated proportion of women examined in comparison with the total woman population in given age might range from 10 to 20%. Even if this proportion of followed may not be correct, the decreased morbidity for cervical cancer in Slovakia during the last decade might be at least tenfold. Furthermore, **Table 1** also shows that at least 6% (by minimal rate 263/3070) but not more than 12% (by maximal rate 466/3943) of smears which had been scored LSIL progressed into the stage of HSIL. For the above-mentioned minimal rate, the intermediate MKCH category was not taken into account; for the maximum rate, it has been split (modified) into corresponding Bethesda categories as explained above. Thus, regardless to any imperfections of both calculations, which may arise from comparison of the Tables 1 and 4, our data point at an increased incidence of newly emerging LSIL cases. Namely, the average positive rate among the smears, which was in the range of 1.5–1.9% during the last 6-years period, has reached 3.5% in the year 2015 (an increase of 180%). As already suggested in our previous paper [14], and confirmed by others, the probability of transition from LSIL and/or ASC-H cases into HSIL strongly depends on the presence of HPV as detected by one of the available HPV DNA tests [15, 16]. The great majority of the ASCUS cases and up to 85% of LSIL cases (especially in the absence of HPV DNA) might undergo spontaneous healing as shown in next paragraph.

2. The role of human papillomavirus (HPV) in the pathogenesis of cervical dysplasia and cancer

The first mammalian papillomavirus (PV) was described by Shope and Hurst [17], who characterized the transmissible nature of cutaneous papillomas arising in wild cottontail rabbits. The narrow host range of PVs in culture to sites with stratified squamous epithelia that is either cornified (skin) or non-cornified (mucosa) was overcome by introducing molecular technics such as the DNA extraction, the polymerase chain reaction (PCR), and vDNA sequencing allowing to identify the genes of the PV DNA regarding to the function of corresponding proteins. The papillomaviruses (PVs) comprise a group of non-enveloped epitheliotropic DNA viruses that predominantly induce benign lesions of the skin (warts) and mucous membranes (condylomas). Some PVs have also been implicated in the development of epithelial malignancies, especially in the cancer of uterine cervix, certain tumors of urogenital tract, and upper airway cancers [18]. Due to given relationships, an increasing amount of information has accumulated from sequencing results of various PV DNAs. Later on, the PVs were classified according to the host species they infect, so that the PVs of human origin were designated as human PVs (HPV). Officially recognized by the International Committee on the Taxonomy of Viruses (ICTV), the former *Papovaviridae* family now falls into two separate families, *Papillomaviridae* and *Polyomaviridae* [19]. The reason being the missing helicase motif in the HPV E1 protein, a domain stretching longer than about 230 amino acids (aa) within the analogous non-structural HPV polypeptide, which otherwise has some similarity with the SV40 T-antigen, the parvovirus NS1 protein, and with a planarian virus-like element [20].

Among the most extensively studied HPV genomes, nearly 100 genotypes were described based on the at least 90% nucleotide homology of sequence encoding one of 2 structural capsid proteins (the L1 protein sequence). The L1 ORF is the most conserved gene within the genome and has therefore been used for the identification and classification of new HPV types corresponding to later characterized species is shown in **Table 5**. It should be mentioned that sorting into species and genus has some theoretical and/or scientific importance, but for practical reasons, the old genotype classification is still in use (**Table 6**). A new HPV isolate is recognized as such, if its complete genome has been cloned and sequenced to determine in which extent the L1 ORF differs from the closest known HPV genotype. If a more than 10% bp difference can be found that is a distinct genotype. Differences between 2 and 10% homology define a subtype and <2% difference reveals a variant. The closely related HPV types HPV-2 and 27, HPV-6 and 11, and HPV-16 and 31, which cause common warts, genital warts, and cervical cancer, respectively, are excellent examples of numerous consistencies between phylogeny and pathology. Furthermore, the HPV genotypes could have been distinguished as high risk (HR) and low risk (LR) according to their ability to transform cells, due to their relationship to cervical dysplasia and/or cancer, and according to their frequency. The squamous carcinoma (SCa) cells and/or the cells in *epidermodysplasia veruciformis* (EV) harbor multiple genome copies of specific HPV types, especially HPV5 and HPV8, but also of HPV14, HPV20, and a few others [21–23]. Their transcripts have been described in several the so-called EV-associated SCa cells [24]. In 2009, HPV5 and HPV8 were classified by IARC as "possibly carcinogenic" in EV patients [25].

Genus	**Properties**	**Species**	**Genotype(s)**	**Clinical significance**
Alphapapillomavirus	Mainly	*1*	HPV32, HPV42	Benign lesions, oral or genital mucosa, LR
	mucosa but also skin lesions;	2	HPV3, HPV10 HPV28, HPV29 HPV78, HPV94	genotypes, benign cutaneous or mucosal lesions,
	conserved E5 ORF within the ERL* ;	*3*	HPV61, HPV72, HPV81, HPV83, HPV84	LR genotypes, mucosal lesions
	HR genotypes immortalize	*4*	HPV2, HPV27, HPV57	Skin warts (common), frequently benign, LR genotypes,
	keratinocytes,	*5*	HPV26, HPV51, HPV69, HPV82	HR genotype, mucosa lesions
		6	HPV30, HPV53, HPV56, HPV66	HR genotypes, mucosa lesions, some are LR genotypes

Genus	Properties	Species	Genotype(s)	Clinical significance
		7	HPV18, HPV39,	HR genotypes, mucosal lesions
	E5 ORF is		HPV45, HPV59,	
	different		HPV68, HPV70,	
		8	HPV7, HPV40,	LR genotypes, butcher warts, skin and
			HPV43	mucosa
		9	HPV16, HPV31,	HR genotypes, mucosal lesions
			HPV33, HPV35,	
			HPV52, HPV58,	
			HPV67	
		10	HPV6, HPV11,	LR genotypes, rarely verrucous carcinoma
			HPV13, HPV44,	
			HPV73, HPV74	HR genotypes, mucosal (cervical) lesions
		11	HPV34, HPV73	(dysplasia and carcinoma)
		13	HPV54	LR genotype, mucosal lesions
		15	HPV71	LR genotype, mucosal lesions
Betapapillomavirus	Latent	1	HPV5, HPV8,	Mainly benign cutaneous lesions
	infection		HPV12, HPV14	
	possible in		HPV19, HPV20	
	general		HPV21, HPV25	
	population		HPV36, HPV 47,	
			HPV93,	
		2	HPV9, HPV15,	Commonly associated with EV,
			HPV17, HPV22,	mucosal lesions and detection of vDNA in
			HPV23,HPV37,	immunosuppression,
			HPV38,HPV80	most frequently LR genotypes
		3	HPV 49, HPV75,	LR genotypes, benign cutaneous
			HPV76	
		4	Candidate types 60	Pre-malignant cutaneous
		5	and 88	Pre-malignant cutaneous
Gammapapillomavirus		1	HPV4, HPV65	Cutaneous lesions, intracytoplasmic
			HPV95	homogenous inclusion bodies
		2	HPV48	Cutaneous lesions
		3	HPV50	Cutaneous lesions
		4	HPV60	Cutaneous lesions

Genus	Properties	Species	Genotype(s)	Clinical significance
		5	HPV88	Cutaneous lesions
Nu-papillomavirus	Several not assigned ORFs,	1	HPV41	Bening as well as malignant cutaneous
Mu-papillomavirus	Human PV, inclusion bodies specific	1 2	HPV1 HPV63	Heterogenous cytoplasmic inclusions, filamentary cytoplasmic inclusions, LCR/URR has 982 bp

[1] According to deVilliers et al. [30]; [2] epidermodysplasia verruciformis. * ERL = the DNA segment between E and L ORFs.

Table 5. Classification of papillomaviruses and the list of their important genotypes.

Disease	Frequent association	Rare association
Skin infection		
Deep plantar warts	1, 2	4, 63
Common warts	2, 1	4, 26, 27, 29, 41, 57, 65, and 77
Butcher's warts	7, 2	1, 3, 4, 10, and 28
Epidermodysplasia verruciformis (ER)*	2, 3, 5, 8, 9, 10, 12, 14, 15, and 17	19, 20, 21, 22, 23, 24, 25, 36, 37, 38, 47, and 70
Skin carcinoma associated with ER	**5** and **8**	
Anogenital infection		
Condyloma acuminatum	6, 11	30, 42, 43, 44, 45, 51, 54, 55, 70
Intraepitelal dysplasia (CIN I a CIN II/III)	6**, 11**, **16**, **18**	(**16**, **18**, 74, 86) 6, 11, **26**, **31**, **33**, **35**, **39**, 42, 43, 44, **45**, **51**, **52**, 53, **56**, **58**, **66**, **73**, and **82**
Carcinoma *in situ*; and invasive carcinoma	**16**, **18**, **31**, **45**	**33**, **35**, **39**, **51**, **52**, **56**, **58**, 59, **66**, **67**, **68**, 73, and 82
Recurrent laryngeal papilloma	6, 11	
Conjuctival papilloma	6, 11, and **16**	

* Congenital skin lesion with high sensitivity to HPV infection.
** Mainly in CIN I/LSIL, CIN II and/or non-invasive forms CINIII/HSIL and/or CIN III+/HSIL.
[#] According to Bonnez [31].

Table 6. Clinical relevance of high-risk (in bold) and low-risk HPV genotypes according to their frequency.

The HPV virions are small non-enveloped capsids 55 nm in size and of icosaedral symmetry. They are composed of 72 subunits formed by 2 structural proteins (L1 and L2, L = late), which are synthesized at the late intervals of productive replication cycle. The viral double-stranded DNA (vDNA) has about 8 kilobase pairs (kbp); it encodes 7 or 8 non-structural polypeptides, designated E1–E8 (E = early). The transcription of viral mRNA is directed clockwise under the control of two promoters, namely the early promoter (P_{97}) and the late promoter (P_{670}) sequence. In between the initiation codon for the transcription of E1 polypeptide ORF (open reading frame) and the stop codon for the L2 capsid protein ORF, an approximately 1.1 kbp long control repeat (LCR) is situated that contains the origin of vDNA replication as well as several binding sites for the binding of viral E2 and/or E1 regulatory proteins (**Table 7**). In addition to the motifs for down-regulation of the productive replication cycle (on the basis of a feedback mechanism), the LCR (also referred to as the URR, upstream regulatory region) contains enhancer sites for attachment of cellular transcription cofactors promoting the binding of cellular RNA polymerase to accomplish viral mRNA synthesis.

Protein	MW	Properties and function
E1	68–76 kDa	Binds to the regulatory long control repeat (LCR/URR) upstream from the E6/E7 ORF promoters. Forms a heterodimer with E2, associates with H1 histones and with cyclins, especially with cyclin E.
E2	40–58 kDa	Activates viral mRNA transcription, binds to the LCR/URR sequence, associates with the E1 protein; acts as cofactor of vDNA replication; operates at distribution of newly copied vDNA molecules during cell division (also in latency). Suppresses the expression of E6/E7 proteins and interacts with the L2 capsid polypeptide (especially at productive virus replication). Induces apoptosis.
E3	10–17 kDa	Function unknown.
E4		Associates with the L1 capsid polypeptide and facilitates virion formation (during productive replication); co-localizes with cytokeratins being produced in the medium and upper spinous layers.

[1] Long control repeat/upstream regulatory region.

Table 7. Basic functions of HPV-coded early (non-structural) polypeptides involved in the replication and latency.

Protein	Molecular weight	Properties and function
E5	10 kDa	Increases and prolongs the activities of receptors interacting with external growth factors such as EGF and/or PDGF2 by binding to their cytoplasmic domain. Inhibits the acidification of endosomes, binds to ATPase within the membranes of vacuoles and increases the stability of the engulfed EGF/EGFR complexes. Activates cellular transcription factors such as AP1* and signal transmission mediating proteins such as c-Jun** and/or c-Fos.
E6	16–18 kDa	Binds to the pivotal cell division regulator p53 (cellular anti-onc protein), enhances its degradation by ubiqitination (most efficiently acting are the E2 from HPV16 and/or HPV18 genotypes).
E7	10–14 kDa	Binds to the retinoblastoma (Rb) protein (its p107 and p130 forms) , which regulate cellular DNA transcription via binding or release of the transcription initiation factor E2F (in response to phosphorylation of the Rb associated *cdk* complex). Activates mainly cyclins A and E,

Protein	Molecular weight	Properties and function
		especially influencing the translocation into nucleus of the transcription cofactor AP1. Activates the histone deacetylase (HDAC) acting at the level of the so-called epigenetic regulation of transcription by removing its blockade.

[1] Epidermal growth factor [2] Platelet-derived growth factor, * Activator protein 1, * Cellular ju-na-na *** Cyclin-dependent kinas.

Table 8. Basic functions of the HPV-coded early (non-structural) oncoproteins.

The E2 polypeptide was initially described as a transcriptional activator [26] capable to initiate viral transcription through the E2 recognition elements located within early promoter (for HPV16, it is the above mentioned P_{97}, while alternatively, for HPV18, it is the P_{105}). As described below in more detail, tumorigenesis is mediated by an integrated HPV DNA fragment, encompassing the E6 and E7 genes exerting transformation activity (**Table 8**). During productive (vegetative) virus replication in human squamous epithelial cells, the essential activities displayed either by the HPV type 16 P_{97} or by the HPV type 18 P_{105} promoters can be repressed by the full-length E2 polypeptide, which binds to one of the four E2 binding sites upstream of either P_{97} or P_{105} [27]. The E2 protein also facilitates long-term persistence of HPV genome in host cells by episomal maintenance providing a mechanism ensuring the distribution of viral genome within the dividing epithelium and its segregation into daughter cells [28, 29]. This can be achieved due to the association of E2 with the mitotic spindles, when it interacts with condensed mitotic chromatin and thereby ensures that the viral genome (which duplicates within the dividing host cell during cellular DNA synthesis) gets attached to nuclear envelope at anaphase and reforms during telophase. The duplication of viral genome during mitosis is accomplished by means of the cellular DNA polymerase, which becomes modified by another early HPV-coded protein, the El polypeptide. The E1 is required for both the initiation and elongation of viral DNA synthesis being accomplished by the cellular DNA polymerase complex by means of its ATPase and DNA helicase activities. The E2 can complex with E1 to strengthen its affinity for binding to the origin of vDNA replication. The papillomavirus E2 protein has several well-characterized regulatory functions affecting viral transcription, viral DNA replication as well as long-term plasmid maintenance. In contrast to the duplication of HPV DNA, which is the main strategy to ensure long-term persistence of viral genome, in the course of acute virus replications, the necessary point is to generate many genome copies which will be packaged into virions. Why that process occurs only in the terminally differentiated cells of the upper squamous epithelium layer and in the benign vegetative vDNA replication, is not known. The switch in question may involve the presence or absence of cellular cofactors expressed in the differentiating keratinocytes, i.e. only within the cytokeratin forming upper squamous epithelium layer. As described later, these cells, if previously proliferating papilloma cells. The mechanisms regulating the switch from plasmid maintenance to vDNA replication not known. This switch may envolve the presence or absence of cellular cofactors expressed in the differentiating keratinocytes, thus is occurs only within the cytokeratin forming upper squamous epithelium layer. As described later, these cells, if previously infected within the lower squamous epithelium layer, then show typical morphology, the so-called koilocytes. Clearly, the relatively increased levels of HPV proteins such as E1 or E2 (or their modifications) may change the appearance of terminally differentiating keratinocytes. One might anticipate that the vegetative DNA replication occurs bi-directionally, through a theta structure intermediate or by a rolling circle mode, which is the principle of vDNA replication in general. Finally, the virion assembly must take place in the nuclei of terminally differentiated keratinocytes, which also contributes to koilocyte formation. The nascent capsids might randomly attach to the HPV DNA, and are further stabilized by the formation of disulfide bonds between conserved cysteines on adjacent L1 monomers acquiring resistance to proteolytic digestion. Taken together, as result of productive replication, the virions form large aggregates within the nuclei of infected keratin forming upper squamous epithelium cells, which then regularly show koilocytosis [32], but rarely reveal cytoplasmic inclusion bodies (see **Table 5** for details).

The newly produced HPV virions do not appear outside of squamous epithelium cells, and its productive replication is closely bound to the suprabasal, mainly medium and upper slayer of dividing keratinocytes. At infection, the HPV virions preferentially bind to heparan sulfate proteoglycans (HSPGs) on the basement membrane or to the basal stem cells, which may be exposed to environmental influence at sites of epithelial trauma or permeabilization. The differentiating squamous epithelium cells cannot become infected. To achieve selective infection of basal differentiating squamous epithelium cells, the initiation of infection preferentially requires attachment to the basal stem cells layered at the basal membrane of stratified squamous epithelium [33–35]. The basement membrane-bound virion undergoes a conformational change of its L2 capsid protein that exposes a highly conserved N-terminal peptide motif to cleavage by furin or the closely related pro-protein convertase [36]. There is a remarkably long delay of 1–3 days between the capsid cell surface binding and its penetration resulting in the onset of viral genome transcription. Itself the internalization of capsids as starts from the attachment to cell surface until the uncoating process begins lasts at least 2–4 h and is very asynchronous. The endocytosis as well as the consequent transmembrane trafficking of HPV capsids is not fully understood. Penetration of engulfed capsids may be initiated either from the acidified late endosomes, in which the L2 conformation change takes place, or by clathrin-dependent uptake [37]. The penetrated virions are transported from the internal membrane surface by involutions called vilopodia, namely from their leading edge to the central cell body via actin-directed retrograde flow [38]. Classical observations testify that there is extremely difficult to isolate and propagate any HPV types in conventional human cell cultures [39].

During the last decade, several details of HPV induced continuous host cell proliferation have been elucidated. It became clear that three non-structural HPV-coded oncoproteins, namely E5, E6, and E7 (**Table 8**) are involved in host cell immortalization, which later on, under the conditions of continuous host cell division results in malignant transformation. It should be mentioned that the transformation as such is a multistep process, launched by the virus-coded oncoproteins as suggested the "hit and run" hypothesis. The E5 protein enhances the sensitivity of HPV carrier cells to external proliferative stimuli, such as the epidermal growth factor [40]. It also binds to the growth factor receptors, for example, to the platelet growth factor receptor (PDGFR), and activates the signal transmission in a ligand-independent manner [41, 42].

Because the integrated vDNA regularly encompasses just the ORFs of E6 and E7 oncoproteins along with the closely positioned LCR sequence, a continuing and increased expression of E6/E7 proteins occurs which seriously affects the regulation of host cell division in direction of its down-regulation [43, 44]. The E6 polypeptide binds the pivotal cell division inhibiting p53 protein [45], while E7 polypeptide binds the retinoblastoma (Rb) protein and the cyclin inhibitory proteins p27 and p21 [46]. The HPV-coded oncoproteins E6/E7, when expressed in significant amounts, continuously drive the host cell from the phase G1 to phase S (synthesis), in which the replication of cell DNA proceeds in an unlimited manner. Noteworthy that immortalization and the process of cancerogenesis are not the same, since the latter is much more complex being related to several chromosomal alterations and to increased number of *c-myc* gene copies (probably arisen due to repeated host cell DNA sequence transpositions), a finding even proportional to the grade of HPV driven dysplasia [47]. In low-grade dysplasias (such as CIN I/LSIL), only a restricted number of the HPV oncogenes is expressed.

Nevertheless, E6 and E7, which have several other activities (**Table 8**), appear to be the main drivers for the progression to high-grade dysplasia and later on to cancer, by orchestrating a series of pathogenic changes. Both are transcribed from the same major early promoters located within the LCR region of their genome. As a rule, the expression of the episomal (not yet integrated) HPV genome is restricted to E6 and E7 polypeptides, which are present in the parabasal, lower layer of squamous epithelium. Here, the viral genome undergoes a regulated duplication along with the host cell proliferation, which is under physiological conditions regulated by corresponding stimuli. The E6 protein is expressed at substantially lower levels than E7, and in early LSIL lesions, since the level of E7 may be more limited than that of E6. Noteworthy, both genes are expressed from a single promoter (latency associated and different from the above-mentioned vegetative ones); their transcripts are alternatively spliced by a post-translation mechanism determining as well as regulating their relative level within the carrier host cell. Integration of the HPV DNA fragment into cellular DNA via non-homologous recombination represents a key change towards immortalization that appears to stabilize the high expression of E6/E7, which, in turn, becomes frequently associated with more severe lesions. Integration may still not occur in great majority of CIN I/LSIL lesions, but is present by an increased rate in HSIL/CIN II and/or CIN III lesions, and is the most frequent in pre-invasive cancer (Ca *in situ*). As a rule, whoever, the integrated E6/E7 ORF containing the HPV DNA fragment is at high probability found in the CIN III lesions. The frequency of viral DNA integration may vary with the HPV genotype, being more frequent for the high-risk (HR) genotypes such as HPV18 and/or HPV16.

The integration of vDNA and/or its fragment occurs due to interruption of its sequence, which can appear at many sites throughout the genome, but is found preferentially at fragile genomic sites, which undergo nicking and cutting in association recombination and/or translocation events of the host cell genome. In certain cases, practically the rest of whole genome may be deleted, so that only the E6 and E7 ORFs remain intact and ready for the transcription along with the nearby located LCR sequence, containing the crucial promoter and enhancer signals lying upstream of the integration site [48]. In a given *in vitro* immobilized keratinocyte culture, the integration process usually involves only one locus or a few loci. The E6/E7 ORF transcription slowly increases due the loss of the feedback block provided by the viral E1 and E2 proteins, which ORFs had been either deleted or at least disrupted. This situation permits the constant expression of high levels of the undesired E6 and E7 mRNA molecules [49]. Consistent with the multistep nature of tumorigenesis, cervical cancers may show additional cytogenetic alterations as compared with adjacent high-grade dysplastic and/or carcinoma *in situ* lesions.

Low-grade dysplasia may be caused by infection with either low-risk (LR) or high-risk (HR) HPV. Persistent (i.e., long-term) infection with a HR HPV type, which occurs in a minority of infected women, is the most important risk factor for developing CIN III or pre-invasive cancer (CIN III+). However, the magnitude of the risk depends not only on the given HPV type, but even more on a HR variant within the given type (compare **Table 6**). In practical terms, HPV persistence usually means that the same HPV genotype can be recovered from at least two or more subsequently taken genital samples obtained over a period of 4–12 months. Persistent infection may clear spontaneously, but less likely it does so in the course of longer duration. Taken together, only some persistent infections progress to CIN III, and subsequently to invasive cancer, but the HR HPV16 infections so such outcome much more likely than other HPV types. The distinct biologic effects of HR E6 and E7 may present at least a partial explanation of the differences in the likelihood of low-grade dysplasia progression, which presence may not be consistently associated with the same probability of the progression to high-grade lesion. Thus, most genital HPV infections are self-limited, and the majority would clear within 12 months.

Taken together, the HPV genome persists within transformed host cells in two different forms: as a non-integrated (episomal) circularized full-length vDNA and, less frequently, as a linear and integrated vDNA sequence. There should be mentioned that during long-term latency, the integration of HPV DNA may occur due to the linearization of the persisting circular vDNA molecule. At integration, the HPV DNA chain gets either interrupted or partially deleted, preferentially at nt 3362–3443 of the E2 ORF [50, 51], usually within the E2 gene ORF [52]. The mixed (episomal as well as integrated) vDNA distribution pattern seems the most prevalent physical state of HPV16 DNA found in ASCUS-graded smears (atypical cells of unknown significance), but can also be detected in cervical scrapings which do not reveal dysplastic changes. This indicates that HPV infection may not always cause dysplasia of the squamous epithelium cells. The prevalence of the integrated HPV DNA sequence over the episomal molecules then appears in a proportion of ASCUS-graded smears (sometimes characterized by ASC-H cells) and in a proportion of LSIL smears, but later on becomes clearly prevalent in the HSIL-grade smears and, of course, in cervical cancer. Women with the prevalence of integrated HPV DNA were almost 10 years older than those with a predominating episomal HPV DNA pattern, which points to a higher risk of HPV infection in women aged over 35 years [53].

3. Overexpression of the p16/INK4A regulatory polypeptide in dysplastic and/or proliferating cells

The aim of our further considerations was to assess the role of p16/INK4A (inhibitor kinase) protein, which is, as a rule, overexpressed in cells revealing increased E7 polypeptide production. The p16/INK4A (inhibitor kinase) polypeptide is a cellular regulatory protein, which inhibits the cyclin-dependent kinases (especially cdk4 and cdk6) associated with cyclins D and/or E. These kinases, if activated, phosphorylate the retinoblastoma phosphoprotein (pRb) complex, which in turn, releases the transcription factor E2F, which is bound in inactive form in non-dividing cells. Under physiological conditions (in normal cells), the Rb protein liberated from the disrupted complex has a feedback effect on p16 expression [47]. Since the E2 polypeptide binds to LCR, the presence of E2 in cells carrying the episomal (i.e., non-integrated) HPV DNA may efficiently control the transcription of mRNA encoding the E6/E7 oncoproteins [54]. In contrast, in cells which carry the integrated HPV genome, the E2 polypeptide production stops, since the E2 ORF becomes disrupted. Therefore, the E2 but also the E1 proteins (both

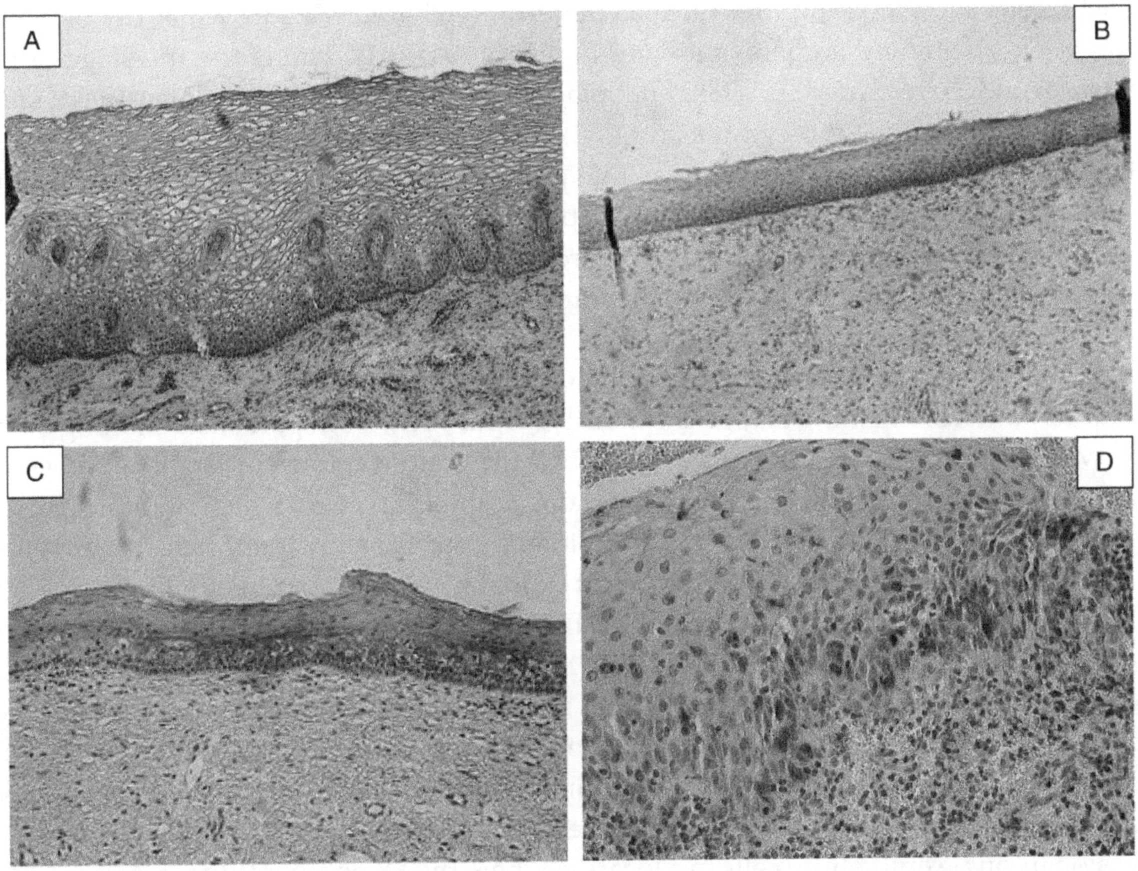

Figure 1. Different patterns of positive p16 staining in CIN I/LSIL. Upper line: continuous staining of p16 antigen of low (A) and/or high intensity (B) confined to the lower spinous layer and/or to the transit amplifying cells, which are situated in parabasal location just adjacent to the p16 negative basal stem cells. No dysplasia can be seen. Line below: staining of p16 antigen in a thin layer of dysplastic cells at parabasal area showing signs of HPV infection such as koilocytes (in the left, C). Bottom in the right (D): progressed dysplasia of the basal layer in part involving the stem cells, which cannot be clearly recognized.

closely involved in the maintenance of long-term latency) may be missing in dysplastic and/or HPV-transformed cells. Unlike to transformed cells, their production becomes down-regulated in the late phase of vegetative (productive) virus replication cycle. It can be stated that in HPV transformed cells, the expression of p16/INK4A protein increases proportionally to elevated levels of the increasing expression of the virus-coded E7 polypeptide, since both rise in the absence of E2 protein [55–58]. The p16/INK4 mRNA more stable and is present in higher levels in the cells in which the HPV DNA sequence had been integrated [59]. The quantification real-time–polymerase reaction (qRT PCR) is useful to identify the levels of transcripts encoding the p16 polypeptide in cervical smears of patients obtained for diagnostic purpose, an approach which is more tedious as the antigen staining, but is similarly sensitive and occasionally may yield more confident results. The p16 mRNA was present in 30% of LGSL but in 75% of HGSIL cases reaching a rate of 85.7% in squamous cell carcinoma cases [60].

The Bethesda scoring system, originally destined for vaginal/cervical smears [1988/1989], has been later adopted for the cervical biopsies at histologic examination. This has happened regardless to the fact that pathologists already had their own nomenclature, which is still in use for cervical biopsy grading widely known as cervical intraepithelial neoplasia (CIN). The dysplastic cells showing a diploid nuclear pattern are characterized by the loss of polarity, crowding, overlapping disorganization, and anisocytosis [61]. Therefore, the stage of CIN I dysplasia cannot be regarded for a truly neoplastic process. At cytological level, the dysplastic cells show altered nuclear-to-cytoplasm (N/C) ratio as well as wrinkling and thickening of nuclear membrane (**Table 4**) so that any CIN I grade changes may correspond to the entity of LSIL [62]. In mild forms of CIN I/LSIL, the dysplastic cells occupy the parabasal layer only but form a continuous zone within the lower third of cervical squamous epithelium, in the so-called lower squamous layer along with the transit amplifying cells, which early dysplasia can be better recognized by the p16 antigen staining (**Figure 1**). Summing up the results of p16 antigen staining in biopsy sections graded CIN I/LSIL, Yildiz et al. [63] could distinguish the continuous parabasal staining of higher intensity (**Figure 1B**), from parabasal staining of lower intensity (**Figure 1A**). In addition, they described the scattered form of positive p16 staining of single and/or small groups of upper squamous epithelium cells, which do not correspond to the suprabasal layer of lower squamous epithelium or the transit epithelium cells (**Figure 2D**). The production of p16 protein to an extent stainable with the commercially available anti-p16 monoclonal antibody (for example the CINTec histology kit) has been attributed to the stimulation of CDKN2A gene (encoding the p16 protein) by the stimuli activated via alternative receptor pathways regulating the transient reactive cell proliferation. This situation should be strongly distinguished from dysplasia, where the cell growth regulation undergoes some kind of dysregulation (for example, by the viral oncogenic polypeptide E7) that causes the switch to an autonomic growth due to repeated cell divisions. Thus, the increased p16 expression in single epithelium cells in a location where the E7 polypeptide may not be present may be related to HPV infection. Noteworthy, older textbooks before the introduction of p16 staining [64] referred to the histological picture of chronic cervicitis characterized by with hyperemia and round cell (lymphocyte) infiltration of the underlying connective tissue in addition to the reactivity and dilution would also influence the p16 antigen staining results ranging from clearly negative to false positive for above-mentioned reasons (**Figure 3**). During the last years, several big companies introduced automatic staining procedures, which on one hand standardized the staining intensity as well as its color, but on other hand, new staining variations appeared between different laboratories. Therefore, in cases suspicious for CIN I/ LSIL, or if thep16 staining reveals a faint reactivity or shows a distribution other than parabasal, or does not correspond to a dysplastic cells area as seen in a parallel HE stained section, the

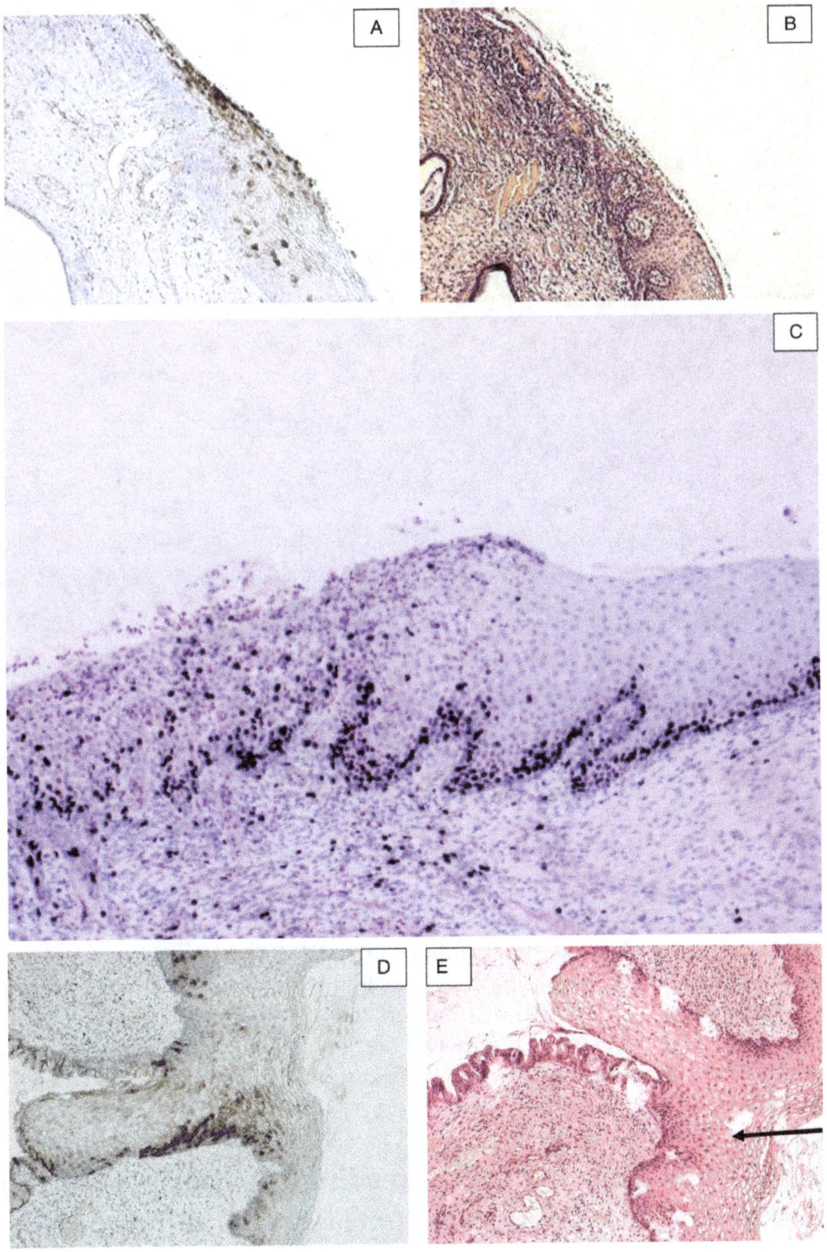

Figure 2. Metaplasia and/or focal dysplasia suspicious for CIN I /LSIL. Line above (A and B; C in the middle): transition of squamous epithelium into a metaplastic area. The cells positive for p16 antigen correspond to the foci of metaplasia (confluent staining), but single p16 positive squamous epithelium cells can be seen as well (A). The area of metaplasia is rich of scattered Ki-67 positive nuclei, while the regularly lined positive nuclei belong to the basal stem cells (C). The line below depicts a reactive proliferation of squamous epithelium (D and E) growing into the cervical gland at the squamocolumnar junction. The positive p16 staining is not precisely parabasal, but corresponds to an initial focus of dysplasia within the lower and/or medium squamous layers (shown by arrow at HE staining). The otherwise dispersed p16 antigen positive squamous cells may be unrelated to HPV infection.

prognostic value of positive p16 staining should be interpreted along with the outcome of the HPV DNA test.

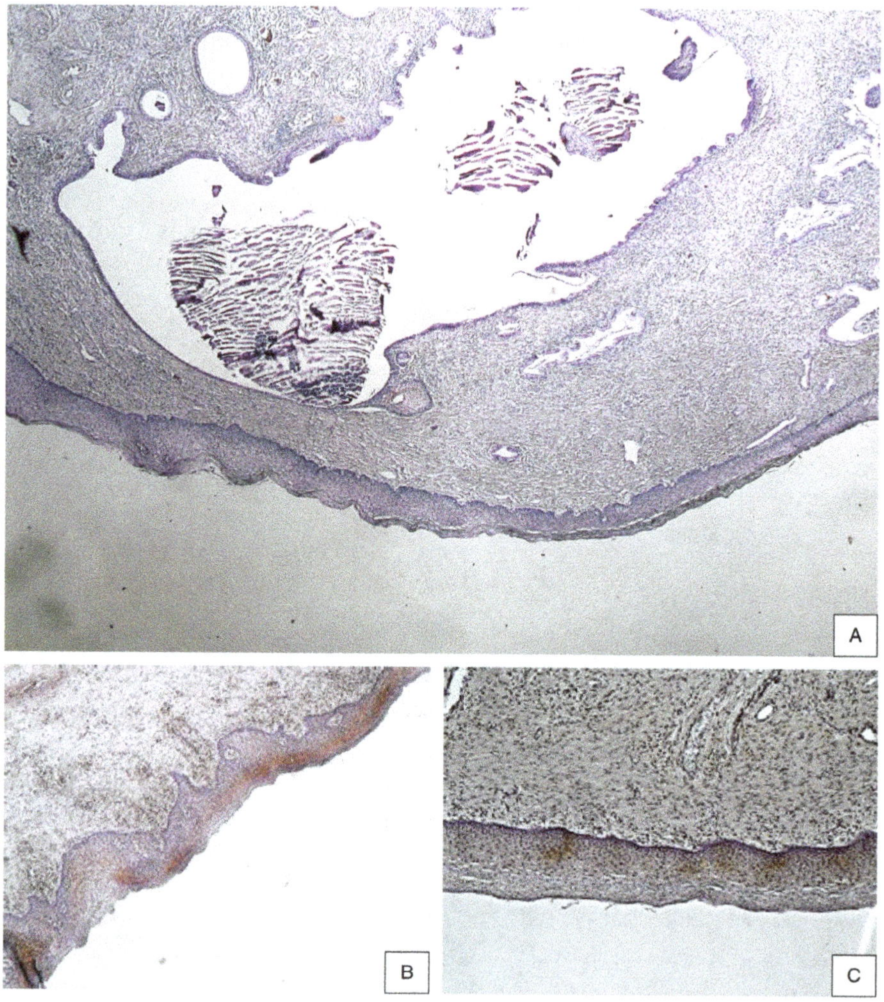

Figure 3. Examples of either negative (A, upper line) and/or midzonal (lower line, B and C) p16 antigen staining. Both examples show non-parabasal location of the p16 positive cells in the upper (rather than in the lower) squamous layer. The staining is of nearly confluent (B) or focal (C) distribution and often corresponds to the localization of koilocytes. Therefore, it is suggestive to accompany cases of productive (vegetative) HPV replication. Such pattern of p16 antigen staining may be suspicious of low-grade lesion (CIN I/LSIL), but should be combined with the HPV DNA test in order to obtain a precise diagnosis.

If dysplastic cells occupy at least one half (exceeding one third) of the original squamous epithelium thickness (but not the whole epithelium layer), the appropriate designation is CIN II. The p16 antigen staining is therefore useful to meet the diagnosis of CIN II/HSIL, since it allows to estimate the precise thickness of dysplasia involving the squamous epithelium (**Figure 4**). In contrast, at the stage of CIN III/HSIL, the dysplastic cells can fully replace the original epithelium (**Figure 5**). At progressed stage, the intensive staining of p16 polypeptide can be found within the nuclei of dysplastic cells as well as in their cytoplasm. The dysplastic cells in question show enlarged nuclei of ovoid shape, which are not equal in size. Since the presence of p16 antigen is a hallmark for distinguishing the immortalized and/or dysplastic cells, at first glance, the site of outgrowth and/or proliferation of squamous epithelium into cervical glands can be detected. The decreased availability of functioning Rb protein due to overexpression of E7 polypeptide, not only leads to increased p16 production, but also explains the higher frequency of nuclei positive for Ki-67 protein, a marker of cell division [65]. For more precise grading of the SIL lesions by the Ki-67 antigen staining, Kruse et al. [66] suggested to count the number of positive nuclei per 100 μm epithelium thickness starting from the parabasal zone (stratification index). The authors in question found a satisfactory correlation of 83% with the dysplastic squamous epithelium cells as seen in HE stained sections, but they also noticed that parallel sections may not fully correspond to the previously cut block level. Furthermore, as seen at our example of the CIN III/HSIL pattern shown on **Figure 5C** and **5D**, while the p16 antigen staining involves the whole dysplastic cell layer, in the Ki-67 stained section the calculation of stratification index may be less convenient. Taken together, staining of parallel sections for Ki-67 and p16 antigens confirmed the usefulness of both markers, even though the p16 marker is more suitable for practical reasons. On the other hand, the frequent zonal distribution of p16 reactivity fits well with the extent of dysplasia CIN I lesion encompassing less than one third of stratified epithelium. In the CIN II-graded lesion, the dysplastic cells encounter the half or nearly two thirds of squamous epithelium (**Figure 4**), while in the CIN III lesion a diffuse distribution of dysplastic cells involves the whole thickness of the original squamous epithelium layer. Therefore, at least in biopsies, the staining for p16 antigen alone has recently emerged as a reliable diagnostic marker suitable for quick orientation and relevant demonstration of the extent dysplasia as well as for the search of potentially invasive growth of squamous cell carcinoma cells penetrating the basement membrane (**Figure 6**).

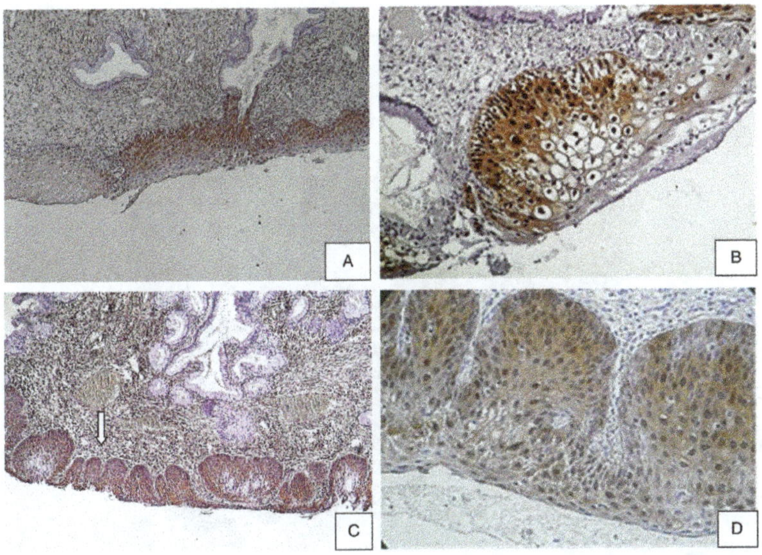

Figure 4. Examples of different CIN II lesions and of the corresponding p16 antigen staining. Upper line (A and B): confluent staining of p16 antigen at transition from stage CIN I (in the left half of the Figure) into stage CIN II (in the right half of same Figure 1A). Figure 1B: The p16 positive dysplastic cells involve the lower and the medium squamous layers but still not the whole epithelium; numerous koilocytes can be seen in the in-close vicinity of the p16 antigen positive dysplastic epithelium cells. Bottom line (C and D): Extensive dysplasia involves the lower and medium squamous cell layers, but is still absent at thin superficial layer of flat granular cells. The distribution of p16 antigen staining

corresponds to transition from CIN II into CIN III (the area enlarged at D is pointed by arrow). As shown in detail (D), a few koilocytes may be still found.

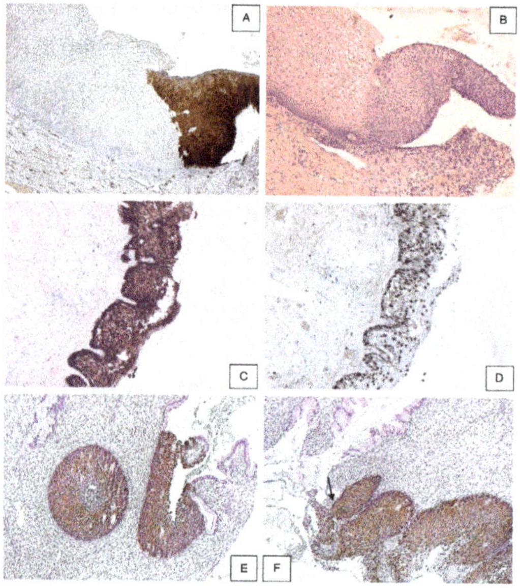

Figure 5. High degree of dysplasia (CIN III/HSIL) which occupies the entire epithelium layer and carcinoma *in situ*. Line above: Transition of squamous epithelium into dysplasia as shown by HE (B) and by p16 antigen staining (A). Middle line: The CIN III/HSIL as seen by p16 and Ki-67 antigen staining (C and D). While the p16 positive dysplastic cells occupy the whole epithelium, the nuclei of dividing cells are either round shaped and of regular size (basal stem cells closely at the basement membrane) or show an irregular ovoid shape of varying in size (dispersed at whole dysplastic layer but not each cell is positive). Bottom line: Carcinoma *in situ* proliferates into the surrounding connective tissue (cells p16 positive) and into a cervical gland replacing the cylindric epithelium but still keeping the basement membrane intact (E). The entirely dysplastic epithelium is positive for the p16 antigen; it shows loss of squamous differentiation along with extensive proliferative growth, but with the basement membrane preserved (F, no invasion at the arrow area).

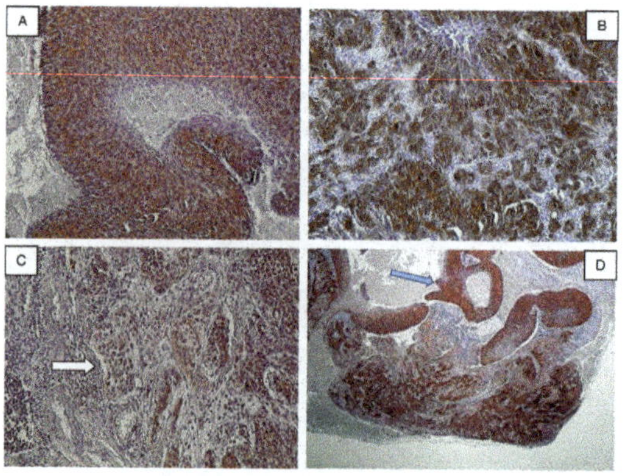

Figure 6. Carcinoma *in situ* (A) versus the invasive growth of spinocellular carcinoma (B) as related to the expression of p16 polypeptide. Dysplastic cells, forming the carcinoma *in situ* (A) as well as the non-differentiated malignant cells of invasive spinocellular carcinoma (B), are strongly positive for p16 and showing cytoplasmic as well as nuclear staining. After disrupting the basement membrane, groups of carcinoma cells grow not only within the surrounding connective tissue, but invade some capillaries and/or small venules as well as lymphatic vessels (C, arrow). At low power view, the origin of invasion can be recognized (D, arrow).

Nevertheless, any such comparisons may suffer from possible imprecision, since the repeatedly stained a tendency to worse grading at the primary evaluation of HE results. Namely, 3% of Ki-67 stained sections were graded CIN I rather than CIN II as described in HE stained sections. Alternatively, 14% cases graded CIN III in the HE stained sections were interpreted CIN II according to the Ki-67 staining. A similar tendency to worse grading from the evaluation, the HE stained sections only was found by us in p16 staining [14]. According to our experience, the viewing of parallel sections stained for p16 as well as Ki-67 antigen markers is of great help at confirming the extent of dysplasia seen in CIN II and/or CIN III HSIL-graded sections. In addition, it contributes to the correct evaluation of CIN I/LSIL lesions among which the reactive and other non-neoplastic staining patterns should be distinguished [67].

According to Dray et al. [68], the CIN II/HSIL- and/or CIN III/HSIL-graded lesions were found in 40.8% of cervical biopsies, while 14.3% showed the mild CIN I/LSIL lesion; the rest of 45% revealed a range of non-dysplastic (inflammatory or reactive) changes. In the latter group, the focal and weaker midzonal or superficial p16/INK4A immunostaining, suggestive of episomal HPV infection, was noted in 10% of biopsies. As shown in our statistics concerning biopsies in the year 2015 examined at the Pathology Diagnostic Center in Martin (Pathology 2, bottom line in **Table 11**), the definitely positive CIN I/LSIL lesions were seen in 36% of biopsies (90 out of 250). These lesions showed parabasal dysplasia within the lower third of squamous epithelium as well as koilocytes among adjacent squamous cells rarely involving the upper squamous layer (**Figure 1**). A proportion of suspicious CIN I/LSIL cases revealed focal dysplasia which, as a rule, correlated with the non-continuous p16 antigen positivity of squamous epithelium (**Figure 2**). The CIN II- and/or CIN III-grade HSIL lesion was detected in 37% of biopsies (89/250). The former showed dysplasia along with positive p16 staining involving about the half of squamous epithelium (**Figure 4**), while by the latter, the entire squamous epithelium layer was strongly positive for the p16 antigen (**Figure 5**). In CIN II cases involving more than one third of squamous epithelium, in the lower as well as in upper squamous layers occasional koilocytes found (**Figure 4B** and **4D**). In clearly CIN III-graded cases, the p16 positive dysplastic cells not only have replaced the whole squamous epithelium but also showed extensive proliferative growth either into the cervical glands or into the underlying connective tissue still with the basement membrane preserved (**Figure 5E** and **5F**). Nevertheless, similar proliferative growth might be occasionally found in CIN II/LSIL-graded cases (**Figure 4A–4C**), but very rarely, even in the CIN I/LSIL focal lesion. (**Figure 2D** and **2E**). In general, the increasing incidence of the combined p16/Ki-67 staining indicates more severe lesions: It may be positive by 26.8% of normal histology (missing dysplasia) cases, by 46.5% in CIN I histology, by 82.8% of CIN II, and/or by 92.8% of CIN III-graded histology [69]. In our hands, squamous epithelium showing no dysplasia was found in 55 out of 250 cases (20%) in biopsies of the Pathology Department 2, but only 10% of biopsies in the Pathology Department 1 (**Table 11**). The findings in the absence of dysplasia fall into at least 2 groups (**Figure 3**): (1) p16 negative cases showing neither dysplasia nor p16 antigen presence, and (2) cases of positive p16 immunostaining in the non-dysplastic areas of squamous epithelium, especially in its midzonal location, which does clearly differ from the parabasal distribution of p16 antigen. The p16 positive staining in the absence of dysplasia should be always examined for HPV DNA presence, and otherwise, the diagnosis can be regarded either for incomplete or at least imprecise from the point of view future prognosis. Although there is good evidence that p16/INK4A immunostaining correlates with the severity of cytological/histological abnormalities, the reproducibility might be limited also because of the insufficiently standardized interpretation of p16 staining results [70].

4. The diagnostic value of cervical smears in carcinoma prevention

As already mentioned in Introduction, due to examination of cervical smears in Slovakia during the last decade, the absolute number of cervical carcinoma cases as well as the morbidity rate has considerably decreased. Preventive cytological examination, which started in our country from 2006, and became especially frequent in the last 5–6 years (compare **Table 1**) in part explains this favorable development. As shown in **Table 4**, in just one out of 10 diagnostic centers serving for the population of approximately 2 million Slovak women in the age from 15 to 60 years, over 37,000 PA smears were enrolled from about 34,000 women were examined.

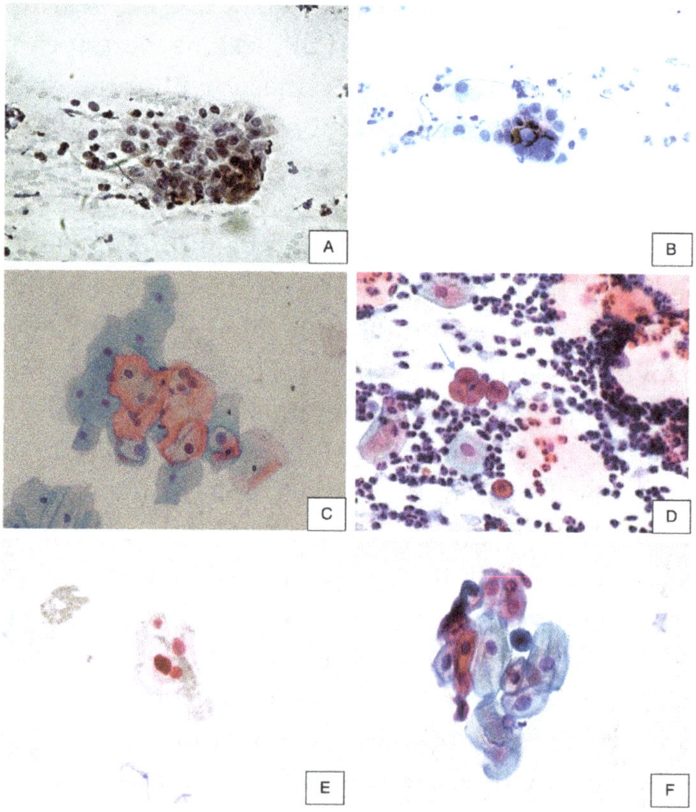

Figure 7. ASCUS- and/or LSIL-graded smears handled by the conventional PA method and stained for p16 antigen (A, B) in comparison with the appearance of atypical and/or abnormal squamous cells as seen after Liqui-PREP staining (C, D, E, and F). The upper line in the left depicts a group of atypical squamous epithelium cells with enlarged nuclei (A) in comparison with a group of abnormal cells-graded LSIL (B), both stained for p16 antigen. The middle line in the right (D) shows inflammation and metaplasia with a group of abnormal epithelium cells scored LSIL (pointed by arrow), while in the middle line left a group of atypical cells with enlarged nuclei can be seen (ASCUS) some of which being suggestive for LSIL (C) . The smear in the right, bottom line shows atypical cells along with the presence of koilocytes (F). In the bottom line left (E), one of the Ki-67 positive abnormal squamous cells shows faint p16 antigen staining in the cytoplasm (simultaneously stained for p16 as well as Ki-67 antigens).

A positive rate of 4.6% experienced in our particular screening is in accord with the data previously reported from the US [16]. Despite of the success of mass screening based on the relatively simple PAP technique, improved cytological tests such as liquid-based cytology (Liqui-PREP) were introduced to achieve more precise reading. The new approach resulted in a significant decrease of low-quality samples [71], when allowing to identify and distinguish the atypical epithelium cells allowing to identify and better distinguish the atypical epithelium cells at their better visualization, which may be of great advantage especially for the recognition of LSIL cases (**Figure 7**).

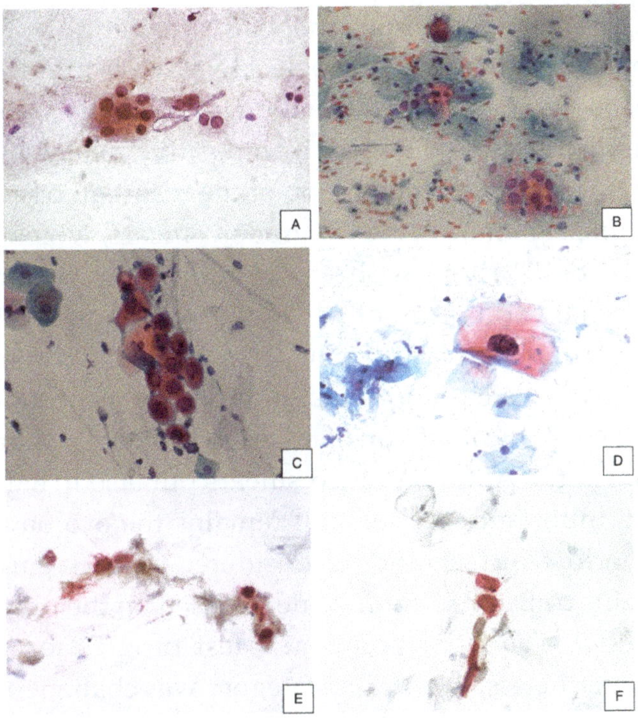

Figure 8. Examples of HSIL-graded smears: Above, in the left (A): The conventional PAP staining is of relatively good quality achieved using the CYNTec staining kit for p16 antigen detection (positive). The rest (B, C, and D) of smears were handled by liquid-based cytology and shows either groups or single dysplastic cells-graded HSIL (B, C) and/or HSIL+ (at D, a single dysplastic cell with an extremely large hyperchromatic nucleus is shown suggestive of carcinoma *in situ*). The bottom line (E and F) shows groups of distorted (shrunken) dysplastic epitelium cells stained with the anti/p16/anti-Ki-67 MoAb mix (nuclei dark purple, cytoplasm contains many p16 antigen brown granules).

As mentioned above, the Bethesda Committee classification [72] and the suggested definitions were later on slightly improved reaching the state which has become widely accepted [73]. Comparisons among laboratories showed that the diagnosis of ASCUS (atypical squamous cells of undetermined significance) may be often used just to avoid clear-cut decision making. Therefore, the principle has been be that this diagnostic category should not exceed 5–6% of the total number of smears investigated. As stressed by Geisinger et al. [74], the main criterion for the clear definition of SIL is the increased size of nucleus (<3 fold for ASCUS, >3 fold in LSIL), increased intensity of chromatin staining and its altered internal structure (finely granular chromatin structure and slight hyperchromasia in ASCUS, coarse chromatin and definitely visible hyperchromasia in LSIL reports claimed the relative value of p16 staining in

ASCUS smears, which may be positive in cases designated as p16 reactive ASC. The proportion of p16 negative smears was reported for the highest in ASCUS (40%) and the lowest in HSIL (5%) specimens [75, 76]. According to Grapsa et al. [77], the p16 staining is weak in LSIL (compare **Figure 7A**), but strong in HSIL cases (**Figure 8A** and **8B**). Thus, the faint p16 staining argues against the diagnosis of LSIL, while p16 overexpression along with high levels of p53 favors the process of malignant transformation of the atypical squamous epithelium cells.

According to Shin et al. [78], the p16 antigen was found in 66.7% of ASCUS and 70% of LSIL cases, confirming that detection of p16/INK4A protein can be used as adjunct test especially at liquid-based cytology. However, several authors noticed a high degree of false p16 reactivity within otherwise negative smears, especially in those containing atrophic cells [79]. They also stressed that in such smears, the number of single p16 reactive atypical cells per the total cell number of cells may not be significant. Such situation is less likely to appear in biopsy sections, where typical confluent distribution of p16 antigen positive cells at the parabasal epithelium layer is of essential help for correct interpretation of the result. In our previous paper [14], we focused our interest on unclear and/or ASCUS-graded smears, which were found HPV DNA positive by a probability of 8–10%, but have been p16 antigen positive with a higher probability ranging from 32 to 61%. The wide range of p16 antigen false positivity of atypical cells was found associated with the staining procedure itself, since the CYN-Tec cytology staining kit showed more clear-cut results, allowing to distinguish the proportion of really p16 antigen positive, but HPV unrelated atypical cells on hand, from artificially stained ones on other hand. It should be stressed that in the ASCUS-graded smears but also in a great proportion of LSIL scored smears the most important criterion still remains the evaluation of nuclear changes, such as the altered N/C ratio, which should be considered for each particular p16 reactive cell. The diagnosis of ASC gains some prediction value, if based on the presence of a few HSIL-like cells (the so-called ASC-H). The latter points at a fast progression to HSIL from the very beginning (**Figure 8**). Nevertheless, the ASC-H category was challenged by other investigators as being problematic, since the morphologic difference in the appearance of such single metaplastic and/or neoplastic cell is not always clear and opens the way to false positive as well as false negative diagnoses [80–82]. Nuclear hyperchromasia and irregular nuclear membrane contours count as the most reliable diagnostic feature in the so-called pre-neoplastic atypia. The presence of such cells in the smears possibly corresponds to the dysplastic cells in histological sections [83], which, however, cannot be present in the smear in the case of CIN I/LSIL (compare **Figure 1**), but may be already easily collected in the cases of CIN II/HSIL (compare **Figure 4**). For better orientation in the most uncertain cases, a short course of local estrogen cream therapy followed by repeated PA tests has been suggested for helpful [84].

According to our experience, the relatively high percentage of p16 reactive atypical cells causing false positive LSIL grading appears in smears if handled by the conventional PA method. Therefore, the LBC should be preferred at repeated examination of patients which had been selected according to the classical Papanicolaou diagnostic system (when scored PA IIIa/IIIb roughly corresponding ASCUS and/or LSIL, as well as PA IV corresponding to HSIL and/or even PA V). The advantage of recently introduced improved diagnostic approach can be demonstrated on the results from the Cytology Laboratory (CL) of the St. Elisabeth Cancer

Institute (SECI) in Bratislava obtained within the years 2012–2013. The total number of gynecological cytology samples enrolled during the given period was 17,272, which corresponds to approximately 46% of samples examined at the Cytology Laboratories of Alpha medical presented in **Table 4**. While **Table 4** shows the positive rate of the screening from samples enrolled by practitioners, the Cancer Institute samples were submitted by specialists to whom the positively screened patients were sent for further care and/or treatment. Therefore, the diagnostic approach met was more complex combining the LBC technic (for example the Liqui-PREP kit) along with the detection of HPV DNA in nearly 53% of samples reflects the advantage of the interpretation of results, which have been achieved by comparison of both methods (**Table 9**). When considering the fact there was no logical need to request the HPV DNA test in the majority of negative cases enrolled (out of these 28% were tested for HPV only) then in becomes clear that the number of smears complete by DNA testing prevailed not only in essentially inevitable cases, such as ASCUS and LSIL, but by average the HPV DNA was tested by a proportion of 52.3% of all smears examined. When considering all the important facts mentioned, then the complete (dual examination) approach has been applied in 68% of ASCUS/LSIL cases (shown in bold type). It comes from **Table 10** that the HPV positive rates ranged from 27 to 33% in ASCUS and/or LSIL cases, respectively, indicating that the probability of further progression in these mild lesions could be quite low. In contrast, by the HSIL-graded smears the HPV DNA test was positive in 92% of cases. The same was true for the combination of positive HPV test with the p16 antigen staining. This was seen by 32% of LSIL-graded cases, in which the probability of progression was then relatively high, since as has been such transition really may occur by up to 15% of LSIL cases (citácia), which means that each second such double positive LSIL case might progress into HSIL. As our statistics concerns, this was really the case, but by a lower probability equal to one out of three LSIL cases. Byun et al. [85] conducted a comparative study including the p16 INK4a/Ki-67 double staining as well as the L1 capsid protein immunostaining along with human papillomavirus (HPV) DNA detection and typing in 56 ASC-H or LSIL-H cases diagnosed by LBC stained smears came to the conclusion that their approach was sufficient to predict CIN II+ and/or CIN III+ later on diagnoses at histological examinations of biopsies obtained from patients who underwent conization. Further interesting considerations are coming from the comparison of the biopsies subsequently resulting from the previous cytological diagnostic based their histological grading made at different Pathology Departments. While in the Diagnostic Center at the Pathology in Martin revealed that the probability of negative and/or non-neoplastic findings (including false positive and/or reactive staining) was approximately 22%. In contrast, the probability of the occurrence of the same result at the Pathology Department of the Oncology Institute in Bratislava was slightly below 10% only (**Table 11**). This difference in the negative scoring of CIN lesions in cervical biopsies reflects a better forecast based on a complex diagnostic approach, involving the use of LBC technology at repeated examination of cervical smears with contemporary HPV DNA tests along with the staining of smears for at least two serological markers. We believe that the cytological diagnosis should reflect a better degree of cooperation between clinicians and laboratory workers. As seen according to the presented algorithm, the suggested minimum of 2 or 3 colposcopic sessions may be satisfactory for precise diagnosis (**Figure 9**). In positive cases (i.e., those graded over PA III according to conventional Papanicolaou system), the repeated smear taken should be handled by the LBC-based technic and stained for at least two markers (p16 and Ki-67 and tested HPV DNA presence.

Cytology	Completed	Not completed	Total examined
Non-suspicious	63 (28%)	225	288
ASCUS	**139 (59%)**	96 (41%)	235
ASC-H	**5 (63%)**	3	8
LSIL	**304 (68%)**	143 (32%)	447
HSIL	124 (53%)	108 (47%)	232
SCa	0	4	4
Total	**635 (52.3%)**	**579**	**1214**

Abbreviations: LBC—liquid-based cytology; HPV—human papilloma virus; ASCUS—atypical squamous cells of undetermined significance; ASC-H—Atypical squamous cells-cannot exclude high-grade squamous intraepithelial lesion; LGSIL—Low-grade squamous intraepithelial lesion; HGSIL—High-grade squamous intraepithelial lesion; SCa—squamous cell carcinoma.

* The CL is a part of the Pathology Department of the St. Elisabeth Cancer Institute, which also is a teaching center of Slovak Postgraduate University in Bratislava

** Negative.

*** HPV DNA not tested.

Table 9. LBC examinations of cervical smears during the period of 2012–2013 at the CL of the St. Elisabeth Cancer Institute, Bratislava.

Cytological diagnosis	Number		Antigenic markers			HPV DNA test	
		Per cent*	p16 positive	Ki-67 positive	p16+/ Ki-67+	Positive alone	p16+/HPV+
Negative*	63	9.9	0	0	0	3	0
ASCUS	139	21.9	87 (63%)	7	4	38 (27%)	21 (15%)
ASC-H	5	0.8	2	2	2	2	2
LSIL	304	47.9	268 (88%)	66	114	99 (33%)	97 (32%)
HSIL	124	19.5	120 (96%)	106	103	114 (92%)	112 (90%)
SCa	0	0	0	0	0	0	0
Total	635	100%	477	181	223	256 (40%)	232 (37%)

LBC—liquid-based cytology; HPV—human papilloma virus; ASCUS—atypical squamous cells of undetermined significance; ASC-H—Atypical squamous cells-cannot exclude high-grade squamous intraepithelial lesion; LSIL—Low-grade squamous intraepithelial lesion; HGSIL—High-grade squamous intraepithelial lesion; SCa—squamous cell carcinoma.

* Calculated from the total completed examinations.

** Scored as non-suspicious, see also in **Table 9**.

Table 10. The completed LBC-based cervical smears according to staining procedures and correlated with the HPV DNA test result.

Cytological diagnosis	Diagnosis at biopsy						Examination
	Non-neoplastic**	CIN I	CIN II	CIN III	SCa	Number total	
ASCUS	20	12	2	4	0	38	Histology
ASC-H	3	0	2	0	0	5	Histology
LSIL	0	56	0	0	0	56	Histology
HSIL	0	4	60	76	0	140	Histology
SCa	0	0	0	0	4	4	Histology
Total (Pathology 1)	**23 (9.4%)**	**72 (30%)**	**64 (26%)**	**80 (33%)**	**4 (1.6%)**	**243 (100%)**	Histology
Example shown at	Figure 2**, Figure 3	Figure 1	Figure 4	Figure 5	Figure 6		
Pathology 2	**55 (22%)**	**90 (36%)**	**46 (18%)**	**52 (21%)**	**7 (3%)**	**250 (100%)**	Histology
		3/11 (27%)		**7/8 (88%)**			HPV DNA

LBC—liquid-based cytology; HPV—human papilloma virus; ASCUS—atypical squamous cells of undetermined significance; ASC-H—Atypical squamous cells-cannot exclude high-grade squamous intraepithelial lesion; LGSIL—Low-grade squamous intraepithelial lesion; HGSIL—High-grade squamous intraepithelial lesion; SCa—squamous cell carcinoma; CIN—cervical intraepithelial neoplasia and its grading.

* Concerns the biopsies examined at CL of St. Elisabeth Cancer Institute.

** Includes the reactive not-dysplastic lesions, such as false positive p16 staining as well as the p16 negative (normal) squamous epithelium.

*** The data concern the Diagnostic Center of Pathology Ltd, Alpha medical, Martin.

\# Important notice: even though the proportion of patients in which the HPV DNA was tested at The Pathology center was relatively low (12 and 15%, respectively), the application of a complex approach Figure 9 proven the prevalence of HPV DNA presence by CIN III/HSIL.

Table 11. Correlations between cytology and biopsy during the same time period of 2013–2014 in two different Pathology Departments.

Diagnosis	Sample number	HPV (all types)		HR HPV genotypes			HR total
		Negative	Positive	HPV16	HPV 18	Not frequent**	
ASCUS/LSIL	520	329	191	59	18	114	191 (34%)
HSIL	45	19	26	2	0	24	26 (57%)
Not determined	932	608	302	93	21	120	(25%)

* Department of Clinical Microbiology, Alpha medical Ltd, Ružomberok, suitable to recognize the genotypes.

** HPV types 31, 33, 35, 39, 45, 51, 52, 56, 58, 59, 66, 68.

Table 12. Results of HPV DNA testing by means of the Cobas 4800 equipment*.

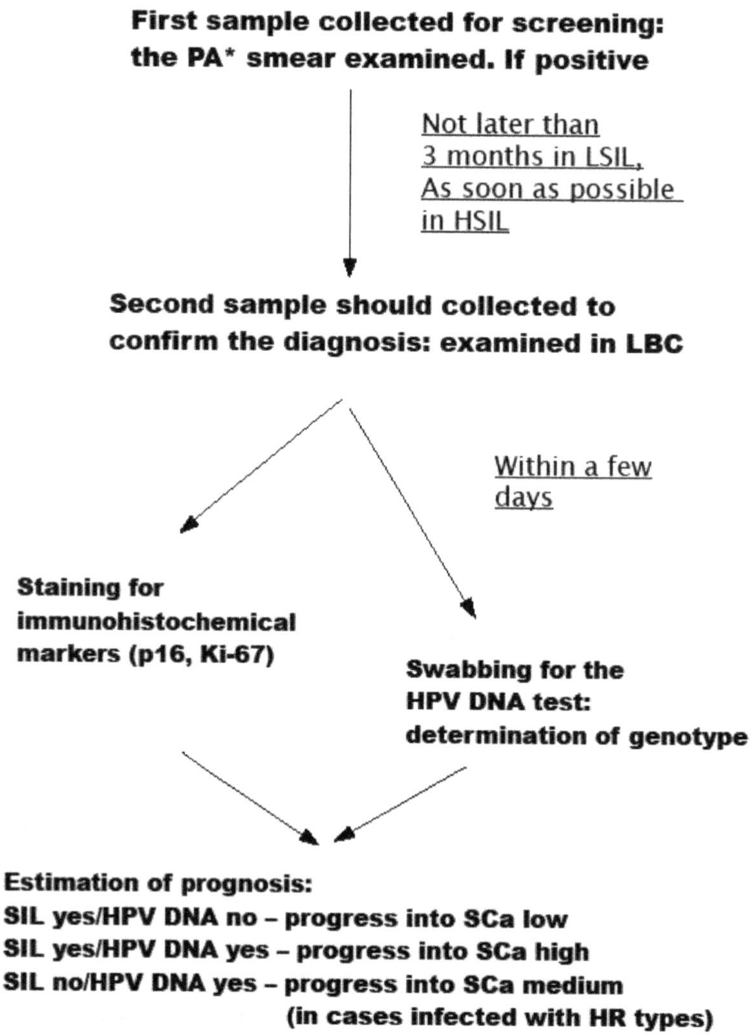

Figure 9. A simple algorithm allowing to assess the precise diagnosis of dysplasia and to estimate its prognosis (all the basic information shown should be at disposal for exact decision making).

5. HPV DNA detection in association with cytological and histological examinations

In countries where cytological diagnostic is widely used for screening, the most useful option is to use HPV DNA testing especially for getting more reliable information allowing to lengthen safely the next smear examination interval [86]. In general, the DNA tests are based either on DNA/DNA hybridization (using labeled complementary DNA probes), or on amplification of vDNA by polymerase chain reaction (PCR) as well as on DNA/RNA hybridization (using complementary RNA probes) followed by visualization of the labeled hybrid signal. Early approaches utilized various modifications of the vDNA to DNA probe hybridization tests, such as in situ hybridization and/or various blotting techniques [87]. To improve the PCR method, multiple primers for L1 and/or E1 gene amplifications have been introduced, aiming to identify the most frequent genotypes (i.e., HPV 6, 11, 16, and 18) in a single-tube reaction [88]. The principle of multiple genotype amplification was further modified using general primers (GPs), which flank the strongly conserved regions located either on L1 and/or E1 ORFs, enabling detection of a wide spectrum of genotypes [89]. The GPs annealed not only to the ORFs of genotypes, which they had been designed for, but also to some another which sequence was not known at that time (later on these were identified as HPV 13, 30, 31, 45, and 51). The consensus or general primer GP5+/GP6+ based procedure became widely used, since it enabled the differentiation between several HR and LR HPV genotypes in a single assay [90, 91]. The GP-PCR technique became further improved in order to detect more genotypes (at least 14 HR HPV along with the 6 frequent LR HPV genotypes). In addition, it was modified in order to visualize the reaction product by enzyme linked immunosorbent assay, that is ELISA [92]. The high-risk types being assessed this way were, as a rule, HPV 16, 18, 31, 33, 39, 45, 51, 52, 56, 58, 59, 66, and 68, and the low-risk ones were at least HPV 6, 11, 40, 42, 43, and 44. Further improvements of GPs allowed their annealing to the DNA of additional genotypes, such as HPV 26, 30, 53, 70, 73, 82, and 83, in order to increase the number of routinely detectable genotypes to 27 out of the 40 possible mucosal human papillomavirus types [93]. Additional consensus primers, having been introduced for L1 ORF amplification, were further modified to avoid synthesis of irreproducible fragments [94]. The latter primer set (PGMY07/11) increased the number of multiple HPV genotype infections detected by adding the rare genotypes such as HPV 26, 35, 42, 45, 52, 54, 59, 66, and 73. Any routine HR versus LR HPV testing may be influenced by the DNA extraction technic, namely depending whether a recommended manual extraction procedure or an automated extraction protocol supplied by the manufacturer of given equipment was used [95]. To avoid the methodic variations, automated vDNA extraction was recommended for HPV genotyping by both, the classical PCR (GP5/GP6 primers) as well as for the real-time PCR-based quantitative TaqMan assay. Further modification of HPV detection in the direction of immunochemistry has resulted into an assay omitting vDNA amplification, while introducing the labeled signal amplification instead. In a latter assay, the denatured vDNA was hybridized under high stringency conditions to single-stranded RNA probes either for LR genotypes (at least 6, 11, 42, 43, and 44) and/or for HR genotypes (at least 16, 18, 31, 33, 35, 45, 51, 52, and 56). The RNA/DNA hybrid complex was then bound to microplates (or tubes) coated with an alkaline phosphatase conjugated monoclonal antibody, able to capture the specific RNA/DNA hybrid [96]. The reaction is then visualized by addition of the chemilumiscent substrate, in which emission light is amplified and measured in a luminometer; the results are expressed in relative light units (RLU). This method is referred to as hybrid capture (HC). At its beginning HC showed lower sensitivity, as compared to as few as 10–100 vDNA copies (about 100 fg HPV DNA) were detectable per 1 ml sample when using the classical PCR. The recent HC2-based high-risk HPV DNA test (Qiagen), which was previously used in the Alpha medical laboratory as well, detects 13 HR genotypes (HPV 16, 18, 31, 33, 35, 35, 39, 45, 51, 52, 56, 58, and 68) at a sensitivity of 1–2 pg/ml (i.e., about 100,000 HPV DNA copies/ml). Another variation of this assay can be also used for detection of at least 5 LR genotypes (HPV 6, 11, 42, 43, and 44). Recio et al. [97] used the first generation HC test for investigating the HPV DNA presence in patients with ASCUS, LSIL, HSIL, and carcinoma *in situ* smears, the latter being used as a relevant standard. Altogether 44% of patients were tested positive, mainly for HR HPV genotypes. The authors concluded that testing of HPV DNA by the HC method is helpful for clinical diagnostic. Monsenogo et al. [90] reported that the HC2 test as compared in 470 patients with the PCR-based Roche Amplicor HPV test, reached an agreement of 96.2%; only 18 cases were found discordant. It should be mentioned that the Amplicor HPV test identifies the PCR-amplified vDNA by means of 13 HR-HPV genotype probes and that the vDNA is being obtained from cervical cells collected into a transport medium [98]. In patients revealing ASCUS smears, both tests for HPV DNA showed a positive rate of 42.3%, while in patients showing LSIL smears, the HPV DNA positive rate was 66.3 and/or 66.8%, respectively, depending on the test performed (the PCR-based test seemed in this case even less sensitive). In patients with HSIL smears, the DNA was positive in both tests at the highest rate of 92.8%.

The HC2 high risk HPV DNA Test takes advantage of the Hybrid Capture 2 (HC2) technology; it is a nucleic acid hybridization assay with signal amplification that utilizes microplate chemiluminescent detection for the qualitative detection of 13 high-risk HPV types (16, 18, 31, 33, 35, 39, 45, 51, 52, 56, 58, 59, 68) in cervical specimens. Specimens containing the target DNA hybridize with a specific HPV RNA probe. The resultant RNA:DNA hybrids are captured onto the surface of a microplate well coated with antibodies specific for RNA:DNA hybrids. Immobilized hybrids are then reacted with alkaline phosphatase conjugated antibodies specific for the RNA:DNA hybrids and detected with chemiluminescent substrate. Several alkaline phosphatase molecules are conjugated to each antibody. Multiple conjugated antibodies bind to each captured hybrid resulting in substantial signal amplification. In contrast to the HC technology, the Cobas® 4800 Human Papillomavirus (HPV) Test is a qualitative *in vitro* test for the detection of human papillomavirus in cervical specimens. The test utilizes amplification of target DNA by the polymerase chain reaction (PCR) and nucleic acid hybridization for the detection of 14 high-risk HPV types in a single analysis. The test specifically identifies HPV16 and HPV18 while concurrently detecting the other high-risk types (31, 33, 35, 39, 45, 51, 52, 56, 58, 59, 66, and 68) at clinically relevant infection levels. The Cobas® 4800 HPV Test primers define a sequence of approximately 200 nucleotides within the polymorphic L1 region of the HPV genome. An additional primer pair would target the human β-globin gene (330 bp amplicon) to provide a process control. A pool of HPV primers present in the Master Mix is designed to amplify HPV DNA from 14 high-risk types (16, 18, 31, 33, 35, 39, 45, 51, 52, 56, 58, 59, 66, and 68). The detection of amplified DNA is performed during thermal cycling using oligonucleotide probes labeled with four different fluorescent dyes. The amplified signal from twelve high-risk HPV types (31, 33, 35, 39, 45, 51, 52, 56, 58, 59, 66, and 68), is detected using the same fluorescent dye, while HPV16, HPV18, and β-globin signals are each detected with their own dedicated fluorescent dye. Fluorescent oligonucleotide probes bind to polymorphic regions HPV and human β-globin gene within the sequence defined by primers.

Summing up, the DNAs can be distinguished according to (1) the ability to identify a pool of high-risk HPV types, with or without genotypization of the most common high-risk viruses (i.e., HPV16 and 18) or (2) to detect a broad spectrum of oncogenic and non-oncogenic HPVs along with individual genotyping. While the assays of the first group are mainly used in screening programs, where there is no clinical benefit from the knowledge of specific HPV types, the assays of the second group are primarily used in HPV surveillance studies and to monitor the eventual spreading of particular viral types in vaccinated women [99]. The HPV16 and HPV18 genotyping, for its high specificity, have been included in the US guidelines for the triage of HPV positive and cytology negative women [100]. In general, the probability of developing precancerous (HSIL) lesions was high in women who were LSIL as well as DNA positive; a lower, but still medium probability for developing cancer was found in HPV DNA positive, but by cytology negative women. The lowest probability was noted in HPV negative but ASCUS/LSIL positive cases. Similar findings were observed in the Microbiology Department of Alpha medical (**Table 12**) showing that the positive rate of HR genotypes was the highest in HSIL cases, the closet in cases with not precisely determined diagnosis. As stressed by Mandelblatt et al. [101], screening of HPV plus patients with LSIL tests within 2 years appears to save lives and is more reasonable than performing the cytology test alone. Another large cohort study in US (performed from 2003 to 2005) found that women aged less than 30 who have ASCUS-grade smears showed HPV positive rate at 53% [102]. On the other hand, women older than 30 years with NIL PAP test were HPV (HC2) positive at a rate of 9%. Since ASCUS smear diagnosis is a clinical and prognostic challenge, it should be combined with HPV testing and repeatedly investigated to show whether or not the transition to HSIL occurs [103]. Also in this follow up, a relatively low proportion (6.7%) of ASCUS positive patients developed HSIL or cancer. Among the patients with HSIL smears, up to 98% was found HPV 565 DNA positive; theoretically such women harbor the integrated incomplete genome in the cervical tissue. It was concluded that the residual specimens collected from routine cervical cytology in ASCUS cases could provide additional information about the HPV DNA status that is of substantial help by identifying those patients, who are likely to develop HSIL, especially if they test positive for the HPV DNA presence.

Acknowledgements

The authors thank Dr. J. Hybenová the Head of the Department of Clinical Microbiology, Alpha medical Ltd, Ružomberok (for her kind advice), as well as Mrs. J. Papanová and Mrs. S. Drahošová from the Pathology Diagnostic Center, Martin, Alpha medical, Slovakia, for their helpful assistance.

Author details

J. Rajčáni[1*], K. Kajo[2,3], O. el Hassoun[1], M. Adamkov[1,4] and M. Benčat[1]

*Address all correspondence to: viruraj@savba.sk

1 Pathology Ltd, Diagnostic Center, Alpha Medical Ltd, Záborského 2, 03601 Martin, Slovak Republic

2 Pathology Ltd, Diagnostic Laboratory, Alpha medical Ltd, Banská Bystrica, Slovak Republic

3 Department of Pathology, St. Elisabeth Cancer Institute, Bratislava, Slovak Republic

4 Department of Histology, Jessenius Medical Faculty, Comenius University, Martin, Slovak Republic

References

[1] Aurelian L, Kessler II, Rosenheim NB, Barbour G. Viruses and gynecologic cancers: herpesvirus protein (ICP 1 OIAG-#), a cervical tumor antigen that fulfills the criteria for a marker of carcinogenicity. Cancer. 1981, 48:455–471.

[2] Petersen EE, Böcker JF, Schmitt M, Wimhöfer G, Hillemanns HG. Carcinoma of the uterine cervix and herpes simplex virus type 2. Investigations on the causal relationship. Geburtshilfe Frauenheilkd. 1975, 35(2):98–107.

[3] Maitland NJ. The aetiological relationship between herpes simplex virus type 2 and carcinoma of the cervix: an unanswered or unanswerable question? Cancer Surv. 1988, 7(3):457–6.

[4] zur Hausen H. Human papillomaviruses and their possible role in squamous cell carcinomas. Top Microbiol Immunol. 1977, 78:1–30.

[5] Yamakawa Y, Forslund O, Chua KL, Dillner L, Boon ME, Hansson BG. Detection of the BC 24 transforming fragment of the herpes simplex virus type 2 (HSV-2) DNA in cervical carcinoma tissue by polymerase chain reaction (PCR). Acta Pathol Micrfobiol Immunol Scand. 1994, 102(1–6):401–406.

[6] Salcedo BMMP, da Silveira GPG. Immunohistochemical expression of p16 and herpes simplex virus type 2 in squamous intraepithelial lesions and cervical cancer. Rev Bras Ginecol Obstet. 2008, 30(2):61–6.

[7] Luff RD. The Bethesda system for reporting cervical vaginal cytologic diagnoses. Report of the 1991 Bethesda workshop. Hum Pathol. 1992, 23:719–721.

[8] Apgar BS, Yoschnik L, Wright TC. The 2001 Bethesda system terminology. Am Fam Physician. 2003, 68(10):1992–1998.

[9] Abali R, Bacanakgil BH, Celik S, Aras O, Koca P, et al. Histolopathological correlation of cervical squamous cell abnormalities detected on cevical cytology. Turk J Pathol. 2011, 27:1414–148.

[10] Sosič GM, Babič G, Dimitrijevič A, Mitrovič S, Varjačič M, et al. Correlation between cervical cytopathology and histopathological cervical biopsy findings according to the Bethesda system. Ser J Exp Clin Res. 2014, 15(4):205–216.

[11] Abati A, Geisewinger KR, Raab SS, Stanley MW, Silverman JF (eds). Modern Cytopathology, Churchill Livingstone, 2003.

[12] Nayar R, Wilbur C (eds). The Bethesda System for Reporting Cervical Cytology, 3rd ed., 321 p. Springer Verlag, Heidelberg 2015. ISBN 978-3-319-11074-5.

[13] Kállay J. Karcinóm krčka meternice (Cervical carcinoma). In: Kaušitz J, Altáner Č (eds.), Onkológia (Oncology). Veda, Publishing House of SAS, Bratislava, 2003, 659 p. ISBN 80-224-0711-9.

[14] Rajčáni J, Adamkov M, Hybenová J, Jackuliak J, Benčat M. Diagnostic role of p16/INK4A protein in Human Papillomavirus (HPV) induced cervical dysplasia. Cent Eur J Biol. 2010, 5(5):554–571.

[15] Kulasingan SL, Hughes JP, Kiviat NB, Mao C, Weiss NS, Kuypers JM, et al. Evaluation of human papillomavirus in primary screening for cervical abnormalities. Comparison of sensitivity, specificity and frequency referral. JAMA. 2002, 288:1749–1757.

[16] Patterson B, Takahashni H. Recent advances in cervical cancer screening. Am J Clin Pathol. 2006, 2(3):1–2.

[17] Shope RE, Hurst EW. Infectious papillomavirus of rabbits with a note on the histopathology. J Exp Med. 1933, 58:67–624.

[18] Howley PM, Schiller JT, Lowy D. Papillomaviruses. In: Knipe DM, Howley PM (eds.), Field's Virology, 6th ed. Kluver W, Lippincott WW, Philadelphia, 2013, pp. 1662–1703. ISBN-10: 1-4511-0563-0.

[19] Fauthquet V, Mayo CM, Maniloff MAJ, Desselberger U, Ball LA. Family Papillomaviridae, Virus Taxonomy, 8th Report of the ICTV, Elsevier-Academic Press, 2005, pp. 239–249.

[20] Rebrikov DV, Bogdanova EA, Bulina ME, Lukyanov SA. A new planarian extrachromosomal virus-like element revealed by subtractive hybridization. Mol Biol. 2002, 36:813–820.

[21] Orth G. Epidermodysplasia verruciformis: a model for understanding the oncogenicity of human papillomaviruses. Ciba Found Symp. 1986, 120:157–174.

[22] deOliveira WR, He Q, Rady PL, Hughes TK, Neto CF, Rivitti EA, Tyring SK. HPV typing in Brazilian patients with *epidermodysplasia verruciformis*: high prevalence of EV-HPV 25. J Cutan Med Surg. 2004, 8(2):110–115.

[23] Dell' Osteetal V, Azzimonti B, DeAndrea M, Mondini M, Zavattaro E, et al. High beta-HPV DNA loads and strong seroreactivity are present in epidermodysplasia verruciformis. J Investig Dermatol. 2009, 129(4):1026–1034.

[24] Pfister H, TerSchegget J. Role of HPV incutaneous premalignant and malignant tumors. Clin Dermatol. 1997, 15(3):335–347.

[25] Bouvard V, Baan R, Straif K, Grosse Y, Secretan B, ElGhissassi F, BenbrahimTallaa L, Guha N, Freeman C, Galiche TL, Cogliano V. Group W.H.O.I.A.f.R. o.C.M.W. A review of human carcinogens—part B: biological agents. Lancet Oncol. 2009, 10(4):321–322.

[26] Spalholz BA, Yang YC, Howleay PM. Transactivation of bovine papillomavirus transcriptional regulatory element by the E2 gene product. Cell. 1985, 42:183–191.

[27] Bernard BA, Bailley C, Lenoir MC, et al. The human papillomavirus 18 (HPV 18) E2 gene product is a repressor of the HPV 18 regulatory region in human keratinocytes. J Virol. 1989, 63:4317–4324.

[28] Piirsoo M, Ustav E, Mandel T, et al. Cis and trans requirements for stable episomal maintenance of the BPV-1 replicator. EMBO J. 1996, 15:1–11.

[29] Skiadopoulos MH, McBride AA. Bovine papillomavirus type 1 genomes and the E2 transactivator protein are closely associated with mitotoic protein. J Virol. 1998, 72:2079–2088.

[30] de Villiers E-M, Fauquet C, Broker C, Bernard H-U, zur Hausen H. Classification of papillomaviruses. Minireview. Virology. 2004, 324:17–27.

[31] Bonez W. Papillomaviruses. In: Richman V, Whitley D, Whitley R (eds.), Clinical Virology, 2nd ed., ASM Press, Washington, 2002, pp. 557–596.

[32] Doorbar J. The papillomavirus life cycle. J Clin Virol. 2005, 32:S7–S15.

[33] Johnson KM, Kines RC, Roberts JN, et al. Role of heparan sulfate in attachment to and infection of the murine female genital tract by human papillomavirus. J Virol. 2009, 83:2067–2074.

[34] Kines RC, Thompson CD, Kowy DR, et al. The initial steps leading to papillomavirus infection occur on the basement membrane prior to cell surface binding. Proc Natl Acad Sci USA. 2009, 106:12,180–12,184.

[35] Doorbar J, Quint W, Banks L. The biology of the life cycle of human papillomaviruses. Vaccine. 2012, 30 (Suppl. 5):55–70.

[36] Day PM, Schiller JT. The role of furin in papillomavirus infection. Future Microbiol. 2009, 4:1255–1262.

[37] Day PM, Lowy DR, Schiller, JT. Papillomaviruses infect cells via a clathrin-depedent pathway. Virology. 2003, 307:1–11.

[38] Schiller JT, Daz PM, Kines RC. Current understanding of the mechanism of HPV infection. Gynecol Oncol. 2010, 118:S12–S17.

[39] Meyers C, Laimins LA. *In vitro* systems for the study and propagation of human papillomaviruses. Curr Top Microbiol Immunol. 1994, 186:199–215.

[40] Martin P, Vass W, Schiller JT. The bovine papillomavirus E5 transforming protein can stimulate the transforming activity of EGF and CSF-1 receptors. Cell. 1989, 59:21–23.

[41] Petti L, DiMayo D. Activation of the platelet derived growth factor receptor by the bovine papillomavirus E5 protein. EMBO J. 1991, 40:845–855.

[42] Petti L, DiMayo G. Stable association between the bovine papillomavirus E5 transforming protein and the b receptor for platelet derived growth factor in stably transformed and acutely transfected cells. J Virol. 1994, 74:3582–3592.

[43] Dyson N, Howley PM, Munger K, Harlow E. The human papillomavirus 16 E7 oncoprotein is able to bind the retinoblastoma gene product. Science. 1989, 243:934–993.

[44] Werness BA, Levine AJ, Howley PM. Association of human papillomavirus types 16 and 18 E6 proteins with p53. Science. 1990, 248:76–79.

[45] Scheffner M, Huibregtse JM, Vierstra RD, Yoshihara M, Sumiri K, Kayiyama G, et al. The HPV-16 and E6-AP complex functions as a ubiquitin-protein ligase in the ubiquitinations of p53. Cell. 1993, 75:495–499.

[46] Golijow CD, Abba MC, Mouron SA, Gomez MA, Doulot FN. C-myc gene amplification detected preinvasive intraepithelial lesions. Int J Gynecol Cancer. 2001, 11:492–465.

[47] Li Y, Nichols MA, Shay JW, Xiong Y. Transcriptional repression of the D type cyclin dependent kinase p16 by retinoblastoma susceptibility gene product pRb. Cancer Res. 1994, 54:6078–6082.

[48] Schwartz E, Freese UK, Gissman L, et al. Structure and transcription of human papillomavirus sequences in cervical carcinoma cells. Nature. 1985, 314:111–114.

[49] Gillison ML. Human papillomavirus –associated head and neck cancer is a distinct epidemiologic, clinical and molecular entity. Sem Oncol. 2004, 31:2269–2282.

[50] Matsukura T, Kol S, Sugase M. Both episomal and integrated forms of human papillomavirus type 16 are involved in invasive cervical cancers. Virology. 1989, 172:63–72.

[51] White A, Livanos FM, Tlsty TD. Differential disruption of genomic integrity and cell cycle regulation in normal human fibroblasts by the HPV oncoproteins. Genes Dev. 1994, 8:666–677.

[52] Choo K-B, Pan C-C, Han S-H. Integration of human papillomavirus type 16 into cellular DNA of cervical carcinoma. Preferential deletion of the E2 gene and invariable retention of the long control region and the E6/E7 open reading frames. Virology. 1987, 161:259–261.

[53] Kulmala SM, Syrjanen SM, Gyllensten UB, Shabalova IP, Petrovichev N, Syrjanen KJ, et al. Early integration of high copy HPV 16 detectable in women with normal and low grade cervical cytology. J Clin Pathol. 2006, 59:513–517.

[54] Kalantari M, Karlsen F, Kritensen G, Holm R, Hagmar B, Johansson B, et al. Disruption of the E1 and E2 reading frames of HPV16 in cervical carcinoma is associated with poor prognosis. Int J Gynecol Pathol. 1998, 17:146–153.

[55] Klaes R, Friedrich T, Spitkovski D, Ridder R, Rudy W, Petri K, et al. Over expression of p16/INK4A as a specific marker for dysplastic and neoplastic epithelial cells of the cervix uteri. Int J Cancer. 2001, 92:276–284.

[56] Murphy N, Ring M, Killalea AG, Uhlmann V, O'Donovan M, Mulcahy F. Cervical dyskaryosis: CIN and cGIN in cervical biopsies and ThinPrep smears. J Clin Pathol. 2003, 56:56–63.

[57] Murphy N, Ring M, Heffron CC, King B, Killalea AG, Hughes C, et al. p16/INK4a, CDC6 and MCM5: predictive biomarkers in cervical preinvasive neoplasia and cervical cancer. J Clin Pathol. 2005, 58:525–534.

[58] O'Neill CJ, McCluggage WG. The p16 expression in the female genital tract and its value in diagnosis. Adv Clin Pathol. 2006, 13:8–15.

[59] Jeon S, Lambert PF. Integration of HPV 16 DNA into the human genome leads to increased stability of E6/E7 mRNAs: implications for cervical carcinogenesis. Proc Natl Acad Sci USA. 1995, 92:1654–1658.

[60] Janučišová V, Kapustová I, Žubor P, Slezák P, Kajo K, et al. The p16INK4A mRNA transcripts in cervical smear with different degress of dysplasia. Čas Gynek. 2012, 77(3): 245–250.

[61] Jacobs A, Kristensen PB, Poulsen HK. Flow cytometric classification of biopsy specimens from cervical intraepithelial neoplasia. Cytometry. 1983, 4:166–169.

[62] Wright TC, Kurman RJ. A critical review of the morphologic classification systems of preinvasive lesions of the cervix: the scientific basis of the paradigm. Papillomavirus Rep. 1994, 5:175–181.

[63] Yildiz IZ, Usubutun A, Firat P, Kucukali T. Efficiency of immunohistological p16 expression and HPV typing in cervical squamous intraepithelial lesion grading and review of p16 literature. Pathol Res Pract. 2007, 203:445–449.

[64] Robboy SJ, Duggan MA, Kurman R. The female reproductive system. In: Rubin E, Farber J (eds.), Pathology, 2nd ed., JB Lippincott, Philadelphia, 1994, pp. 908–971, ISBN 0-397-51047-0.

[65] Kruse AJ, Baak JPA, deBruin PC, Jiwa M, Snijders WP, Fons G, et al. Ki-67 immunoquantitation in cervical intraepithelial neoplasia (CIN): a sensitive marker for grading. J Pathol. 2001, 196:48–54.

[66] Kruse AJ, Baak JPA, Janssen EA, Bol MG, Kjellerod KH, Fianne B, et al. Low and high risk CIN I and II lesions: prospective predictive value of grade, HPV and Ki-67. J Pathol. 2003, 199:462–470.

[67] Keating JT, Cviko A, Rietdorf S, Quade M, Sun D, Duensing S, et al. K-67, cyclin E and p16/INK4 are complementary surrogate biomarkers forhuman papillomavirus-related cervical neoplasia. Am J Surg Pathol. 2001, 25:884–891.

[68] Dray M, Russell P, Dalrymple C, Wallman N, Angus G, Leong A, Carter J, Cheerala B. p16(INK4a) as a complementary marker of high-grade intraepithelial lesions of the uterine cervix. I: experience with squamous lesions in 189 consecutive cervical biopsies. Pathology. 2005, 37(2):112–124.

[69] Wentzensen N, Schwartz L, Zuna RE, Smith K, Mathews C, Gold MA, Andy Allen R, Zhang R, Terence Dunn S, Walker JL, Schiffman M. Performance of p16/Ki-67 immunostaining to detect cervical cancer precursors in a colposcopy referral population. Clin Cancer Res. 2012, 18(15):4154–4141.

[70] Tsoumpou I, Arbyn M, Kyrgiou M, Wentzensen N, Koliopoulos G, Martin-Hirsch P, et al. The p16(INK4a) immunostaining in cytological and histological specimens from the uterine cervix: a systematic review and meta-analysis. Cancer Treat Rev. 2009, 35:210–220.

[71] Cenda MT, Demir N, Sezer O, Doganay L, Ortac R. Clinical results of the liquid cytology tool, liquid PREP, in comparison with conventional smears of detection of squamous abnormalities. Asian Pac J Cancer Prev. 2009, 10:399–402.

[72] National Cancer Institute (NCI) Workshop. The 1988 Bethesda system for reporting cervical/vaginal cytologic diagnoses. JAMA. 1989, 262:931–934.

[73] Solomon D, Thomas PA, Lenel JC, Moriarti A, O'Connor D, Prey M, et al. The 2001 Bethesda system terminology for reporting results of cervical cytology. JAMA. 2002, 287:2114–2119.

[74] Geisinger KR, Raab SS, Stanley MW, Silverman JJ, Abati A. Modern Cytopathology, Churchill-Livingstone, New York, 2004, pp. 83–196.

[75] Nieh S, Chen Su-F, Chu T-Y, Lai H-CH, Fu E. Expression of 16INK4A in Papanicolaou smears containing atypical squamous cells of undetermined significance from uterus cervix. Gynecol Oncol. 2003, 91:201–208.

[76] Guo M, Hu L, Baliga M, He Z, Hughson MD. The predictive value of p16INK4 and hybrid capture 2 human papillomavirus testing hot high grade cervical intraepithelial neoplasia. Am J Clin Pathol. 2004, 122:894–901.

[77] Grapsa D, Frangou-Plemenou M, Kondi-Pafiti A, Stergiou E, Nicolopoulou-Stamati P, Patsouris E, Chelidonis G, Athanassiadou P. Immunocytochemical expression of P53, PTEN, FAS (CD95), P16INK4A and HPV L1 major capsid proteins in ThinPrep cervical samples with squamous intraepithelial lesions. Diagn Cytopathol. 2014, 42(6):465–475. DOI: 10.1002/dc.23003

[78] Shin EK, Lee SR, Kim MK, Kang EJ, Ju W, Lee SN, et al. Immunocytochemical staining of p16ink4a protein as an adjunct test in equivocal liquid base cytology. Diagn Cytopathol. 2008, 36:311–319.

[79] Duncan L, Jacob S, Hubbard E. Evaluation of p16INK4a as a diagnostic tool in the triage of Pap smears demonstrating atypical squamous cells of undetermined significance. Cancer Cytopathol. 2008, 114:34–48.

[80] Dressel DM, Wilbour DC. Atypical immature squamous metaplastic cells in cervical smears: association with high grade squamous intraepithelial lesions and carcinoma of the cervix. Acta Cytol. 1992, 36:630–631.

[81] Hatem F, Wilbur DC. High-grade squamous cervical lesions following negative Papanicoulaou smears: false negative cervical cytology or rapid progression. Diagn Cytopathol. 1995, 12:135–141.

[82] Gupta DK, Komaromi-Hiller G, Raab SS. Interobserver and intraobserver variability in the cytologic diagnosis of normal and abnormal metaplastic squamous cells in PAP smears. Acta Cytol. 2001, 45:697–703.

[83] Abati A, Jaffurs W, Wilder AM. Squamous atypia in the atrophic cervical vaginal smear. Cancer Cytopathol. 1998, 84:218–225.

[84] Wright TC, Cox JT, Massad LS. 2001 consensus guidelines for the management of women with cervical cytological abnormalities. JAMA. 2002, 287:2120–2129.

[85] Byun SW, Lee A, Kim S, Choi YJ, Lee YS, Park JS. Immunostaining of p16INK4a/Ki-67 and L1 capsid protein on liquid-based cytology specimens obtained from ASC-H and LSIL-H. J Med Sci. 2013, 10(12):1602–1607. DOI: 10.7150/ijms.6526

[86] Cuzick J, Arbyn M, Sankaranarayanan R, Tsu V, Ronco G, Mayrand MH, Dillner J, Meijer CJ. Overview of human papillomavirus-based and other novel options for cervical cancer screening in developed and developing countries. Vaccine. 2008, 19(8):K29–K41. DOI: 10.1016/j.vaccine.2008.06.019

[87] Rando FF. Nucleic acid hybridization as a diagnostic tool for the detection of human papillomaviruses. Adv Exp Med Biol. 1990, 263:89–109.

[88] Anceschi MM, Falcinelli C, Pieretti M, Cosmi EV. Multiple primer pairs polymerase chain reaction for the detection of human papillomavirus types. J Virol Methods. 1990, 28:59–65.

[89] van den Brule AJ, Snijders PJ, Gordijn RL, Becker OP, Maijer CJ, Walboomers JM. General primer-mediated polymerase chain reaction permits the detection of sequenced and still unsequenced human papillomavirus genotypes in cervical scrapes and carcinomas. Int J Cancer. 1990, 45:644–649.

[90] deRoda-Husman AM, Walboomers JMM, van den Brule AJC, Meijer CJLM, Snijders PJF. The use of general primers GP5 and GP6 elongated at their 3′ ends with adjacent highly conserved sequences improves human papillomavirus detection by polymerase chain reaction. J Gen Virol. 1995, 76:1057–1062.

[91] Jacobs MV, de Roda Husman AM, van den Brule AJC, Snijders PJF, Walboomers JMM. Group specific differentiation between high and low risk human papillomavirus

genotypes by general primer-mediated PCR and two cocktails of oligonucleotide probes. J Clin Microbiol. 1995, 33:901–905.

[92] Jacobs MW, Snijders PJF, van den Brule AJC, Helmhorst TJM, Meijer CJLM, Walboomers JMM. A general primer GP5+/GP6+-mediated PCR enzyme immunoassay method for rapid detection of 14 high risk and 6 low risk human papillomavirus genotypes in cervical scrapings. J Clin Microbiol. 1997, 35:791–795.

[93] Schmidt M, Dondog B, Waterboer T, Pawlita M. Homogenous amplification of general human alpha papillomavirus by PCR using a novel broad-spectrum GP5+ and GP6+ primers. J Clin Microbiol. 2008, 46:1050–1059.

[94] Gravitt PE, Peyton CL, Alessi TQ, Wheeler CM, Coutlee F, Hildesheim A, et al. Improved amplification of genital human papillomaviruses. J Clin Microbiol. 2000, 38:357–361.

[95] Oevestad IT, Janssen EA, Beak JP. The effect of different DNA isolation methods on the outcome of high risk HPV testing. Indian J Pathol Microbiol. 2007, 50:733–739.

[96] Reid R, Lorincz AT. Human papillomavirus tests. Bail Clin Obstet Gynecol. 1995, 9:65–103.

[97] Recio FO, Srivastava S, Wong C, Hempling RE, Eltabakh GH, Piver MS. The clinical value of digene hybrid capture HPV DNA trstiny in a referral-based pc. Eur J Gynaecol Oncol. 1998, 19:203–208.

[98] Monsenogo J, Bohbot JM, Pollini G, Krawec C, Vincent C, Merinargues I, et al. Performance of the Roche AMPLICOR human papillomavirus test in prediction of cervical intraepithelial neoplasia (CIN) in women with abnormal PAP smear. Gynecol Oncol. 2005, 99:160–168.

[99] Tornesello ML, Buonaguro L, Giorgi-Rossi P, Buon FM. Viral and cellular biomarkers in the diagnosis of cervical intraepithelial neoplasia and cancer. BioMed Res Int. 2013, Article ID 519619: 10. DOI: 10.1155/2013/519619

[100] Moyer VA. Screening for cervical cancer: US preventive services task force recommendation statement. Ann Intern Med. 2012, 156(12):880–891.

[101] Mandelblatt JS, Lawrence WF, Womack SM, Jacobson D, Yi B, Hwang YT, et al. Benefits and costs of using HPV testing to screen for cervical cancer. JAMA. 2002, 287:2372–2387.

[102] Datta SD, Koutsky LA, Ratelle S, Unger ER, Shlay J, Weather B, et al. Human papillomavirus and cervical cytology in women screened for cervical cancer in the United States, 2003–2005. Ann Intern Med. 2008, 148:557–559.

[103] Manos MM, Kinney WK, Hurley LB, Sherman ME, Shieh-Ngai J, Kurman RJ, et al. Identifying women with cervical neoplasia using human papillomavirus DNA testing and equivocal Papanicolaou results. JAMA. 1999, 281:1605–1610.

2

Pathogenesis of Human Papillomavirus – Immunological Responses to HPV Infection

G. Hossein Ashrafi and Nadia Aziz Salman

Abstract

Papillomavirus is an oncogenic virus which infects mucosal and cutaneous epithelia where it induces benign hyperproliferative lesions. Few studies have been conducted on the causative factors associated with the development of cancer. Infections by high-risk human papillomaviruses (HPVs) have been implicated as causative agents in a variety of cancers such as anogenital, and head and neck cancers. HPVs appear to have evolved mechanisms resulting in escape from host immune surveillance and delay of resolution of infection. The HPV E5 oncoprotein is one of the possible effectors that allows the virus to escape from host immune system through the downregulation of surface classical major histocompatibility complex class I (MHC I) and not the nonclassical MHC I. Lack of classical MHC I in infected cells expressing E5 would allow evasion of cytotoxic T lymphocytes (CTLs) killing and thus establishment and persistence of viral infection.

In this chapter we discuss the process of immunomodulation by HPV and review our recent discoveries on the association of HPV with cancers and its implication in medicine.

Keywords: cancer, HR-HPV, E5, MHC I, CTL

1. Introduction

The global cancer burden is markedly increasing and is thus a leading cause of death, second only to cardiovascular disease [1–3]. Based on the most recent available data collected by the international agency for cancer, an estimated 14.1 million new cancer cases and 8.2 million cancer-related deaths occurred in 2012, compared with 12.7 million and 7.6 million, respectively, in 2008 [4].

The human body is dependent on regulated cell division and elimination which forms homeostasis within the body. Certain genes play vital roles in regulating the cell cycle. These genes are grouped into three categories, tumour suppressor genes (TSGs), proto-oncogenes and DNA repair genes. Any alteration in these groups of genes downregulates the cell control mechanisms and ultimately causes cancer cell development and malignant transformation [5]. Genetic changes in the progression of cancer typically affect two different types of genes, oncogenes (e.g., *Ras*) and TSGs (e.g., P53 and pRB). Both of the oncogenes and TSGs encode many kinds of proteins that play a key role in cancer induction. These genes control cell growth and proliferation, and mutations in these genes can contribute to the development of cancer.

Despite of the evolving medical significance of cancers, few studies have been conducted to identify the possible risk factors that implicated in the initiation of cancer. However, there are well-established risk factors that have been identified for its association with the development of cancer such as clinical, genetic and epidemiological factors. In addition, biological agents have been implicated in various cancers including viruses, bacteria and parasites.

Viruses have been the most studied in their relation to tumour formation. They are thought to be associated with 15–20% of all human cancers worldwide of which about 80% are cancers of the cervix and liver [6, 7]. Viruses have evolved multiple strategies to transform host cell. One common route is to alter the expression of cellular genes by integration of the viral genome into the cellular DNA. Viruses also help cause malignancy by introducing an oncogene into a cell to disrupt the regulation of cell division [8–10].

Infectious agents have been implicated, either as direct carcinogens or as promoters. Viral infections, in particular, human papillomaviruses (HPVs) are recognised as carcinogenic agents in humans and are responsible for a significant share of the global cancer burden [7, 11, 12].

HPVs are small double-stranded DNA oncogenic viruses of approximately 8 kbp. HPVs are ubiquitous in the human population, and occasionally infection leads to cervical cancer. Although the body is working to get the infection under control, HPVs infect and disturb cutaneous and mucosal epithelial cells of the anogenital tract, hands or feet which can lead to a variety of diseases with a range of severities depending on the types of HPV infection.

To date, over 100 different types of HPV have been identified, and about one-third of these infect epithelial cells in the genital tract. The type HPV family is divided into two categories: low-risk HPVs and high-risk HPVs (HR-HPVs). The low-risk HPV types such as HPV 6 and HPV 11 commonly cause benign genital warts (condylomas). These lesions can regress even without treatment [13], due to cell-mediated immune responses [14]. While the high-risk types of HPV which include HPV 16, 18, 31, 35 and 45 are associated with the development of anogenital cancers and found in up to 99% of all cervical carcinomas [15, 16]. These HR-HPV types cause benign genital epithelial hyperproliferative lesions, such as low-grade premalignant cervical intraepithelial neoplasia (CIN I). In most premalignant cases, lesions can regress even without treatment. However, in a limited number of cases, the lesions persist or progress to invasive cancer due to the lack or ineffective immunological responses.

It has been reported that the low-grade CIN I would progress to high-grade lesion (CIN III) and eventually invasive cervical cancer [17]. Consequently, the associations of the HPV infection in the development of cancer are an area of ongoing interest.

2. The host immune evasion by HPV

The papillomaviruses are small double-stranded DNA viruses which belong to the papillomaviridae family [6]. HPVs infect cutaneous or mucosal epithelial cells initiating benign or cancerous lesions that depend on the HPV types. The lifecycle, oncogenic characteristics and molecular-based evidence of HR-HPVs are suggestive of a causal role for cancer. HPV infections are normally cleared by the immune system; however, the persistence of HPV could trigger a progression to malignant lesion in the presence of other risk factors. For instance, it is well documented that the persistent infection of the cervix with HR-HPV types 16 and 18 is an initiating event of the cervical cancer [18, 19]. Therefore, the establishment, persistence of HR-HPV infection and evasion of the host immune system are necessary for premalignant lesions to initiate and progress towards squamous carcinoma [20–22].

The host immune response mechanism plays a significant role in controlling and limiting HPV infection. The suppression of HPV-induced lesion depends on the host inflammatory reaction and penetration of lymphocytes to the infected tissue [14]. Thus, the prevalence of HPV-induced lesions is higher in immunosuppressed individuals such as transplant recipients or human immunodeficiency virus (HIV)-infected patients [23, 24].

Lack of HPV clearance and persistence of viral infection for many months are necessary before the onset of an immune response. The reasons of this fact are still unknown. And perhaps one of the most important ongoing questions in the field of papillomavirus research is the latency of the host immune response in eliminating the virus in immunocompetent hosts as well as immunosuppressed hosts.

The nonlytic feature of HPV is one of the explanations for evading the recognition of HPV infection. HPV does not lyse the infected cell or cause viremia, and this will reduce the exposure of viral antigen to cell-mediated immunity and consequent lack of inflammation. HPV life cycle characterised by the physical evasion from the immune cells' recognition through HPV restoration and protection within infected cells' nuclei [25, 26]. Additionally, HPV has the ability to downregulate major histocompatibility complex class I (MHC I) and disrupt the interferon (IFN) pathway. HPV facilitates this mechanism using early oncoproteins, E5, E6 and E7, which have the ability to interfere and actively participate to the downregulation of host immune system. The role of E6 and E7 is to inhibit the production of IFN in natural killer (NK) cells or the expression of transporter associated with antigen processing (TAP) [27, 28].

E5 oncoprotein downregulates surface MHC class I by retaining it in the Golgi apparatus (**Figures 1** and **2**) [20, 29]. Downregulation of MHC class 1 has been observed with E5 from different PVs, including HPV-85 and HPV-16 (**Figure 3**), indicating that key functions of E5 are conserved between the PV species and HPV types [21].

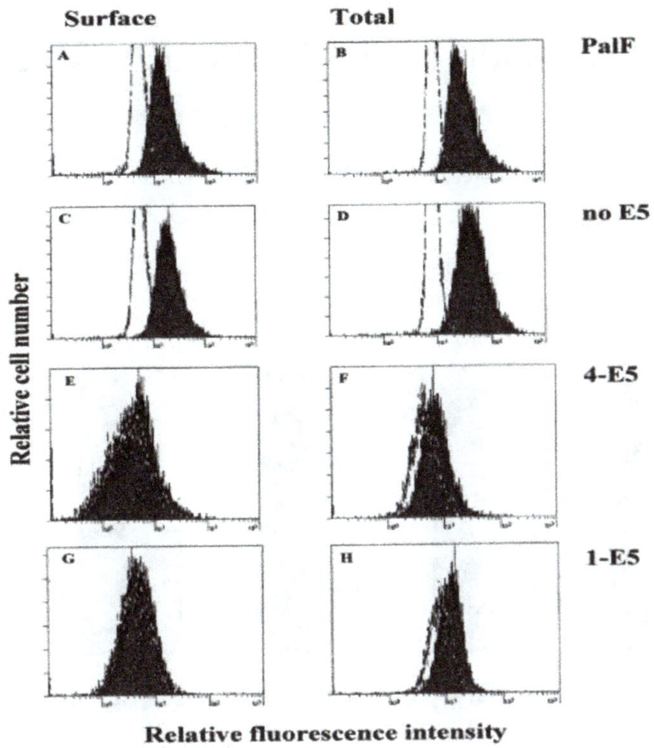

Figure 1. The expression of MHC I in control and transformed PalF cells using Define FACS as "Fluorescence-activated cell sorting" (**A and B**), control cells (**C and D**), 4-E5 transfected cells (**E and F**) and 1-E5 transfected cells (**G and H**) were incubated with anti MHC 1 antibody. Surface MHC I (**A, C, E and G**) and total MHC I (**B, D, F and H**) [**29**].

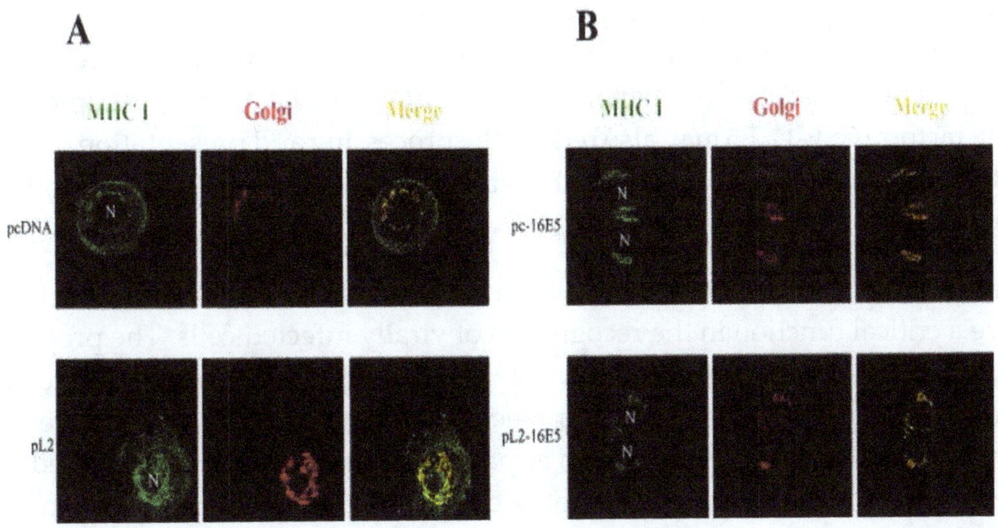

Figure 2. Visualisation of the GA and MHC I. HaCaT cells carrying empty vectors or cells expressing HPV-16 E5 were costained with anti-HLA class I antibody (mAb W6/32) and anti-golgi GM130 antibody (mAb 4A3) and analysed using Leica TCS SP2 fluorescence confocal microscopy. Representative cells are shown. (**A**) Control HaCaT cells carrying either pcDNA or pL2 empty vector. (**B**) HeCaT cells expressing HPV-16 E5 in either pcDNA (pc-16E5) or pL2 (pL2-16E5). N = nucleus [**20**].

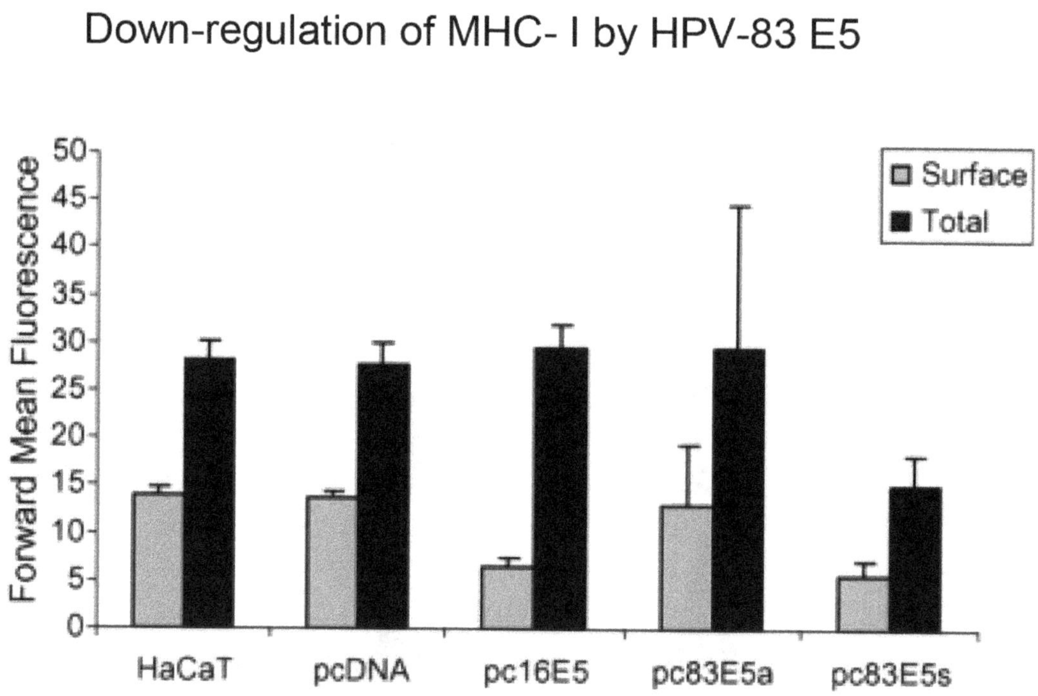

Figure 3. Total and surface expression of MHC-I using FACS analysis in normal HaCaT cells transfected with pcDNA (empty vectors), pcHPV16E5, HPV83-E5a (antisense orientation) and HPV83-E5s (sense orientation) [**21**].

E5 is the smallest HPV oncogenic protein that is located in the membranes of the endoplasmic reticulum (ER) and Golgi apparatus of the transformed cells. This hydrophobic protein is a structure of 83 amino acids in HR-HPV type 16, is expressed before the onset of viral replication. E5 contribute to cell transformation through interaction with several cellular proteins, including the epidermal growth factor receptor (EGF-R), the human receptor for colony stimulating factors (CSF-1). E5 may also reduce the processing and presentation of viral antigen through the interaction with 16 kDa subunit of the vacuolar H^+-ATPase acidification of endosome [30].

The human MHC class I molecules are known as human leukocyte antigen (HLA) system, which have a critical function in the recognition of virally infected cells. The proteasomes and other cytoplasmic proteases are playing a role in viral protein degradation into short chain peptides of 8–10 amino acids long. HLA molecules and intracellular viral antigenic peptides complex are transported through the Golgi apparatus to the cell surface of infected cells where it is presented and recognised by the cytotoxic $CD8^+$ T cells. The activated cytotoxic T lymphocytes (CTLs) are able to destroy the infected cell through the mechanism of apoptosis that mediated either by granulate exocytosis (perforin and granzymes) or by Fas-Fas ligand interaction [26].

High frequency of virus-specific CTLs is a characteristic of persistent viral infection such as cytomegalovirus (CMV) and Epstein-Barr virus (EBV), however low frequency of HPV-specific CTL has been detected in CIN III and cervical cancer patients [31, 32].

$CD4^+$ T helper lymphocytes (Ths) are able to identify foreign antigens that presented on MHC class II molecules (antigen-MHC II complex). MHC class II molecules are mostly expressed on professional antigen presenting cells (APCs) such as dendritic cells, macrophages and B cells, but they can also be expressed on the epithelial cells (target for HPV) by IFN treatment.

T helper cells are capable of secreting cytokines that allow the proliferation and maintenance of cytotoxic lymphocytes. Additionally, they play a role in activation of B cells for antibody production, as well as dendritic cells for antigen presentation. Th cells potentially have an important role in cell-mediated immunity against HPV infection. The reactivity of HPV-restricted Th cells was found in patients with a persistent papillomavirus infection [33, 34].

While E6 and E7 are presented throughout the course of the HPV infection, their functions are necessary for the maintenance of a transformed status. Expression of E5 takes place in the early stage of papillomavirus infection and in the deep layers of the infected epithelium. Ashrafi et al. [29] were the first to report that E5 protein of HPV downregulates the classical HLA (A and B) but not the nonclassical HLA-E. This potentially allows the cell to escape CTL and also NK cells' killing [20].

The downregulation of MHC class I by E5 oncoprotein allows the infected cell to evade cell-mediated immune response and this potentially enables other HPV oncoproteins in the establishment and persistence of virus infection. Interestingly, it has been reported that the oncogenic E5 also inhibits the Fas receptor [35] and HLA II [36]. This strongly indicates that E5 might have additional major role in negatively regulating the immune response.

The downregulation of MHC I is an imperative mechanism to evade CTL-mediated immune clearance, however, the lack of surface MHC I will activate NK cells to attack and destroy the infected cells. Human NK cells express surface receptors (NKRs) that interact with HLA class I molecules, including killer cell immunoglobulin-like receptors (KIRs) that mainly recognise classical HLA-C and also C type lectin receptors which identify nonclassical HLA-E molecule. In the absence of classical HLA-C and non-classical HLA-E, NK-mediated cell lysis would be inhibited due to the recognition of MHC class I molecules by their inhibitory receptors. Consequently, certain viruses, including HIV and CMV, have the ability to escape both CTL and NK cells' killing. HIV-negative proteins (Nef) and CMV US3/UL40 proteins have evolved to selectively downregulate HLA (A and B), the main presenters of peptides to CTLs, but not HLA-C or nonclassical HLA-E [37, 38].

3. HR-HPVs and cancers

HR-HPV types are considered as the most important aetiological factors for many types of cancers such as cervical cancer. The risk of cervical cancer has increased in parallel with the incidence of certain genotypes of HR-HPV. Therefore, the presence of these genotypes indicates a significant risk factor for the initiation and progression of almost 90% of cervical cancer cases [18].

Despite the medical significance of HR-HPV infection, there is still a lack of information on the incidence of cancers that are caused by different HR-HPV genotypes in different populations. An investigation on the incidence and distribution of HR-HPV genotypes in cervical cancer patients confirmed the presence of additional high-risk types (HPV-45 and HPV-39) other than common types (HPV-16 and HPV-18) [19].

Being a sexually contagious virus, HPV virus has the ability to spread through sexual and skin-to-skin contact. HR-HPVs have also been found to be the causative agents for almost up to half of vaginal, penile, anal and oral cancers. These findings suggest that HR-HPV virions might be spread from the original infected site to other organs and lead to cancer development in various organs [18].

To date, studies on the role of HPV in breast carcinogenesis have generated considerable controversies and it is still not clear whether HPV infection is implicated in breast cancer pathogenesis [39]. HPV infection is a sexually transmissible disease, and most breast cancers originate from mammary duct epithelia. Therefore, the relationship between HPV and breast cancer is imperative for many reasons. The exposure of the mammary ducts to the external environment increases the risk of HPV infection. Our unpublished data have shown the presence of HR-HPV types of viral DNA other than 16 and 18 in freshly collected human breast cancer tissue and this provides a solid basis to advance research in a crucial health problem affecting women.

These initial findings support the association of HPV and breast cancer and highlight possible causative agents of breast cancer. Therefore, further research is required to investigate whether HR-HPV infection plays a role in the pathogenesis of breast cancer. The information gained will pave the way to better awareness of breast cancer risk factors other than those recognised to date.

4. Conclusions

Identification of HPV pathogenesis offers means of therapeutic intervention targeted against HPV oncoproteins (E5, E6 and E7) which will facilitate early lesion eradication. This will also provide results central to our understanding of HPV pathogenesis and help elucidate early events in HPV infection that may determine persistence and disease development.

Moreover, our findings on the presence of high-risk HPV-39 and HPV-45 types in cervical cancer other than types 16 and 18 [19] and the presence of different types of HR-HPV in breast cancer will postulate a need for further assessment of the influence of current prophylactic vaccination programs that is protective against the two most common oncogenic papillomaviruses, HPV-16 and HPV-18, but not against other high-risk mucosal HPVs detected in our studies.

Viral carcinogenesis and cancer prevention are rapidly developing sectors of this field, and the future translation of this chapter lead to a faster resolution of HPV infection, and with obvious advantages for all HPV-affected patients, and in particular for individuals affected by early HPV-related cancer diseases.

Author details

G. Hossein Ashrafi[1*] and Nadia Aziz Salman[2]

*Address all correspondence to: h.ashrafi@kingston.ac.uk

1 Cancer Study Group, SEC Faculty, Kingston University London, Kingston Upon Thames, UK

2 School of Life Science, Pharmacy and Chemistry, SEC Faculty, Kingston University London, Kingston Upon Thames, UK

References

[1] Jemal A, Bray F, Center MM, Ferlay J, Ward E, Forman D (2011). Global cancer statistics. CA: A Cancer Journal for Clinicians. 61(2), 69–90.

[2] Kochanek KD, Xu J, Murphy SL, Minino AM, Kung HC (2011). Deaths: final data for 2009. National Vital Statistics Report. 60, 1–166.

[3] Murphy SL, Xu J, Kochanek KD (2012). Deaths: preliminary data for 2010. National Vital Statistics Report. 60, 1–69.

[4] Cancer Research UK (2012). UK Cancer Incidence and Mortality (2010) Summary, May 2012 [Online]. Available at http://publications.cancerresearchuk.org [accessed 8 February 2016].

[5] Alberts B, Johnson A, Walter P, Lewis J, Raff M, Roberts K (2008). Molecular biology of the cell. 5th edn., New York: Garland Science (Chapter 20; Cancer, pp 1230–1256).

[6] zur Hausen H (2002). Papillomaviruses and cancer: from basic studies to clinical application. Nature Reviews Cancer 2, 342–350.

[7] Parkin DM (2006). The global health burden of infection-associated cancers in the year 2002. International Journal of Cancer 118, 3030–3044.

[8] DiMaio D, Lai CC, Klein O (1998). Virocrine transformation: the intersection between viral transforming proteins and cellular signal transduction pathways. Annual Review of Microbiology 52, 397–421. Review.

[9] Murakami Y, Saigo K, Takashima H, Minami M, Okanoue T, Bréchot C, Paterlini-Bréchot P (2005). Large scaled analysis of hepatitis B virus (HBV) DNA integration in HBV related hepatocellular carcinomas. Gut. 54(8), 1162–1168.

[10] Arias-Pulido H, Peyton CL, Joste NE, Vargas H, Wheeler CM (2006). Human papillomavirus type 16 integration in cervical carcinoma in situ and in invasive cervical cancer. Journal of Clinical Microbiology. 44(5), 1755–1762.

[11] zur Hausen H (2009). Papillomaviruses in the causation of human cancers – a brief historical account. Virology 384, 260–265.

[12] Thun MJ, DeLancey JO, Center MM, Jemal A, Ward EM (2010). The global burden of cancer: priorities for prevention. Carcinogenesis. 31, 100–110.

[13] Nasiel K, Roger V, Nasiell M (1986). Behaviour of mild cervical dysplasia during long-term follow-up. Obstetrics and Gynecology. 67, 665–669.

[14] Coleman N, Birley HD, Renton AM, Hanna NF, Ryait BK, Byrne M, Taylor-Robinson D, Stanley MA (1994). Immunological events in regressing genital warts. American Journal of Clinical Pathology. 102, 768–774.

[15] Walboomers JM, Jacobs MV, Manos MM, Bosch FX, Kummer JA, Shah KV, Snijders PJ, Peto J, Meijer CJ, Muñoz N (1999). Human papillomavirus is a necessary cause of invasive cervical cancer worldwide. Journal of Pathology 9, 12–19.

[16] Muñoz N, Bosch FX, de Sanjosé S, Herrero R, Castellsagué X, Shah KV, Snijders, PJF , Meijer CJLM (2003). Epidemiologic classification of human papillomavirus types associated with cervical cancer. The New England Journal of Medicine 348, 518–527.

[17] Klaes R, Woerner SM, Ridder R, Wentzensen N, Duerst M, Schneider A, Lotz B, Melsheimer P, von KnebelDoeberitz M (1999). Detection of high-risk cervical intraepithelial neoplasia and cervical cancer by amplification of transcripts derived from integrated papillomavirus oncogenes. Cancer Research. 59, 6132–6136.

[18] zur Hausen H (2008). Papillomaviruses – to vaccination and beyond. Biochemistry (Moscow). 73(5), 498–503.

[19] Haghshenas MR, Golini-moghaddam T, Rafiee A, Emadeian O, Shykhpour A, Ashrafi GH (2013). Prevalence and type distribution of high-risk human papillomavirus in patients with cervical cancer: a population-based study. Infectious Agents and Cancer. 8, 20.

[20] Ashrafi GH, Haghshenas MR, Marchetti B, O'Brien P, Campo MS (2005). The E5 protein of human papillomavirus type 16 selectively down-regulates surface HLA class I. International Journal of Cancer. 113, 276–283.

[21] Ashrafi GH, Brown D, Fife KH , Campo MS (2006). Down-regulation of MHC class I is a property common to papillomavirus E5 proteins. Virus Research. 120, 208–211.

[22] Ashrafi GH, Haghshenas MR, Marchetti B, Campo MS (2006). The E5 protein of human papillomavirus type 16 HLA class I and interacts with the heavy chain via its first hydrophobic domain. International Journal of Cancer. 119, 2105–2112.

[23] Halpert R, Fruchter RG, Sedlis A, Butt K, Boyce JG, Sillman FH (1986). Human papillomavirus and lower genital neoplasia in renal transplant patients. Obstetrics and Gynecology 68, 251–258.

[24] Petry KU, Scheffel D, Bode U, Gabrysiak T, Köchel H, Kupsch E, Glaubitz M, Niesert S, Kühnle H, Schedel I (1994). Cellular immunodeficiency enhances the progression of human papillomavirus-associated cervical lesions. International Journal of Cancer. 57, 836–840.

[25] O'Brien PM, Campo MS (2003). Papillomaviruses: a correlation between immune evasion and oncogenicity? Trends in Microbiology 11, 300–305.

[26] Seifert U, Marañón C, Shmueli A, Desoutter JF, et al (2003). An essential role for tripeptidyl peptidase in the generation of an MHC class I epitope. Nature Immunology 4, 375–379.

[27] Barnard P, McMillan NA (1999). The human papillomavirus E7 oncoprotein abrogates signaling mediated by interferon-alpha. Virology 259, 305–313.

[28] Nees M, Geoghegan JM, Hyman T, Frank S, Miller L, Woodworth CD (2001). Papillomavirus type 16 oncogenes downregulate expression of interferon-responsive genes and upregulate proliferation-associated and NF-kappaB-responsive genes in cervical keratinocytes. Journal of Virology. 75, 4283–4296.

[29] Ashrafi GH, Tsirimonaki E, Marchetti B, O'Brien PM, Sibbett GJ, Andrew L, Campo MS (2002). Down-regulation of MHC class I by papillomavirus E5 oncoproteins. Oncogene. 21, 248–259.

[30] Venuti A, Paolini F, Nasir L, Corteggio A, Roperto S, Campo MS, Borzacchiello G (2011). Papillomavirus E5: the smallest oncoprotein with many functions. Molecular Cancer. 10, 140.

[31] Evans EM, Man S, Evans AS, Borysiewicz LK (1997). Infiltration of cervical cancer tissue with human papillomavirus-specific cytotoxic T-lymphocytes. Cancer Research. 57, 2943–2950.

[32] Nimako M, Fiander AN, Wilkinson GW, Borysiewicz LK, Man S (1997). Human papillomavirus-specific cytotoxic T lymphocytes in patients with cervical intraepithelial neoplasia grade III. Cancer Research 57, 4855–4861.

[33] de Gruijl TD, Bontkes HJ, Peccatori F, Gallee MP, et al (1999). Expression of CD3-zeta on T-cells in primary cervical carcinoma and in metastasis-positive and -negative pelvic lymph nodes. British Journal of Cancer. 79, 1127–1132.

[34] Welters MJ, de Jong A, van den Eeden SJ, et al (2003). Frequent display of human papillomavirus type 16 E6-specific memory t-helper cells in the healthy population as witness of previous viral encounter. Cancer Research. 63, 636–641.

[35] Kabsch K, Alonso A (2002). The human papillomavirus type 16 E5 protein impairs TRAIL- and FasL-mediated apoptosis in HaCaT cells by different mechanisms. Journal of Virology. 76, 12162–12172.

[36] Zhang B, Li P, Wang E, Brahmi Z, Dunn KW, Blum JS, Roman A (2003). The E5 protein of human papillomavirus type 16 perturbs MHC class II antigen maturation in human foreskin keratinocytes treated with interferon-gamma. Virology. 10, 100–108.

[37] Cohen GB, Gandhi RT, Davis DM, Mandelboim O, Chen BK, Strominger JL, Baltimore D (1999). The selective downregulation of class I major histocompatibility complex proteins by HIV-1 protects HIV-infected cells from NK cells. Immunity. 10, 661–671.

[38] Kasper MR, Collins KL (2003). Nef-mediated disruption of HLA-A2 transport to the cell surface in T cells. Journal of Virology. 77, 3041–3049.

[39] Simões PW, Medeiros LR, SimõesPires PD, Edelweiss MI, Rosa DD, Silva FR, Silva BR, Rosa MI (2012). Prevalence of human papillomavirus in breast cancer: a systematic review. International Journal of Gynecological Cancer. 22(3), 343–347.

3

High-Risk Human Papillomavirus and Colorectal Carcinogenesis

Ala-Eddin Al Moustafa, Noor Al-Antary and Amber Yasmeen

Abstract

Colorectal, colon and rectal, cancer is the third most common malignancy in both men and women worldwide. Colorectal carcinogenesis is a complex, multistep process implicating environmental and lifestyle factors in addition to gene mutation and viral infections. On the other hand, it is well established that human papillomaviruses (HPVs) infection play a crucial role in certain types of human carcinomas including cervical and head and neck (HN); as roughly 96% and 30% of these cancers are positive for high-risk HPVs, respectively. Moreover, it has been reported that the presence of high-risk HPVs is associated with vascular invasion, lymph node metastases, and tumor size in cervical and HN cancers. Recently, several investigations pointed-out that high-risk HPVs are present in around 70% of human colorectal cancers. Likewise, our group has demonstrated that E6/E7 oncoproteins of HPV type 16 convert noninvasive and nonmetastatic human cancer cells to invasive and metastatic form. Accordingly, it is evident that high-risk HPVs are present in human colorectal cancers where they could play an important role in the development of these malignancies. In this chapter, we will discuss the presence and role of high-risk HPVs in human colorectal carcinogenesis and metastasis; particularly, the interaction between E5 and E6/E7 oncoproteins of high-risk HPVs in colorectal malignancies, which has been linked with the initiation and progression of these tumors.

Keywords: colorectal cancer, high-risk HPVs, E5 & E6/E7 oncoproteins, cancer initiation, cancer progression

1. Introduction

Colorectal cancers (CRCs) colon and rectal, are the most common malignancies, accounting for approximately 1.36 million new cases worldwide every year [1]. These cancers are characterized by a marked propensity for local invasion and lymph node metastases. Thus, the overall 5-year-survival rate for patients diagnosed with colorectal cancers is approximately 60% worldwide and has not significantly improved over the past decade [2]. Colorectal carcinogenesis is a complex, multistep process involving environmental, demographic, and lifestyle factors in addition to gene alterations and viral infections. The highest incidence of CRCs is observed in Western Europe, North America, Australia as well as in some Middle-Eastern countries [3, 4]. It is notable also that although the rate of this disease is relatively lower in sub-Saharan African communities, South America, and Asia; however, CRCs are gradually increasing due to assimilating life style and dietary habits of Western countries [3–5]. Additionally, around two-thirds of CRC patients will develop distant metastases during the course of their illness, which is the main cause of cancer-related death of this disease [6].

Although, human papillomaviruses (HPVs) have been established as etiological agents of invasive cervical cancer, as generally 96% of these cancers are positive for high-risk HPVs [7–9]. However, persistent infection with high-risk HPVs is necessary but not sufficient for the development of malignant lesions [10, 11]. Furthermore, it was pointed-out that high-risk HPVs have carcinogenic effects at several other anatomical sites in women and men such as head and neck (HN) as well as colorectal [12–15]. These studies and others showed that high-risk HPVs are present in roughly 30% and 70% of HN and colorectal cancers, respectively, especially in their invasive form [14, 15]. Accordingly, we recently investigated the incidence of high-risk HPVs in CRCs in the Syrian population; our data revealed that 54% of human CRCs in Syria are positive for high-risk-HPVs; this was accompanied by an expression/overexpression of Fascin, Id-1, and P-cadherin genes [16], which are major regulators of cell invasion and metastasis [17–19]. Meanwhile, we revealed that E5 and E6/E7 oncoproteins of high-risk HPVs could cooperate together to enhance cancer progression through the deregulation of several key controller genes of the epithelial–mesenchymal transition (EMT) event [7, 20, 21]. It is clear that CRCs and especially their invasive forms are major health problems wherein high-risk HPVs infection can play important roles in the development of these malignancies as well as their metastasis via EMT. In this chapter, we will overview the presence and contributions of high-risk HPVs in CRC initiation and progression.

2. Colorectal cancers

CRCs are the most prevalent cancers worldwide, along with lung and breast cancers, they are one of the deadliest diseases today [22]. For instance, in the United States, CRCs are the third leading cause of cancer death in both sexes and the second overall in men and women combined [23, 24]. At current rates, approximately 5–6% of individuals will develop colon or rectum cancer within their lifetime [23]. These malignances are most common in Europe with

432,000 new cases reported annually in men and women combined, and the second most common cause of cancer deaths in Europe [22, 25]. In general, it is the second leading cause of cancer-related mortality worldwide and the third most commonly diagnosed malignant disease [26].

The prognosis of patients with colorectal cancer has slowly but steadily improved during the past decades in many countries. A 5-year relative survival has reached almost 65% in high-income countries, such as Australia, Canada, the USA, and several European countries, but has remained less than 50% in low-income countries [27–29]. Relative survival decreases with age, and at young ages, it is slightly higher for women than for men [30]; taking into consideration that the stage at diagnosis is the most important prognostic factor.

Colorectal carcinogenesis is common in the elderly; as approximately 90% of new colorectal cancers are diagnosed in patients over 50 years with the median age of diagnosis being 69 years. Furthermore, the incidence of CRCs dramatically rises as one ages, regardless of sex and racial background [26]. Although, it is well-known that patients with colorectal cancer may have a range of symptoms that include occult blood loss, rectal bleeding, change in stool caliber, unintentional weight loss, or have signs of bowel obstruction or perforation.

There are many risk factors for the development of colorectal cancer, one of which is colonic polyps. Pathologic entities include tubular adenoma, tubulovillous adenoma, villous adenoma, hyperplastic polyp, sessile serrated adenoma, sessile serrated polyp, and traditional serrated adenoma. In addition, some hamartomatous polyps are considered premalignant lesions [31]. Among precancerous polyps adenomatous and advanced adenomatous polyps that have polyp size >10 mm, in addition to villous/tubulovillous histological features, or having high-grade dysplasia (HGD), are found to have an increased prevalence and incidence in the elderly [26], and have a potential to progress to invasive adenocarcinomas [26, 32]. HGD is associated with larger size, villous morphology, *TP53* mutation, and deletion of a region of chromosome 18q. Chromosomal instability can be demonstrated in late precursor adenomas. In this sequence, *APC* mutation is a common early event, while the serrated lesions commonly have *BRAF* or *KRAS* mutation [31]. Other risk factors include diet and lifestyle (such as consumption of red meat, smoking, excessive alcohol, weight gain, etc.) as well as advancing age [23, 26].

For the most part, colorectal cancer arises sporadically, however, few cases are associated with inherited syndromes such as familial adenomatous polyposis (FAP; <1% of CRC) where patients exhibit germline mutations in one allele of the adenomatous polyposis (*APC*) tumor suppressor gene, MUTYH-associated polyposis (MAP; rare recessive condition, carrier estimated at ~1%), and Lynch syndrome/hereditary nonpolyposis colon cancer (LS/HNPCC; 2–4% of CRCs) [7, 33].

The usual malignant tumor of the large bowel is a well-to-moderately differentiated adenocarcinoma secreting variable amounts of mucin [34]. In World Health Organization (WHO) classification, a number of histologic variants of this tumor are listed, such as mucinous adenocarcinoma, signet ring cell, medullary, micropapillary, serrated, cribriform comedo-type, adenosquamous, spindle cell, and undifferentiated. The most widely used immunohistochemical markers for colorectal adenocarcinoma are cytokeratin (CK) 20, CK7, and CDX2. The most common immunophenotype of colorectal adenocarcinoma is positivity for CK20 and negativity for CK7 [35]. The CRCs are divided in to four grades. G1 are well-differentiated tumors (usually adenocarcinomas) that have more than 95% glandular structures. Further, G2 are designated as moderately differentiated tumors with 50–95% gland formation. G3 are poorly differentiated tumors with 5–50% gland formation; whereas G4 are highly aggressive and undifferentiated tumors with less than 5% gland formation. Recently, WHO also suggests dividing CRCs into low grade (G1 and G2) and high grade (G3 and G4) categories. The diagnosis of G3 and G4 is relatively consistent, but differentiation between G1 and G2 is associated with a significant degree of inter-observer variability [36, 37] .

As we mentioned above, CRCs are characterized by a marked propensity for invasion and metastasis. About 20% of patients with newly diagnosed colorectal cancer present with distant metastases [38, 39]. The most common location is the liver [38, 40]; however, investigators identified lung metastases in 2·1% of patients newly diagnosed with CRC in a large cancer registry in France [41]. Frequency was nearly three times higher for patients with rectal cancer than for patients with colon cancer. Smaller studies [42–44] have shown isolated lung metastases in 9–18% of patients with rectal cancer; although distant metastases can be identified in other organs including the bone and the brain [38].

As we cited above, lifetime risk of CRCs is estimated to be 5–6% in the general population of Western countries [45, 46]. Although hereditary forms of CRC have been well established; however, most cases are sporadic [47]. Numerous epidemiological studies have identified lifestyle and environmental factors contributing to the occurrence of CRCs [48, 49]. In the past decades, *Helicobacter pylori* and Epstein Barr virus infections have been identified as potential causal factors of gastric cancer [50, 51] and personal communication. A number of studies aimed to assess the possible role of viral infections, such as infection with high-risk HPVs, human polyomaviruses, and human herpesviruses in colorectal carcinogenesis [7, 45, 52, 53]. Thus, in the next paragraph the presence and role of high-risk HPVs in human CRCs will be reviewed.

3. Human papillomaviruses (HPVs)

Papillomaviruses were first identified in rabbits in 1933, and they were found to be involved in transmissible growth of benign papillomas [54]. HPVs were first identified in 1956, and they were associated with a variety of benign growths in humans [55]. However, it was later observed that HPVs, a highly prevalent sexually transmitted infection, have potentially serious health consequences in males and females. HPV infections have received considerable attention in recent years. So far, more than 150 HPV types have been isolated and characterized. While the involvement of HPV in causing benign warts was already known, the first evidence of the association between human cancer and certain HPV types was proposed more than thirty years ago by zur Hausen and his colleagues [56].

The common mode of transmission and acquisition of HPV is by horizontal transmission consequent to sexual activity. Occasionally, HPV may be transmitted through modes other than sexual activity [57–61]. Thus, prevalence sites of HPVs include the epithelium of the vagina, vulva, penis, anal canal, cervix, perianal region, crypts of the tonsils, and oropharynx. Persistent HPV infection is essential for the development of cervical precancerous lesions and cancer. However, this may take a long time, usually a decade or more after the initial infection [62].

HPVs are small, double-stranded DNA viruses that generally infect cutaneous and mucosal epithelial tissues of the anogenital tract. The HPV DNA genome encodes approximately eight open reading frames (ORFs) [52, 62]. It is divided into three functional parts: the early (E) region, the late (L) region, and a long control region (LCR). The E region is important for replication, cellular transformation, and for the control of viral transcription, whereas the L region encodes the structural proteins (L1-L2) that take part in assembly [12]. The LCR is necessary for viral DNA replication and transcription. The seven proteins of the E region are E1, E2, E3, E4, E5, E6, and E7. E1 is necessary for viral DNA replication, while E2 has a role in viral gene transcription and replication. The function of E3 is still not understood. On the other hand, E4 protein interacts with the keratin cytoskeleton and intermediate filaments. Moreover, it facilitates virus assembly and release. The E5 protein interacts with the receptors of growth factors and stimulates cellular proliferation and inhibits apoptosis. E6 induces DNA synthesis, prevents cell differentiation, and interacts with tumor suppressor proteins and repair factors. In fact, E7 induces cell proliferation and interacts with negative regulators of cell cycle and tumor suppressor proteins. E5, E6, and E7 proteins act as oncogenes which are associated with carcinogenesis [12, 20, 63–66] (please see below).

As we mentioned above, over 150 different viral types have been identified, and about one-third of these infect epithelial cells in the genital tract [67]. HPVs are classified as either high risk or low risk. Infections with low-risk types are generally self-limiting and do not lead to malignancy. However, infections with high-risk HPVs (type 16, 18, 31, 33, 35, 39, 45, 51, 52, 55, 56, 58, 59, 68, 73, 82, and 83) are associated with the development of cervical cancers since more than 96% of these cancers are positive for high-risk HPVs [7, 9, 68–70].

It is well known that high-risk HPV early proteins, including E5, E6, and E7 oncoproteins, increase cellular alteration and probably lead to HPV induced carcinogenesis [20, 71–73]. More specifically, the E5 oncoprotein interacts with EGF-R1 signaling pathways (MAP Kinase and P13K-Akt) and proapoptotic proteins [74–76]; and therefore, it can play an important role in cell transformation and tumor formation. On the other hand, E6 and E7 of the high-risk HPV types, such as HPV16, are thought to work together in lesions caused by this virus, since, the two proteins are expressed from bicistronic mRNA [77] and initiated from the viral early promoter (p97). These proteins have functions that stimulate cell cycle progression and both can associate with regulators of the cell cycle [70, 72, 78].

Several studies have shown that the viral E6 protein complements the role of E7 and is thought to prevent the induction of apoptosis in response to unscheduled S-phase entry mediated by E7 [70, 79]. The E6 protein is also involved in the inactivation of p53-mediated growth suppression and/or apoptosis and can also associate with other proapoptotic proteins including Bak [80] and Bax [81]. In addition, E6 stimulates cell proliferation independently from E7 through its C-terminal PDZ-ligand domain [70, 82]. E6-PDZ binding is sufficient to mediate suprabasal cell proliferation [83, 84] and may contribute to the development of metastatic tumours by disrupting normal cell adhesion. On the other hand, the E7 viral is involved with members of the pocket protein family such as pRb, which is well documented. E7 binding to pRb displaces E2F, irrespective of the presence of external growth factors and leads to the expression of proteins necessary for DNA replication [70, 71, 78, 85].

To address the role of E6/E7 genes in high-risk HPV-associated carcinogenesis *in vivo*, transgenic mice have been developed expressing E6/E7 of HPV type 16 individually and together under the human K14 promoter [86, 87]. These transgenic mice developed skin tumors, in general, and cervical cancer with chronic estrogen administration [87, 88]. On the other hand, and to examine the oncogenic properties of E5 *in vivo*, K14-E5 transgenic mice were generated in which the expression of E5 was directed to the basal layer of the stratified squamous epithelia. These mice exhibited the epidermal hyperplasia, aberrant differentiation of the epithelium, and were susceptible to spontaneous skin tumors [89]. Recently, it was reported that K14-E6/E7 transgenic mice have high susceptibility to colorectal cancers and precancerous lesions after dimethylbenz[a]anthracene-treatment, which is a chemical carcinogen that is known to induce squamous cell carcinomas in other sites [90]. These studies show clearly that high-risk HPVs play an important role in cancer initiation and/or progression of several anatomical sites, which could include colorectal, through their E5, E6, and E7 oncoproteins.

4. High-risk HPVs in colorectal cancers

High-risk HPVs have been established as etiological agents of invasive cervical cancer, as more than 96% of these cancers are positive for high-risk HPVs which are the most common viral sexually transmitted infection worldwide [7–9]. Infection with high-risk HPVs is important for the development of premalignant lesions and/or progression of the disease [10, 11]. Additionally, it was revealed that high-risk HPVs have carcinogenic effects at several other anatomical regions in women and men such as HN as well as colorectal [12–15]. These studies showed that high-risk HPVs are present in roughly 30 and 70% of HN and colorectal cancers, respectively, especially in their invasive form [14, 15]. Therefore, several recent studies including one from our group pointed-out that high-risk HPVs are present in human CRCs, specifically types 16, 18, 31, 33, and 35 [7, 12, 15, 16, 52]. Moreover, six recent meta-analysis studies confirmed the presence of high-risk HPVs in human CRCs [70, 91–95]; however, the prevalence of high-risk HPVs varied from one geographic location to another [7, 52]. Meanwhile, it was stated that high-risk HPVs are present especially in the invasive form of these malignancies worldwide [15].

Nevertheless, it is important to mention that high-risk HPV infection alone is not sufficient to induce neoplastic transformation of human normal epithelial cells; the infected cells must undergo additional genetic changes and/or coinfection with another oncovirus to reach full transformation and consequently tumor formation. Based on this fact, we have developed a new model to study the cooperation effect between high-risk HPVs and other oncogenes in human carcinogenesis using human normal epithelial (HNE) cells. In this model, we established that E6/E7 oncoproteins of high-risk type 16 cooperate with the ErbB-2 receptor to induce cellular transformation of HNE cells; this was accompanied by a delocalization of β-catenin from the undercoat membrane to the nucleus in HNE cells. Furthermore, we reported that cyclin D1 is the target of E6/E7/ErbB-2 cooperation via the conversion of β-catenin's role from a cell–cell adhesion molecule to a transcriptional regulator [96]. In parallel, we revealed that D-type cyclins (D1, D2, and D3) are essential for cell transformation induced by E6/E7/ErbB-2 cooperation in human HNE and mouse normal embryonic fibroblast (NEF) cells [96, 97]. Finally, we were able to show that the cooperation effect of E6/E7 with ErbB-2, in human normal epithelial and cancer cells, occurs via β-catenin tyrosine phosphorylation through pp60 (c-Src) kinase activation [98, 99]. Thus, the cooperation between E6/E7 oncoproteins of high-risk HPVs and other oncogenes could occur in colorectal carcinogenesis.

On the other hand, and to determine the role of high-risk HPVs infection in human cancer cells, we examined the effect of E6/E7 of HPV type 16 in two noninvasive human breast cancer cell lines. We reported that E6/E7 of HPV type 16 induce cell invasive and metastatic abilities of the two cell lines *in vitro* and *in vivo*, respectively, in comparison with their wild-type cells [100]. This is accompanied by an overexpression of Id-1, a family member of helix-loop-helix transcription factors which regulates cell invasion and metastasis of human cancer cells [101, 102]. We also demonstrated that E6/E7 oncoproteins upregulate Id-1 promoter activity in human cancer cells. These data suggest that high-risk HPVs could play an important role in the progression of human carcinomas via Id-1 deregulation. Thus, we believe that E6/E7 oncoproteins of high-risk HPVs could play a similar role in the progression of human CRCs.

In order to investigate the role of high-risk HPV infection in human colorectal carcinogenesis, we examined the effect of E6/E7 of HPV type 16 in two human primary normal colorectal "mesenchymal" cell lines, NCM1 and NCM5, which were established in our laboratory [20].

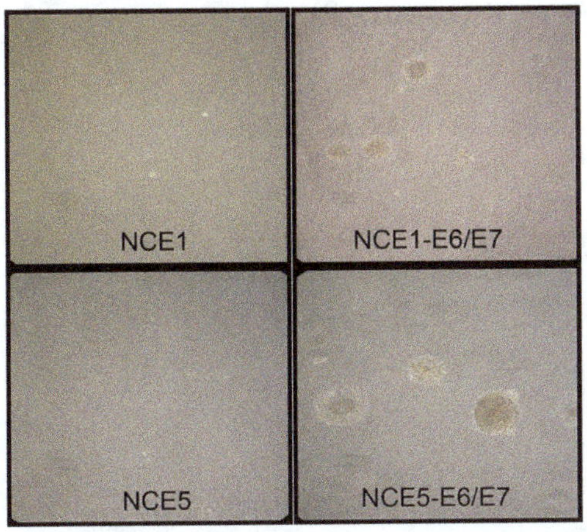

Figure 1. E6/E7 oncoproteins of high-risk HPV type 16 induce cellular transformation in human primary normal colorectal "mesenchymal" cell lines, NCE1, and NCE5 cells [103]. We note that NCE1 and NCE5 cells are unable to grow in soft agar. In contrast, NCE1 and NCE5 cells expressing E6/E7 oncoproteins form colonies in soft agar assay, which is an important characteristic of cancer cells.

We found that the expression of E6/E7 oncoproteins stimulate cell proliferation and induce cellular transformation (**Figure 1**) and migration of NCM1 and NCM5 cell lines. Moreover, our data revealed that E6/E7 of HPV type 16 provoke the upregulation of D-type cyclins and Cyclin E as well as Id-1 in these cell lines [103]. It is important to highlight that there are no other studies regarding the role of E6/E7 oncoproteins of high-risk HPVs in human colorectal cancers. Meanwhile, the function of E5 oncoprotein, in these malignancies, has not been investigated yet.

Additionally, we have recently investigated the incidence of high-risk HPVs in human CRCs in the Syrian population in a cohort of 78 cancer samples using PCR and tissue microarray analyses. We reported, for the first time, that high-risk HPVs are present in 42 samples (53.84%), which represent the majority of invasive colorectal cases; more significantly, our data pointed-out that the most frequent high-risk HPV types in the Syrian population are 16, 33, 18, 35, and 31, respectively. Furthermore, the expression of E6 oncoprotein of high-risk HPVs was found to be correlated with Fascin, Id-1, and P-cadherin expression/overexpression in the majority of cancer tissue samples, which are major regulators of cell invasion and metastasis [17–19, 52]. Our data imply that high-risk HPVs are present in human CRCs, and their presence is associated with invasive and metastatic phenotype [16, 52, 104]. Collectively, these data suggest that high-risk HPVs are present in CRCs and therefore could play an important role in the initiation and progression of these cancers. Thus, we believe that high-risk HPVs can be associated with a subset of colorectal cancers. However, future large-scale multicenter case–control studies with data on risk factors such as lifestyle and sexual behavior are needed; meanwhile, molecular and cellular studies are necessary to determine the role of E5 and E6/E7 oncoproteins in human colorectal cancer and normal cells since it was proposed that E5 can cooperate with E6/E7 oncoproteins to enhance cancer progression of other human malignancies via the EMT event [20, 52]. Thus, we believe that E5 and E6/E7 of high-risk HPVs can cooperate with other oncogenes and/or risk factors such as smoking or alcohol to initiate colorectal cancer; in addition, E5 could cooperate with E6/E7 to enhance cancer progression of this malignancy via the EMT event (**Figure 2**).

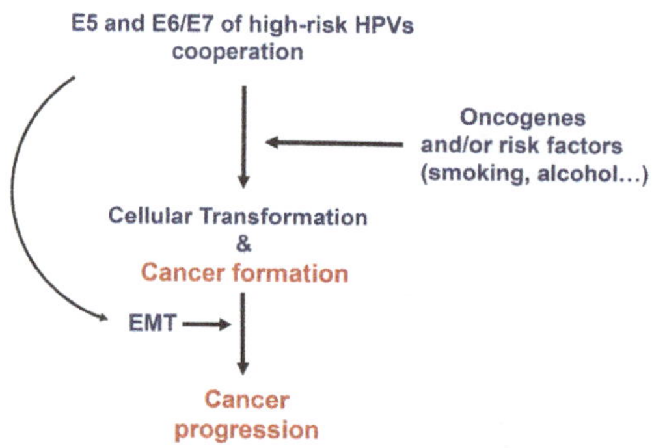

Figure 2. E5 and E6/E7 of high-risk HPVs cooperation and colorectal carcinogenesis. We believe that E5 and E6/E7 of high-risk HPVs can cooperate with other oncogene overexpressions that are linked to lifestyle or/and environmental factors to induce cellular transformation and consequently tumor formation. On the other hand, E5 and E6/E7 together can enhance cancer progression of colorectal cancer via the initiation of the epithelial-mesenchymal transition (EMT) event .

Finally, we think it is important to talk about the prevention strategy of HPV infections and their related cancers, which is essentially based on HPV vaccines. These vaccines are made of virus-like particles (VLPs) that contain inactive L1 HPV proteins—proteins from and specific to each type of HPV viruses [105, 106]. Thus, the quadrivalent vaccine Gardasil (Merck and Co) was developed and approved by the FDA in 2006 for protection against low-risk HPV types 6 and 11, which cause genital warts—and rarely, nongenital warts [107] and high-risk HPV types 16 and 18 [108]. The quadrivalent vaccine will not protect against anogenital disease other than HPV types 6, 11, 16, and 18 [109, 110]. In 2010, the FDA approved the quadrivalent vaccine for the prevention of CRC [106]. The efficacy of prevention of rectal intraepithelial neoplasia in some group of patients is 77.5% [111]. In 2009, a bivalent vaccine (Cervarix; GlaxoSmithKline) was approved for the prevention of HPV infections from high-risk types 16 and 18 [112]. On December 10, 2014, the FDA approved a 9-valent HPV vaccine (Gardasil-9; Merck and Co) that was approved to be given in three intramuscular doses to males 9–15 years of age and females 9–26 years of age [106, 113]. The 9-valent HPV vaccine targets high-risk HPV type 16 (responsible for 50% of cervical carcinogenesis) [114], high-risk HPV type 18 (detected in 20% of cervical cancers) [115], and types 31, 33, 45, 52, and 58, which are responsible for 25% of cervical cancers. Immunizations against low-risk HPV types 6 and 11, which cause genital warts, are also included in the 9-valent vaccine [106, 116]. Approval of the 9-valent vaccine was based on a randomized control study with 14,000 females 16–26 years of age; it noted efficacy of 97% [106]. Therefore, this vaccine will have an important role in preventing HPV infections and their related cancers including colorectal malignancies and their metastasis.

5. Conclusion and perspectives

This chapter presented substantial evidence that high-risk HPVs are present in human CRCs, thereby these viruses, through their E5 and E6/E7 oncoproteins, could play an important role in the initiation and progression of these malignances (Figure 2) [20, 100]. However, we believe that further studies are required to determine the function of E5 and E6/E7 oncogenes in human colorectal normal and cancer cells. Thus, developing new *in vitro* and *in vivo* models, such as cell lines and animal models, are necessary to identify the exact role of these oncoproteins and their potential cooperation in human colorectal carcinogenesis. Such studies can lead to the discovery of new targets to manage these malignances and other human carcinomas related to high-risk HPVs.

Alternatively, and with regards to colorectal malignancies as well as other human carcinomas prevention, we assume that the elimination of a number of known risk factors especially unprotected sexual activity, physical inactivity, smoking, alcohol, high consumption of red meat, and oncovirus infections such as high-risk HPVs could diminish the development of these malignancies and their metastases [20, 23, 26]. Additionally, prevention methodologies of high-risk HPVs using presently available vaccines could greatly reduce high-risk HPVs-associated cancers, including colorectal, and their progression to invasive form, which is responsible for the majority of cancer-related deaths.

Acknowledgements

We are grateful to Mrs. A. Kassab for her critical reading of the chapter. The research works from Dr. Al Moustafa's laboratory is supported by the College of Medicine of Qatar University.

Author details

Ala-Eddin Al Moustafa[1,2,3*], Noor Al-Antary[1] and Amber Yasmeen[4]

*Address all correspondence to: aalmoustafa@qu.edu.qa; ala-eddin.almoustafa@mcgill.ca

1 College of Medicine & Biomedical Research Centre, Qatar University, Doha, Qatar

2 Oncology Department, McGill University, Montreal, Quebec, Canada

3 Syrian Research Cancer Centre of the Syrian Society against Cancer, Aleppo, Syria

4 Segal Cancer Centre, Lady Davis Institute for Medical Research, JGH, McGill University, Montreal, Quebec, Canada

References

[1] Ferlay J, Soerjomataram I, Dikshit R, Eser S, Mathers C, et al. Cancer incidence and mortality worldwide: sources, methods and major patterns in GLOBOCAN 2012. International Journal of Cancer. 2015;136:E359–86.

[2] Rose J, Augestad KM, Cooper GS. Colorectal cancer surveillance: what's new and what's next. World Journal of Gastroenterology. 2014;20:1887–97.

[3] Beg S, Siraj AK, Prabhakaran S, Bu R, Al-Rasheed M, et al. Molecular markers and pathway analysis of colorectal carcinoma in the Middle East. Cancer. 2015;121:3799–808.

[4] Tezcan G, Tunca B, Ak S, Cecener G, Egeli U. Molecular approach to genetic and epigenetic pathogenesis of early onset colorectal cancer. World Journal of Gastrointestinal Oncology. 2016;8:83–98.

[5] Vainio H, Miller AB. Primary and secondary prevention in colorectal cancer. Acta Oncologica. 2003;42:809–15.

[6] Mattar RE, Al-Alem F, Simoneau E, Hassanain M. Preoperative selection of patients with colorectal cancer liver metastasis for hepatic resection. World Journal of Gastroenterology. 2016;22:567–81.

[7] Al Moustafa AE, Al-Awadhi R, Missaoui N, Adam I, Durusoy R, et al. Human papillomaviruses-related cancers. Presence and prevention strategies in the Middle east and north African regions. Human Vaccines & Immunotherapeutics. 2014a;10:1812—21.

[8] de Sanjose S, Diaz M, Castellsague X, Clifford G, Bruni L, et al. Worldwide prevalence and genotype distribution of cervical human papillomavirus DNA in women with normal cytology: a meta-analysis. The Lancet Infectious Diseases. 2007;7:453–9.

[9] Smith JS, Lindsay L, Hoots B, Keys J, Franceschi S, et al. Human papillomavirus type distribution in invasive cervical cancer and high-grade cervical lesions: a meta-analysis update. International Journal of Cancer. 2007;121:621–32.

[10] Begum S, Gillison ML, Ansari-Lari MA, Shah K, Westra WH. Detection of human papillomavirus in cervical lymph nodes: a highly effective strategy for localizing site of tumor origin. Clinical Cancer Research: An Official Journal of the American Association for Cancer Research. 2003;9:6469–75.

[11] Graflund M, Sorbe B, Sigurdardottir S, Karlsson M. HPV-DNA, vascular space invasion, and their impact on the clinical outcome in early-stage cervical carcinomas. International Journal of Gynecological Cancer: Official Journal of the International Gynecological Cancer Society. 2004;14:896–902.

[12] Abramowitz L, Jacquard AC, Jaroud F, Haesebaert J, Siproudhis L, et al. Human papillomavirus genotype distribution in anal cancer in France: the EDiTH V study. International Journal of Cancer. 2011;129:433–9.

[13] Shukla S, Bharti AC, Mahata S, Hussain S, Kumar R, et al. Infection of human papillomaviruses in cancers of different human organ sites. The Indian Journal of Medical Research. 2009;130:222–33.

[14] Umudum H, Rezanko T, Dag F, Dogruluk T. Human papillomavirus genome detection by in situ hybridization in fine-needle aspirates of metastatic lesions from head and neck squamous cell carcinomas. Cancer. 2005;105:171–7.

[15] Varnai AD, Bollmann M, Griefingholt H, Speich N, Schmitt C, et al. HPV in anal squamous cell carcinoma and anal intraepithelial neoplasia (AIN). Impact of HPV analysis of anal lesions on diagnosis and prognosis. International Journal of Colorectal Disease. 2006;21:135–42.

[16] Ghabreau L, Segal ED, Yasmeen A, Kassab A, Akil N, et al. High-risk human papillomavirus infections in colorectal cancer in the Syrian population and their association with Fascin, P-cadherin and Id-1 expressions: a tissue microarray study. Clinical Cancer Investigation 2012; J 1: 26–30.

[17] Ling MT, Wang X, Zhang X, Wong YC. The multiple roles of Id-1 in cancer progression. Differentiation; Research in Biological Diversity. 2006;74:481–7.

[18] Oh SY, Kim YB, Suh KW, Paek OJ, Moon HY. Prognostic impact of fascin-1 expression is more significant in advanced colorectal cancer. The Journal of Surgical Research. 2012;172:102–8.

[19] Van Marck V, Stove C, Jacobs K, Van den Eynden G, Bracke M. P-cadherin in adhesion and invasion: opposite roles in colon and bladder carcinoma. International Journal of Cancer. 2011;128:1031–44.

[20] Al Moustafa AE. E5 and E6/E7 of high-risk HPVs cooperate to enhance cancer progression through EMT initiation. Cell Adhesion & Migration. 2015;9:392–3.

[21] Yasmeen A, Alachkar A, Dekhil H, Gambacorti-Passerini C, Al Moustafa AE. Locking Src/Abl tyrosine kinase activities regulate cell differentiation and invasion of human cervical cancer cells expressing E6/E7 oncoproteins of high-risk HPV. Journal of Oncology. 2010;2010. doi: 10.1155/2010/530130

[22] Binefa G, Rodriguez-Moranta F, Teule A, Medina-Hayas M. Colorectal cancer: from prevention to personalized medicine. World Journal of Gastroenterology. 2014;20:6786–808.

[23] Chan AT, Giovannucci EL. Primary prevention of colorectal cancer. Gastroenterology. 2010;138:2029–43 e10.

[24] Schoen RE, Pinsky PF, Weissfeld JL, Yokochi LA, Church T, et al. Colorectal-cancer incidence and mortality with screening flexible sigmoidoscopy. The New England Journal of Medicine. 2012;366:2345–57.

[25] European Colorectal Cancer Screening Guidelines Working G, von Karsa L, Patnick J, Segnan N, Atkin W, Halloran S, et al. European guidelines for quality assurance in colorectal cancer screening and diagnosis: overview and introduction to the full supplement publication. Endoscopy. 2013;45:51–9.

[26] Day LW, Velayos F. Colorectal cancer screening and surveillance in the elderly: updates and controversies. Gut and Liver. 2015;9:143–51.

[27] Butler EN, Chawla N, Lund J, Harlan LC, Warren JL, et al. Patterns of colorectal cancer care in the United States and Canada: a systematic review. Journal of the National Cancer Institute Monographs. 2013;2013:13–35.

[28] Marin-Gabriel JC, Fernandez-Esparrach G, Diaz-Tasende J, Herreros de Tejada A. Colorectal endoscopic submucosal dissection from a Western perspective: today's promises and future challenges. World Journal of Gastrointestinal Endoscopy. 2016;8:40–55.

[29] Sankaranarayanan R. Screening for cancer in low- and middle-income countries. Annals of Global Health. 2014;80:412–7.

[30] Ballester V, Rashtak S, Boardman L. Clinical and molecular features of young-onset colorectal cancer. World Journal of Gastroenterology. 2016;22:1736–44.

[31] Lochhead P, Chan AT, Giovannucci E, Fuchs CS, Wu K, et al. Progress and opportunities in molecular pathological epidemiology of colorectal premalignant lesions. The American Journal of Gastroenterology. 2014;109:1205–14.

[32] Grady WM, Pritchard CC. Molecular alterations and biomarkers in colorectal cancer. Toxicologic Pathology. 2014;42:124–39.

[33] Sengupta N, Yau C, Sakthianandeswaren A, Mouradov D, Gibbs P, et al. Analysis of colorectal cancers in British Bangladeshi identifies early onset, frequent mucinous histotype and a high prevalence of RBFOX1 deletion. Molecular Cancer. 2013;12:1.

[34] Rosi J, Ackerman L. Surgical Pathology, Mosby Elsevier editors. 10th edition; 2011.

[35] Fleming M, Ravula S, Tatishchev SF, Wang HL. Colorectal carcinoma: pathologic aspects. Journal of Gastrointestinal Oncology. 2012;3:153–73.

[36] Maguire A, Sheahan K. Controversies in the pathological assessment of colorectal cancer. World Journal of Gastroenterology. 2014;20:9850–61.

[37] Al Moustafa AE. Role of high risk human papillomavisus in breast carcinogenesis. In: Satya Prakash Gupta editors. Book Cancer causing Viruses and their Inhibitors. Taylor and Francis Group, CRC Press; Germany, 2014, p. 245–262. ISBN 9781466589773

[38] Brenner H, Kloor M, Pox CP. Colorectal Cancer. Lancet. 2014;383:1490–502.

[39] Leufkens AM, van den Bosch MA, van Leeuwen MS, Siersema PD. Diagnostic accuracy of computed tomography for colon cancer staging: a systematic review. Scandinavian Journal of Gastroenterology. 2011;46:887–94.

[40] Niekel MC, Bipat S, Stoker J. Diagnostic imaging of colorectal liver metastases with CT, MR imaging, FDG PET, and/or FDG PET/CT: a meta-analysis of prospective studies including patients who have not previously undergone treatment. Radiology. 2010;257:674–84.

[41] Mitry E, Guiu B, Cosconea S, Jooste V, Faivre J, et al. Epidemiology, management and prognosis of colorectal cancer with lung metastases: a 30-year population-based study. Gut. 2010;59:1383–8.

[42] Choi DJ, Kwak JM, Kim J, Woo SU, Kim SH. Preoperative chest computerized tomography in patients with locally advanced mid or lower rectal cancer: its role in staging and impact on treatment strategy. Journal of Surgical Oncology. 2010;102:588–92.

[43] Kirke R, Rajesh A, Verma R, Bankart MJ. Rectal cancer: incidence of pulmonary metastases on thoracic CT and correlation with T staging. Journal of computer assisted tomography. 2007;31:569–71.

[44] Tan KK, Lopes Gde L, Jr., Sim R. How uncommon are isolated lung metastases in colorectal cancer? A review from database of 754 patients over 4 years. Journal of Gastrointestinal Surgery: Official Journal of the Society for Surgery of the Alimentary Tract. 2009;13:642–8.

[45] Chen H, Chen XZ, Waterboer T, Castro FA, Brenner H. Viral infections and colorectal cancer: a systematic review of epidemiological studies. International Journal of Cancer. 2015;137:12–24.

[46] Jemal A, Bray F, Center MM, Ferlay J, Ward E, et al. Global cancer statistics. CA: A Cancer Journal for Clinicians. 2011;61:69–90.

[47] Lynch HT, de la Chapelle A. Hereditary colorectal cancer. The New England Journal of Medicine. 2003;348:919–32.

[48] Aykan NF. Red meat and colorectal cancer. Oncology Reviews. 2015;9:288.

[49] Liang PS, Chen TY, Giovannucci E. Cigarette smoking and colorectal cancer incidence and mortality: systematic review and meta-analysis. International Journal of Cancer. 2009;124:2406–15.

[50] Collins D, Hogan AM, Winter DC. Microbial and viral pathogens in colorectal cancer. The Lancet Oncology. 2011;12:504–12.

[51] Wu Q, Yang ZP, Xu P, Gao LC, Fan DM. Association between *Helicobacter pylori* infection and the risk of colorectal neoplasia: a systematic review and meta-analysis. Colorectal Disease: The Official Journal of the Association of Coloproctology of Great Britain and Ireland. 2013;15:e352–64.

[52] Al Moustafa AE, Ghabreau L, Akil N, Rastam S, Alachkar A, et al. High-risk HPVs and human carcinomas in the Syrian population. Frontiers in Oncology. 2014b;4:68.

[53] Coelho TR, Gaspar R, Figueiredo P, Mendonca C, Lazo PA, et al. Human JC polyomavirus in normal colorectal mucosa, hyperplastic polyps, sporadic adenomas, and adenocarcinomas in Portugal. Journal of Medical Virology. 2013;85:2119–27.

[54] Shope RE, Hurst EW. Infectious papillomatosis of rabbits: with a note on the histopathology. The Journal of Experimental Medicine. 1933;58:607–24.

[55] Moore PS, Chang Y. Why do viruses cause cancer? Highlights of the first century of human tumour virology. Nature Reviews Cancer. 2010;10:878–89.

[56] zur Hausen H. Papillomaviruses and cancer: from basic studies to clinical application. Nature Reviews Cancer. 2002;2:342–50.

[57] Edwards S, Carne C. Oral sex and the transmission of viral STIs. Sexually Transmitted Infections. 1998;74:6–10.

[58] Frega A, Cenci M, Stentella P, Cipriano L, De Ioris A, et al. Human papillomavirus in virgins and behaviour at risk. Cancer Letters. 2003;194:21–4.

[59] Gervaz P, Allal AS, Villiger P, Buhler L, Morel P. Squamous cell carcinoma of the anus: another sexually transmitted disease. Swiss Medical Weekly. 2003;133:353–9.

[60] Ho GY, Bierman R, Beardsley L, Chang CJ, Burk RD. Natural history of cervicovaginal papillomavirus infection in young women. The New England Journal of Medicine. 1998;338:423–8.

[61] Sonnex C, Strauss S, Gray JJ. Detection of human papillomavirus DNA on the fingers of patients with genital warts. Sexually Transmitted Infections. 1999;75:317–9.

[62] Prabhu SR, Wilson DF. Human papillomavirus and oral disease—emerging evidence: a review. Australian Dental Journal. 2013;58:2–10; quiz 125.

[63] Antonsson A, Forslund O, Ekberg H, Sterner G, Hansson BG. The ubiquity and impressive genomic diversity of human skin papillomaviruses suggest a commensalic nature of these viruses. Journal of Virology. 2000;74:11636–41.

[64] Hiller T, Iftner T. The human papillomavirus. In: Prendiville W, Davies P, editors. Human Papillomavirus and Cervical Cancer. The Health Professional's HPV Handbook. London and New York: Taylor & Francis; 2004, p. 11–26.

[65] de Villiers EM, Fauquet C, Broker TR, Bernard HU, zur Hausen H. Classification of papillomaviruses. Virology. 2004;324:17–27.

[66] Mammas IN, Sourvinos G, Spandidos DA. The paediatric story of human papillomavirus (Review). Oncology Letters. 2014;8:502–6.

[67] Bernard HU. The clinical importance of the nomenclature, evolution and taxonomy of human papillomaviruses. Journal of Clinical Virology: The Official Publication of the Pan American Society for Clinical Virology. 2005;32 Suppl 1:S1–6.

[68] Castellsague X, Diaz M, de Sanjose S, Munoz N, Herrero R, et al. Worldwide human papillomavirus etiology of cervical adenocarcinoma and its cofactors: implications for screening and prevention. Journal of the National Cancer Institute. 2006;98:303–15.

[69] Zuna RE, Allen RA, Moore WE, Mattu R, Dunn ST. Comparison of human papillomavirus genotypes in high-grade squamous intraepithelial lesions and invasive cervical carcinoma: evidence for differences in biologic potential of precursor lesions. Modern Pathology: An Official Journal of the United States and Canadian Academy of Pathology, Inc. 2004;17:1314–22.

[70] Abbas A, Yang G, Fakih M. Management of anal cancer in 2010. Part 1: overview, screening, and diagnosis. Oncology. 2010;24:364–9.

[71] Doorbar J. Latent papillomavirus infections and their regulation. Current Opinion in Virology. 2013;3:416–21.

[72] Grm HS, Massimi P, Gammoh N, Banks L. Crosstalk between the human papillomavirus E2 transcriptional activator and the E6 oncoprotein. Oncogene. 2005;24:5149–64.

[73] Yuan CH, Filippova M, Duerksen-Hughes P. Modulation of apoptotic pathways by human papillomaviruses (HPV): mechanisms and implications for therapy. Viruses. 2012;4:3831–50.

[74] Kim SH, Juhnn YS, Kang S, Park SW, Sung MW, et al. Human papillomavirus 16 E5 up-regulates the expression of vascular endothelial growth factor through the activation of epidermal growth factor receptor, MEK/ ERK1,2 and PI3K/Akt. Cellular and Molecular Life Sciences: CMLS. 2006;63:930–8.

[75] Oh JM, Kim SH, Cho EA, Song YS, Kim WH, et al. Human papillomavirus type 16 E5 protein inhibits hydrogen-peroxide-induced apoptosis by stimulating ubiquitin-proteasome-mediated degradation of Bax in human cervical cancer cells. Carcinogenesis. 2010;31:402–10.

[76] Suprynowicz FA, Disbrow GL, Krawczyk E, Simic V, Lantzky K, et al. HPV-16 E5 oncoprotein upregulates lipid raft components caveolin-1 and ganglioside GM1 at the plasma membrane of cervical cells. Oncogene. 2008;27:1071–8.

[77] Stacey SN, Jordan D, Williamson AJ, Brown M, Coote JH, et al. Leaky scanning is the predominant mechanism for translation of human papillomavirus type 16 E7 oncoprotein from E6/E7 bicistronic mRNA. Journal of Virology. 2000;74:7284–97.

[78] Munger K, Basile JR, Duensing S, Eichten A, Gonzalez SL, et al. Biological activities and molecular targets of the human papillomavirus E7 oncoprotein. Oncogene. 2001;20:7888–98.

[79] Ghittoni R, Accardi R, Hasan U, Gheit T, Sylla B, Tommasino M. The biological properties of E6 and E7 oncoproteins from human papillomaviruses. Virus Genes. 2010;40:1–13.

[80] Thomas M, Banks L. Inhibition of Bak-induced apoptosis by HPV-18 E6. Oncogene. 1998;17:2943–54.

[81] Magal SS, Jackman A, Ish-Shalom S, Botzer LE, Gonen P, et al. Downregulation of Bax mRNA expression and protein stability by the E6 protein of human papillomavirus 16. The Journal of General Virology. 2005;86:611–21.

[82] Thomas M, Laura R, Hepner K, Guccione E, Sawyers C, Lasky L, et al. Oncogenic human papillomavirus E6 proteins target the MAGI-2 and MAGI-3 proteins for degradation. Oncogene. 2002;21:5088–96.

[83] Nguyen ML, Nguyen MM, Lee D, Griep AE, Lambert PF. The PDZ ligand domain of the human papillomavirus type 16 E6 protein is required for E6's induction of epithelial hyperplasia in vivo. Journal of Virology. 2003a;77:6957–64.

[84] Nguyen MM, Nguyen ML, Caruana G, Bernstein A, Lambert PF, et al. Requirement of PDZ-containing proteins for cell cycle regulation and differentiation in the mouse lens epithelium. Molecular and Cellular Biology. 2003b;23:8970–81.

[85] Doorbar J. The papillomavirus life cycle. Journal of Clinical Virology: The Official Publication of the Pan American Society for Clinical Virology. 2005;32 Suppl 1:S7–15.

[86] Herber R, Liem A, Pitot H, Lambert PF. Squamous epithelial hyperplasia and carcinoma in mice transgenic for the human papillomavirus type 16 E7 oncogene. Journal of Virology. 1996;70:1873–81.

[87] Song S, Pitot HC, Lambert PF. The human papillomavirus type 16 E6 gene alone is sufficient to induce carcinomas in transgenic animals. Journal of Virology. 1999;73:5887–93.

[88] Riley RR, Duensing S, Brake T, Munger K, Lambert PF, Arbeit JM. Dissection of human papillomavirus E6 and E7 function in transgenic mouse models of cervical carcinogenesis. Cancer Research. 2003;63:4862–71.

[89] Genther Williams SM, Disbrow GL, Schlegel R, Lee D, Threadgill DW, et al. Requirement of epidermal growth factor receptor for hyperplasia induced by E5, a high-risk human papillomavirus oncogene. Cancer Research. 2005;65:6534–42.

[90] Stelzer MK, Pitot HC, Liem A, Schweizer J, Mahoney C, et al. A mouse model for human anal cancer. Cancer Prevention Research. 2010;3:1534–41.

[91] Baandrup L, Thomsen LT, Olesen TB, Andersen KK, Norrild B, et al. The prevalence of human papillomavirus in colorectal adenomas and adenocarcinomas: a systematic review and meta-analysis. European Journal of Cancer. 2014;50:1446–61.

[92] Damin DC, Ziegelmann PK, Damin AP. Human papillomavirus infection and colorectal cancer risk: a meta-analysis. Colorectal Disease: The Official Journal of the Association of Coloproctology of Great Britain and Ireland. 2013;15:e420–8.

[93] De Vuyst H, Clifford GM, Nascimento MC, Madeleine MM, Franceschi S. Prevalence and type distribution of human papillomavirus in carcinoma and intraepithelial neoplasia of the vulva, vagina and anus: a meta-analysis. International Journal of Cancer. 2009;124:1626–36.

[94] Lorenzon L, Ferri M, Pilozzi E, Torrisi MR, Ziparo V, French D. Human papillomavirus and colorectal cancer: evidences and pitfalls of published literature. International Journal of Colorectal Disease. 2011;26:135–42.

[95] Machalek DA, Poynten M, Jin F, Fairley CK, Farnsworth A, et al. Anal human papillomavirus infection and associated neoplastic lesions in men who have sex with men: a systematic review and meta-analysis. The Lancet Oncology. 2012;13:487–500.

[96] Al Moustafa AE, Foulkes WD, Wong A, Jallal H, Batist G, et al. Cyclin D1 is essential for neoplastic transformation induced by both E6/E7 and E6/E7/ErbB-2 cooperation in normal cells. Oncogene. 2004;23:5252–6.

[97] Yasmeen A, Hosein AN, Yu Q, Al Moustafa AE. Critical role for D-type cyclins in cellular transformation induced by E6/E7 of human papillomavirus type 16 and E6/E7/ErbB-2 cooperation. Cancer Science. 2007a;98:973–7.

[98] Al Moustafa AE, Kassab A, Darnel A, Yasmeen A. High-risk HPV/ErbB-2 interaction on E-cadherin/catenin regulation in human carcinogenesis. Current Pharmaceutical Design. 2008;14:2159–72.

[99] Yasmeen A, Bismar TA, Dekhil H, Ricciardi R, Kassab A, et al. ErbB-2 receptor cooperates with E6/E7 oncoproteins of HPV type 16 in breast tumorigenesis. Cell Cycle. 2007b;6:2939–43.

[100] Yasmeen A, Bismar TA, Kandouz M, Foulkes WD, Desprez PY, et al. E6/E7 of HPV type 16 promotes cell invasion and metastasis of human breast cancer cells. Cell Cycle. 2007c; 6:2038–42.

[101] Fong S, Itahana Y, Sumida T, Singh J, Coppe JP, et al. Id-1 as a molecular target in therapy for breast cancer cell invasion and metastasis. Proceedings of the National Academy of Sciences of the United States of America. 2003;100:13543–8.

[102] Sikder HA, Devlin MK, Dunlap S, Ryu B, Alani RM. Id proteins in cell growth and tumorigenesis. Cancer Cell. 2003;3:525–30.

[103] Ricciardi R, Ghabreau L, Yasmeen A, Darnel AD, Akil N, et al. Role of E6/E7 oncoproteins of high-risk human papillomaviruses in human colorectal carcinogenesis. Cell Cycle. 2009;8:1964–5.

[104] Al Moustafa AE, Yasmeen A, Ghabreau L, Akil N. Does the Syrian population have to wait for the new generation of human papillomaviruses vaccine? Human Vaccines & Immunotherapeutics. 2012;8:1867–8.

[105] Dochez C, Bogers JJ, Verhelst R, Rees H. HPV vaccines to prevent cervical cancer and genital warts: an update. Vaccine. 2014;32:1595–601.

[106] Handler MZ, Handler NS, Majewski S, Schwartz RA. Human papillomavirus vaccine trials and tribulations: Clinical perspectives. Journal of the American Academy of Dermatology. 2015;73:743–56; quiz 57–8.

[107] Papadopoulos AJ, Schwartz RA, Lefkowitz A, Tinkle LL, Janniger CK, et al. Extragenital bowenoid papulosis associated with atypical human papillomavirus genotypes. Journal of Cutaneous Medicine and Surgery. 2002;6:117–21.

[108] Grimes RM, Benjamins LJ, Williams KL. Counseling about the HPV vaccine: desexualize, educate, and advocate. Journal of Pediatric and Adolescent Gynecology. 2013;26:243–8.

[109] Brown DR, Kjaer SK, Sigurdsson K, Iversen OE, Hernandez-Avila M, et al. The impact of quadrivalent human papillomavirus (HPV; types 6, 11, 16, and 18) L1 virus-like particle vaccine on infection and disease due to oncogenic nonvaccine HPV types in generally HPV-naive women aged 16–26 years. The Journal of Infectious Diseases. 2009;199:926–35.

[110] Goldstone SE, Jessen H, Palefsky JM, Giuliano AR, Moreira ED, Jr., et al. Quadrivalent HPV vaccine efficacy against disease related to vaccine and non-vaccine HPV types in males. Vaccine. 2013;31:3849–55.

[111] Palefsky JM, Giuliano AR, Goldstone S, Moreira ED, Jr., Aranda C, et al. HPV vaccine against anal HPV infection and anal intraepithelial neoplasia. The New England Journal of Medicine. 2011;365:1576–85.

[112] Paavonen J, Naud P, Salmeron J, Wheeler CM, Chow SN, et al. Efficacy of human papillomavirus (HPV)-16/18 AS04-adjuvanted vaccine against cervical infection and precancer caused by oncogenic HPV types (PATRICIA): final analysis of a double-blind, randomised study in young women. Lancet. 2009;374:301–14.

[113] Merck. Patient Information about GARDASIL®92014 (2014) Available at: http://www.merck.com/product/usa/pi_circulars/g/gardasil_9/gardasil_9_ppi.pdf

[114] Ault KA. Epidemiology and natural history of human papillomavirus infections in the female genital tract. Infectious Diseases in Obstetrics and Gynecology. 2006;2006 Suppl: 40470.

[115] Burger RA, Monk BJ, Kurosaki T, Anton-Culver H, Vasilev SA, et al. Human papillomavirus type 18: association with poor prognosis in early stage cervical cancer. Journal of the National Cancer Institute. 1996;88:1361–8.

[116] Hariri S, Unger ER, Schafer S, Niccolai LM, Park IU, et al. HPV type attribution in high-grade cervical lesions: assessing the potential benefits of vaccines in a population-based evaluation in the United States. Cancer Epidemiology, Biomarkers & Prevention: A Publication of the American Association for Cancer Research, Cosponsored by the American Society of Preventive Oncology. 2015;24:393–9.

4

Biotechnologies Involved in Differentiation of Cervical Lesions

Ruxandra Stanculescu

Abstract

The purpose of this paper is to describe the updated biotechnologies approved to be used for identifying precancerous cervical lesions in clinical practice. The paper focuses on the new biotechnologies able to detect human papillomavirus (HPV) such as nucleic acid hybridization assays, signal amplification assays, and nucleic acid amplification. Particular attention is given to the discussion regarding the differences among the biotechnologies used, such as Digene Hybrid Capture test using Hybrid Capture 2 technology and the Cervista HR-HPV assay. The scientific progress is emphasized by new markers such as cycline $p16^{INK4a}$, viral oncoproteins E6 and E7, high-risk (HR) HPV genotyping, and dual test p16/Ki67. The results of the large ongoing studies conducted worldwide highlight these markers' capacity to disclose the differences between transient and transforming HPV infection and mild abnormal cytologies which could spontaneously regress or develop into cancer. Although both screening programs and opportunistic screening concerning cervical cancer are used worldwide, major geographic differences exist nowadays as regards the access to these programs. Finally, to achieve the objective of this study, the recommendations of various guidelines available across Europe, United States, and Australia, as well as the diagnosis tests accessible to women in low-resource countries are presented.

Keywords: Pap's smear, HPV genotyping test, E6/E7 mRNA, $p16^{INK4a}$, dual test $p16^{INK4/Ki67}$

1. Introduction

According to the data reported by GLOBOCAN 2012 (IARC), cervical cancer is included among the leading causes of cancer worldwide. As regards the incidence of cervical cancer, GLOBO-

CAN report underlines that this type of cancer is the fourth most common cancer in women, and the seventh overall. The estimated number of new cases for 2012 is 528,000 [1]. For the same year, the registered number of deaths from cervical cancer was assessed at 266,000 cases. In terms of cervical cancer incidence and death by this disease, there is a major difference between the demographic regions of the world, strongly corresponding with the resource-setting level. Mortality varies 18-fold between various world regions, with rates ranging from less than 2 per 100,000 (in Western Asia, Western Europe, and Australia/New Zealand) to more than 20 per 100,000 (in Melanesia (20.6), Middle Africa (22.2), and Eastern Africa (27.6)) as stated by the GLOBOCAN 2012 report. A valuable consequence of the cervical cancer screening programs' implementation is that the incidence of cervical cancer rate dropped to half or more than half over the past 30 years, especially in countries with high levels of resources. For 2016, according to the American Cancer Society's estimates for cervical cancer in the United States, approximately 12,990 new cases of invasive cervical cancer will be diagnosed and 4120 women will die from cervical cancer. Cervical cancer is extremely rare in women younger than 20 and women over 65 years of age; only 15% of cervical cancer was reported to be identified at these ages. The improvement of collected data quality (statistics, information range) as concerns the occurrence of cervical cancer and the death by this disease is due to the implementation of national screening programs in many countries. Nowadays, more types of cervical cancer screening programs are in place, and a larger number of different biotechnologies are available across the world, which allow to identify early precancerous conditions of the cervix and therefore to obviate progression to cancer. On the other hand, it is very important that clinicians know the usable benefits and potential harms of biotechnologies able to achieve the triage of women with abnormal cytology or to identify cases with high-risk human papilloma virus in the stage of transforming infection. Due to a noteworthy scientific progress, clinicians now have many possibilities for early detection of a cervical lesion that might evolve into cervical cancer. The aim of the new biotechnology procedures is to achieve both high sensitivity and specificity in order to differentiate cervical lesions that may develop into cancer from those which spontaneously regress. Within the frame of this paper are included both the principal methods recommended by clinicians and researchers in cervical cancer field and the benefits and disadvantages of each biotechnology and marker. Our approach is designed so as to be useful especially to gynecologists with a view to a better management of the diagnosis and treatment of precancerous lesions. Hence, this paper explains what attempts should be made in the framework of each chosen biotechnology and what kind of tests increases the accuracy of an early diagnosis with regard to precancerous cervical lesions.

The data collection was performed by literature search, using PubMed, EMBASE, and the Cochrane Library (covering the 2000–2015 time frame), the main subject being detection of Human Papillomavirus Infection and cellular markers for early detection of precancerous cervical lesions. This study makes reference to the results of large studies published worldwide, such as in ATHENA, HERMES, PALMS, KPNC studies, Compass Trial, and the Newsletter on Human Papillomavirus—HPV Today (2015). This paper is structured in three sections. The first one covers different types of biotechnologies able to uncover precancerous and cancerous cervical lesions which are approved for use in medical clinical practice. The second section is dedicated to discussions about the benefits and drawbacks of each biotechnology reported to detect precancerous lesions. At last, attention is paid to recommendations of the overall current guidelines.

2. Biotechnologies able to detect the precancerous and cancerous cervical lesions

A strong contribution to the early detection of precancerous cervical lesions belongs to Papanicolou. The Pap's test has been in place since 1950, when George Papanicolou introduced this method as a cytological test able to detect morphological changes of abnormal cells. Generally, there are three kinds of markers for cervical cancer screening: viral markers, cellular markers, and epigenetic markers, which can identify, alone or in combination, early precancerous cervical lesions.

The laboratory tests able to reveal precancerous and cancerous cervical lesions use cytolological, viral, cellular, and genetic markers such as Pap's test, HPV genotyping test, cellular markers, epigenetic markers, and other markers.

2.1. Pap's test: cytological diagnosis

Papanicolau stain—commonly known as Pap's test—is the best-performing method used for cervical screening. The cytologist analyses, via this test, the exfoliated cervical cells to detect the morphological changes characteristic to neoplasic alterations. The cervical cell samples must be taken within the squamocolumnar junction of the cervix. This area is relatively accessible, making sampling easy, but it is unable to provide information about the lesions within the endocervical canal such as adenocarcinoma precursors [2, 3]. For the same Papanicolou stain, there are two methods that differ in terms of collecting technology: one is used to collect cervical cells (being known as conventional type), and the other is liquid-based (cytology type).

The conventional type uses the fixation of cervical cells of the sample, followed by classic Pap staining (EA 50, Hematoxilina Harris, Orange G, and different concentrations of ethanol). The duration of this procedure is about 45 min.

The liquid-based collection medium biotechnology is deemed more advanced because it is more versatile. Cervical cells are collected by using a cytobrush, which is then introduced into a collection medium (e.g., Cytofast). This method gives the opportunity both to keep the physiological structure and morphology of any kind of cells for 24 months at room temperature and to perform more investigations (e.g., HPV oncotypes, cyclin immunomarkers) [4, 5]. Since 2013, Hospitex Diagnostics highlights that the monolayer slides from liquid-based collection medium are safer, faster and fully representative, in comparison with the conventional smear screening procedure. The interpretation of the cytological results is done according to the Bethesda System Criteria established in 2001. During the past 15 years, a cytological diagnosis which included medical recommendation was possible due to the Bethesda System Criteria.

2.2. Viral markers

The viral markers validated for usage in cervical cancer detection are HPV DNA and HPV genotyping, E6/E7 mRNA, and HPV proteins [6].

First of all, this paper describes, in line with its purpose, the biotechnologies which can be used to become aware of human papillomavirus infection (HPV) and identify the high-risk HPV genotypes (HR-HPV). There are several other technologies able to identify human papillomavirus infection. These methods have different benefits and drawbacks, for which reason a good option should be made to properly choose the individual test or screening program.

One of the following methods should be used to accomplish HPV detection: nucleic acid hybridization assays, signal amplification assays, and nucleic acid amplification [7, 8].

The techniques able to employ radiolabeled nucleic acid hybridization assay to identify HPV infection are Southern blotting, in situ hybridization, or dot blot hybridization.

Signal amplification assays pertain to another biotechnology consisting in two tests known as the Digene Hybrid Capture test which utilizes Hybrid Capture 2 (hc2) technology (by Qiagen) and the Cervista HR-HPV assay (by Hologic) [9].

Nucleic acid amplification methods involve many kinds of methodologies based on microarray analysis, PapilloCheck, polymerase chain reaction (PCR), real-time PCR, Abbott real-time PCR, COBAS 4800 HPV test, HPV genome sequencing, the Linear Array, CLART human papillomavirus, INNO-LiPA, clinical array HPV, Microplate colorimetric hybridization assay, HPV-mRNA detection, HPV viral load quantification and integration.

Many technologies approved in the Unites States and Europe, relying on large population-based studies and randomized trial, recommend using Hybrid Capture 2 test and Cervista test to spot HPV infection. Hybrid Capture 2 test was endorsed by the US Food and Drug Administration (FDA) in 2003 and is able to detect 13 HR-HPV types (16, 18, 31, 33, 35, 39, 45, 51, 52, 56, 58, 59, and 68) or 5 low risk (LR)-HPV types (6, 11, 42, 43, and 44), using specific antibodies' signal amplification and chemoluminescent detection. In 2009, FDA approved the Cervista HR-HPV, which detects 14 HR-HPV types (16, 18, 31, 33, 35, 39, 45, 51, 52, 56, 58, 59, 66, and 68) by using a signal amplification method and a fluorescent signal for detecting specific nucleic acid sequences. In 2009, FDA approved another HPV DNA test, Cervista HPV 16/18, which uncovers HPV 16 and 18 oncogenotypes [10].

In April 2014, FDA approved Cobas HPV test, which is a PCR-based HPV DNA test using the same fluorescent label for the fluorescent signal from 12 HR-HPV and simultaneous recognitions with three separate fluorescent labels of HPV 16, HPV18, and beta-globulin signals.

When applied alone, the detection of HR-HPV DNA does not discriminate between the transient and transforming HPV infections. This differentiation is possible by discerning viral oncoproteins E6 and E7 mRNA and protein expression. The progression from a transient to a transforming HPV infection is identified by the high increase of E6/E7 mRNA expression [11, 12]. These oncoproteins interfere with key cellular cycles that control cell proliferation and apoptosis. E7 disrupts pRb from its binding to E2F, and E6 interferes with p53. Therefore, viral oncoprotein E7 triggers uncontrolled cell cycling and E6 abrogates apoptosis. Two of the most widespread tests of the commercial assays designed to detect HPV E6/E7 mRNA are Pre Tect Proofer (Norchip), which detects five oncotypes of HR-HPV (16, 18, 31, 33, and 45), and APTIMA (GenoProbe) which covers 14 HPV types (16, 18, 31, 33, 35, 39, 45, 51, 52, 56, 58, 59, 66, and 68).

Another HPV assay—known as Qiagen assay (United States)—is an adoption of Digene HC2 assay. The signal amplification assay perceives 14 different HR-HPV oncotypes (16, 18, 31, 33, 35, 39, 45, 51, 52, 56, 58, 59, and 66). The particularity of Qiagen HPV assay consists in the fact that this platform does not require electricity or water, but only needs a limited work space (25×50 cm^2). The result is obtained shortly (2.5 h only).

The main methods used to detect HPV integration are PCR, fluorescence in situ hybridization, and Real-Time PCR. The latter two methods allow calculating the ratio between the levels of E2 and E6/E7 HPV genes. When the HPV is integrated, the viral genome shows a 1:1 ratio between the E2 and E6/E7 genes [13].

2.3. Cellular markers

The cell markers approved by the World Health Organization (WHO) to be used in clinical practice are p16^{INK4a} and dual test p16^{INK4a}/Ki67. Another possible option arises from the ongoing research about a new clinical cell marker concerning the detection of topoisomerase 2α, in cervical cytology slides.

2.3.1. Cellular markers: cyclin p16^{INK4a}

Uncovering of p16^{INK4a} is tightly correlated with HPV integration. In a normal cell, p16^{INK4a} blocks cyclin-dependent kinases (CDK) 4/6. Increased expression of the E6 and E7 oncogenes disrupt cell cycle regulation. In the normal cell, cell cycle progression is activated by CDK 4/6 and partially regulated by p16^{INK4a}. However, because in HPV-transformed cells, cell cycle activation is caused by E7 and not by CDK 4/6, p16^{INK4a} has no effect on the cell cycle activation. Increased expression of p16^{INK4a} in cells driven by viral oncogene-mediated cell cycle dysfunction can be distinguished through cellular immunostaining by immunocytology or immunohistology tests [14]. In brief, p16^{INK4a} is a tumor-suppressor protein and cyclin-dependent kinase (cdk) inhibitor that blocks CDK 4/6-mediated pRb phosphorylation to inhibit E2F-dependent transcription and cell cycle progression. It is obvious that the progression of dysplastic lesions to cancer is highlighted by increased expression of two viral oncogenes, E6 and E7. The last-mentioned oncoprotein, E7, inactivates retinoblastoma gene product (pRB) that inhibits transcription of the cyclin-dependent kinase inhibitor gene p16^{INK4a}. This explains why the overexpression of p16^{INK4a} is similar to the increased activity of E7, and so the overexpression of both p16^{INK4a} and E7 are markers of HPV integration in the genome of the host cell [15]. The cyclin p16^{INK4a} must be evaluated as a stand-alone test and as an adjunct to cytology or HPV testing [16, 17].

The cervical cells are collected similar to those for Pap's smear test. The liquid-based collection medium has the advantage of being able to collect more cervical cells both for Pap's smear, immunocytochemistry tests and for HPV genotyping test. In the current activity, the clinician has the possibility to demand two tests used to identify specific immunocytomarkers, such as p16^{INK4a} alone or the dual test which evaluates, on the same cervical cell, two immunocytomarkers consisting in p16^{INK4a} and Ki67.

Over the past 10 years, the cyclin inhibitor kinase p16^{INK4a} has been identified by immunocytochemistry staining using a CINtec p16^{INK4a} ready-to-use cytological kit (clone E6H4) manufactured by mtm laboratories AG (Heidelberg, Germany). Wentzensen published the morphological characteristics necessary to evaluate the immunocytological expressions of p16^{INK4a} within the cervical cell, both for nucleus and cytoplasm. Therefore, the criteria which must be analyzed are increased nucleus size or increased nucleus/cytoplasmic ratio, irregular nuclear shape, granular or hyperchromatic chromatin with variable cellular morphology, together with the intensity of cytoplasmic staining [18].

There are many models in the published literature that allow identifying the intensity of the immunocytoexpression of p16^{INK4a}. One method used for a correct interpretation of the immunoexpression classified samples as p16^{INK4a}-negative and p16^{INK4a}-positive when positivity was observed for at least two of the aforementioned criteria. On the other hand, to obtain greater accuracy in the slides' interpretation, a scoring system was introduced, which scored the absence and the gradual intensity of the immunocytological expression staining. Therefore, the scoring system assigns 0 point for cases without p16-positive cells (p16–), 1 point for p16-positive cells with changed morphology in the absence of nuclear abnormalities (p16+), 2 points for p16-positive cells with a single nuclear abnormality (p16++), and 3 points for the presence of at least two nuclear alterations within the same cell (p16+++) [18]. In this manner, the physician can establish a correct cytodiagnosis much more accurately.

2.3.2. *Cellular markers: p16$^{INK4a/Ki67}$ dual-stained*

The CINtec PLUS assay (mtm laboratories AG, Heidelberg, Germany) is currently gaining increased credibility; it is a commercially available test which combines the immunostaining of p16^{INK4a} with the immunostaining of Ki67 within the same cervical cell [19].

This methodology allows the cytologist to see, within the same epithelial cell, the nucleus stained red for Ki67 immunoexpression, and both the nucleus and the cytoplasm stained brown for p16^{INK4a} immunoexpression. The test has predictive power to identify the progressive evolution to a higher degree of dysplasia and cancer. Positive dual staining is significant only for cells with modified morphology (atypical cells). Schmidt and other researchers [20] highlight the fact that for a better cytological diagnosis, the most important aspect is the positive dual staining within the nucleus of atypical cells. The evaluation of the p16/Ki67 dual staining could be better ascertained by an automatic reader system that obviates subjectivism.

2.3.3. *Other cellular markers*

Other cellular markers expressed in the S-phase of uncontrolled cellular cycle due to the activity of HPV oncoproteins in the stage of transforming infection include Topoisomerase 2α (TOP2A) and minichromosome maintenance protein 2 (MCM2). These markers could be noticed in SurePath cervical cytology specimens by an indirect polymer-based immunoperoxidase method (ProEx C, TriPath Oncology, Burlington, NC). The cytologist is interested in evaluating the presence of nuclear stain in epithelial cells, and the combination of nuclear staining and abnormal morphology. ProEx C is an immunocytochemical test, able to identify the possibility of proliferative process in women with low-grade cytological abnormalities [21].

There are also many other studies that recommend the immunocytochemical test ProEx C for TOP2A and MCM2 as adjunct test to conventional ASC-US cytology test.

2.4. Epigenetic markers

Nowadays there are ongoing studies about the chromosomal imbalances involved in the development of cervical cancer. Researchers pay attention to the chromosomal changes occurring early in the proliferative process. Epigenetic markers consist in DNA methylation, chromosomal abnormalities, miRNA abnormalities, and proteomics. The literature data reveal that it is about host methylation and viral methylation. Many genes are frequently methylated and remain in a silent stage during carcinogenesis, acting as negative regulators of cellular cell cycle. To identify the increased frequency of DNA, methylation of many genes (e.g., *DAPK, CADM1, TERT, CDH13, MAL*) in the early stage of carcinogenesis may hint that these could be biomarkers for early detection of cervical cancer [22]. Studies were not focused on a single gene only, and therefore, a gene panel was developed (e.g., *CADM/MAL; RAS ßITWST/MGMT*), targeting to improve the possibilities to attain earlier the best triage of HPV-infected cervical lesions. The analysis of viral methylation suggests that the promoter regions of oncoprotein E5 and E7 are more frequently methylated in the later stages of carcinogenesis, and as a consequence these tests allow to detect HGCIN [23].

Cervical cancer recognizes genomic instability manifested by amplification of the same regions, especially 3q/TERC or loss of other regions such as 6q and 11q. These abnormalities in the chromosomal architecture could be used in the triage of HPV-positive women with ASC-US or LSIL conventional cytology [24]. Other biotechnologies including miRNAs with increased or decreased expression, proteomics within cervical–vaginal mucus arise; their target is to discover the best predictive markers to discover, at an early stage, the risk of progress from mild to severe dysplasia and cancer.

3. Biotechnologies and test results: advantages and limitations

3.1. Pap's test: advantages and limitations

Researchers agreed that the advantage of Pap's test consists in its high specificity concerning the detection of women who do not prove to be positive for cervical lesions. On the other hand, Pap's test is limited due to its low sensitivity in identifying women with dysplastic cervical lesion prone to develop into cancer. The studies conducted on women of Europe and North America showed that the sensitivity of the cytology in detecting CIN2+ lesions is only 53%, while other studies reveal a modest sensitivity (60–70%) [25, 26].

An advantage of Pap's test consists in its use for both opportunistic cervical cancer screening and national screening programs. The clinician must know that neither the changes in the terminology of cytology by Bethesda reporting system, nor the novel techniques such as liquid-based cytology do not prove more efficient in terms of the improvement of the sensitivity and specificity of Pap's test [27, 28]. On the contrary, Hospitex Diagnostics' report (2013) highlights that the monolayer slides from liquid-based collection medium are safer, faster, and fully representative in comparison with conventional smears screening procedure. We must admit that the introduction of liquid-based cytology has decreased the number of inadequate slides and allowed to advocate a reflex testing for other viral or molecular markers [29].

A disadvantage of Pap's test is the need to be interpreted by two or more specialists trained in cytology for a more accurate cytologic diagnosis; thereby, the test implies subjectivity in the evaluation of morphology cells [30]. Also, the costs of Pap's test are not negligible by two reasons, the first is the training cost of the specialist reader and the second is the fact that screening based on cytology frequently needs repeated Pap's test during the lifetime. Initially, the Pap's test was recommended at 1-year interval, and this is why Pap testing brings substantial cost burden on the health system [31]. The method of cytological screening is able to perceive the lesions that have a high risk of progression, but this prospect is limited by the fact that when used alone, the method can distinguish neither atypical squamous cells of undetermined significance (ASC-US) lesion, nor low-grade squamous intraepithelial (L-SIL) lesions able to spontaneously go into remission against lesions able to progress. Statistical data have shown that 10–15% cases with ASC-US and LSIL cytology develop CIN3 [32, 33].

3.2. HPV test: advantages and limitations

The disadvantages of Pap's test justify why it is necessary to identify the HR-HPV types. With this aim in mind, researchers are trying to define new marks in order to get more powerful characterizations for cervical cancer prevention.

As regards the time necessary to achieve a result concerning HR-HPV assay, an advantage can be seen in Qiagen platform which needs only 2.5 h, while Digene Hybrid Capture HR-HPV testing needs about 6 h. Therefore, the former platform allows both diagnosis and treatment in a single day.

The disadvantage of HR-HPV assay is that it exposes women to overtreatment, as, when applied alone, HR-HPV assay does not reveal the difference between transient and transforming HPV infections. These features do not make it possible to differentiate women with spontaneous remission of cervical lesions, from women with progressive cervical lesions that develop into cervical cancer. Hence, this triage of women with remission or progress of cervical lesion with HPV infection requires a larger number of investigations such as detection of E6 and E7 mRNA markers whose immunoexpression is a real proof of HPV integration in host cells.

The inconveniences of the three techniques which use radiolabeled nucleic acid hybridization assays to detect HPV infection consist in relatively large amounts of purified DNA, more time-consuming procedures, and low sensitivity of the results of test [8].

The Hybrid Capture 2 system has the added advantage of detecting 13 HR-HPV types and 5 LR-HPV types [34].

Cervista assay shows a high sensitivity and specificity to HPV 16/18 genotyping and 100% sensitivity in the detection of CIN3 [35, 36].

A deep analysis of the published reviews underlines that Hybrid Capture 2 test and Cervista HR-HPV have two limitations concerning both the lack of differentiation between single HPV genotype infections and multiple concurrent HPV genotype infections, and the shortage of a test in relation to quantitative viral load [10]. It is very important for the gynecologists to obtain details about the existence of HPV infection with type 16 or 18, because these types allow for a stratification of the risk with reference to the possibility of developing cervical cancer. Thereby, the detection of HPV 16 or 18 has both the advantage of stratifying the oncologic risk of HPV infection and of providing clinicians with information which is useful in managing the precursors of cervical lesions, taking into account that in situations with persistent infections, the risk of precancerous lesions' progression to cancer is between 10 and 15% in cases with HR-HPV 16/18, and below 3% for all other combined HR types [7].

Abreu and colleagues [7] put forward a concept aiming to classify the necessity of DNA HPV testing. These authors concluded that there are six circumstances which require the test, as follows:

- **a.** triage of women with equivocal or low-grade cytological abnormalities
- **b.** follow-up of women with abnormal screening results who are negative at colposcopy/biopsy
- **c.** prediction of the therapeutic outcome after treatment of cervical intraepithelial neoplasia (CIN)—management of follow-up
- **d.** primary screening for HPV DNA testing, alone or in combination with a Pap's test, envisaging to detect cervical cancer precursors
- **e.** gain valuable information on the persistence of certain HPV types
- **f.** investigations of regional and country-based prevalence of type-specific HPV to provide the baseline values against which the global impact of HPV vaccination can be assessed in the future [7].

3.3. Cellular markers: advantages and limitations

3.3.1. Cycline p16^{INK4a}

The p16^{INK4a} positivity shows that the cervical cells are HPV-infected but could not clearly detect a real progress to cancer. The p16^{INK4a} positivity is correlated with HPV infection but could not allow to discriminate between a HR-HPV or a LR-HPV oncotype infection. On the other hand, the p16^{INK4a} expression is independent of the HPV type, and therefore genotyping is unnecessary. In the context of disruption of cell cycle regulation, the p16^{INK4a} expression by cycling cells is a specific marker of HPV-E7 overexpression or other events that inactivate Rb [15].

The immunoexpression of p16^{INK4a} exists both in the nucleus and cytoplasm, but its intensity is in line with the degree of cervical dysplasia. Only the p16^{INK4a} overexpression within the nucleus of the cell shows a high degree of cervical dysplasia. The presence of low p16^{INK4a} immunoexpression within the cytoplasm could not be related to cervical dysplasia's progress to cancer. Another limitation of this marker is the subjectivism in immunostaining slides' evaluation, despite the above-mentioned criteria and the scoring system proposed by Wentzensen, Samarawardana, and Denton. The evaluation of slides requires special cytologist abilities to detect the morphological abnormalities of cells and interpret the immunoexpression degree p16^{INK4a}. The clinician must take into account the possibility that sometimes the cytologist notices the physiological presence of p16^{INK4a}. In this context, it is necessary to require a morphological evaluation of p16-immunostained cells with the purpose of distinguishing HPV-transformed cells from metaplastic cells [37, 38].

Along with the aforementioned features of cycline p16^{INK4a}, and with the benefits and drawbacks of this test, the conclusion is that it must be evaluated both as a stand-alone test and as an adjunct to cytology or HPV testing. In line with the overall opinion, cyclin p16^{INK4a} is a specific biomarker able to identify dysplastic cervical epithelia in sections of cervical biopsy samples or cervical smears [34]. The meta-analysis of reviews published shows that there is a major heterogeneity in the methods used to identify p16^{INK4a} in samples. As regards the statistical value in detecting CIN2+ lesions, cycline p16^{INK4a} has a sensitivity between 0.59 and 0.96, and a specificity flanked by 0.41–0.96 [17].

3.3.2. Dual test p16^{INK4a}/Ki67: advantages and limitations

Dual test p16^{INK4a}/Ki67 has a better interobserver reproducibility and accuracy in cervical cancer screening compared to stand-alone p16^{INK4a}. As indicated in Kaise Permanente Northern California (KPCN) study, where cancer screening was performed based on HPV and cytology co-testing by p16/Ki67 dual staining in 2400 HPV-positive women, the recommendation to use p16/Ki67 cytologies is feasible in routine cytology laboratories with minimal time of training and easy reproducibility [39, 40].

The evaluation of p16/Ki67 dual staining could be better conducted by an automatic reader system that reduces subjectivism to the highest possible extent.

p16^{INK4a}/Ki67 dual test has a higher sensitivity than Pap's test in identifying high-grade cervical lesions associated with HR-HPV infection and the same specificity as the above-mentioned test.

3.4. Epigenetic markers: advantages and limitations

Despite some extended studies investigating the utility of epigenetic markers, such markers are not yet applied in clinical practice and guidelines do not refer to samples of these biotechnologies. However, the researchers' discoveries as regards this solution proved the utility of epigenetic markers for the triage of HPV-positive women with mild abnormal cytologies. There seems to be an opportunity in the future to self-sample from cervical mucus or vaginal fluid, and such samples could theoretically be investigated with reference to epigenetic markers.

4. Discussion: recommendations of the large studies and worldwide guidelines

Pap's test has limited sensitivity to detect precancerous cervical lesions but has high specificity. Compared to cytological diagnosis by HPV DNA testing, it offers a higher sensitivity and a long-term reassurance as regards the minimal risk of developing cervical cancer in women who were proven to be negative in HPV-DNA testing. Hence, these women are safe as regard a progressive dysplasia and could benefit from a large interval between cytological tests, with extension to 2–3 years of the screening interval [29].

In keeping with the ASC-US/LSIL Triage Study (ALTS)—1998, HPV DNA testing is a viable strategy able to clarify especially ASC-US cytology. In fact, ALTS Study counsels clinicians to manage ASC-US cytologies using three different options: triage by HPV testing as an adjunct to cytology, immediate referral to colposcopy, and conservative management with repeating Pap's test. The triage of ASC-US cytologies has relevant significance, because approximately 10–15% of women with ASC-US cytologies proved to be CIN3 at histopathological exam. The relevance of ALTS study consists in the fact that researchers deem that HPV DNA testing could be achieved only by triage of ASC-US cytologies, while the triage of mildly abnormal cytologies is not possible due to the high number of HR-HPV belonging to this female population [32].

Numerous studies have confirmed that HPV testing demonstrates high sensitivity and lower specificity for detecting high-grade cervical intraepithelial lesions. This poor specificity is explained by the fact that most HPV infections are transient and only a lower number of cases develop transforming infections.

Due to the fact that HPV DNA testing offers higher sensitivity and Pap's testing has higher specificity, researchers have progressed in line with the necessity of developing a new marker able to corroborate high sensitivity and specificity.

Berjeron and colleagues (2010) demonstrated on 500 cases, by using H&E-stained slides, as well as $p16^{INK4a}$-immunostained slides analyzed by the same 12 pathologists, that the diagnosis was improved and the sensitivity increased by about 13% after adding $p16^{INK4a}$ immunostaining. The research results recommend using $p16^{INK4a}$ for clinical practice, because this marker was proved able to identify both CIN1 lesions associated with HR-HPV types and CIN2+ lesions [41].

The papers published in 2010 by Samarawardana and Denton have shown that $p16^{INK4a}$ immunostaining on cytology provides significantly better specificity than HR-HPV for the triage of ASC-US and LSIL cytology cases [42, 43].

In conclusion, the diagnosis accuracy is higher when clinicians suggest one of these options: HPV DNA testing in conjunction with Pap's test or p16^{INK4a} associated with Pap's test for the triage of ASC-US cytologies.

In 2014, ATHENA study results demonstrated that COBAS HPV technology contributes to the ASC-US triage. The researchers' remarks were useful for a new approach of the cervical cancer screening. Hence, ATHENA study highlights the fact that negative intraepithelial lesions (NIEL) on cytological exam proved to be ≥CIN3 on histopathological exam. The careful data analysis of ATHENA study has shown that more than 57% of women aged 25–29 years whose cytological diagnosis is negative for intraepithelial cervical lesion proved to have a histopathological diagnosis ≥ CIN3. This evidence justifies why HR-HPV testing for genotypes 16/18 is more efficient in the primary screening of the cervical cancer compared to the Papanicolou cytology test. Cervical lesions able to progress to cancer could be prevented by the early detection of 16 and 18 HPV genotypes by COBAS HPV technology [44]. This technology is able to simultaneously identify 16 and 18 HPV genotypes (the HPV types that are the most responsible for the progress of dysplastic cervical lesions) associated with other 12 oncogenotypes.

The major contribution of COBAS HPV technology consists in the information that individualization of the 16 or 18 HPV oncoproteins underlines the necessity to change the management of an abnormal middle dysplasia from follow-up strategy with Pap's test repeated in 1 year, to other strategies involving, for example, colposcopy, biopsies.

However, HR-HPV testing alone is not able to distinguish between transient and proliferative HPV infections. In view of the gains and weaknesses proven by research as regards the usefulness of Pap's test and HR-HPV in screening women in order to discover those cervical lesions able to evolve into cancer, it is obvious that attention should also be paid to other biomarkers for increased credibility. Therefore, the progress of research led to the necessity of highlighting an immunomarker capable to increase the sensitivity of Pap's test. The cyclin p16^{INK4a}, both in cytology exam and histology exam, is able to identify the HPV-infected cells and therefore to provide a more accurate diagnosis. As a matter of fact, it is acknowledged that the positivity of p16^{INK4a} is an important feature of high-risk HPV infected cells.

Women tested HPV DNA-positive and with p16^{INK4a} ICC-negative could be safely managed with follow-up HPV DNA testing in 2 to 3 years.

Conversely, the positivity for Ki67 in the cell nucleus is a marker of nuclear proliferation. The intensity of Ki67 immunoexpression increases more strongly in abnormal cells. The advantage of p16^{INK4a} test used alone or within a dual test (p16^{INK4a} and Ki67) is that the high intensity of p16^{INK4a} and Ki67 immunoexpression in the nucleus warns that the cell will develop into cancer. If p16^{INK4a} is positive in the cytoplasm only, there is a transient HPV infection, and the cervical lesion is able to spontaneously regress.

As regards the significance of p16^{INK4a}/ Ki67 dual staining immunohistochemical test, Samarawardana and colleagues showed as early as 2011 that this test has increased its capacity to identify high-grade cervical lesions [45].

The novel data established that the p16^{INK4a}/ Ki67 dual staining by immunocytochemical (ICC) method is a better solution to identify the high-grade cervical lesions associated with HR-HPV infection [46].

Another aspect which must be thoroughly discussed consists in the careful measurement of the sensitivity and specificity of each biotechnology used for the diagnosis of cervical lesions [43].

A meta-analysis performed by Jolien Roelens (2012) highlights that p16^{INK4a} ICC has more accuracy than the HR-HPV test concerning the triage of ASC-US cytology samples. Both tests have similar sensitivities, but p16^{INK4a} ICC has higher specificity than HR-HPV test. In LSIL samples, p16^{INK4a} was more specific, but less sensitive than HR-HPV in the detection of ≥CIN2+ [20]. Over the past 10 years, similar results have been published by well-known researchers such as Izaaks, Denton, Holladay, Wentzensen [14, 43, 48, 49].

The positive p16^{INK4a} ICC test rises Pap's test sensitivity to identify the cervical lesions prone to develop into cervical cancer. Therefore, the intensity of p16^{INK4a} immunoexpression in the nucleus is in relation to the degree of cervical lesion.

In the study conducted by Denton and Bergeron (2010), it was shown that p16^{INK4a} cytology provides significantly better specificity than HR-HPV for the triage of ASC-US and LSIL. Both HPV-testing and p16^{INK4a} immunocytomarker test have similar sensitivity percentage rates, capable to detect high-grade cervical lesions at histopathological exam. In conclusion, the specialists involved in this research field have shown that p16^{INK4a} cytology has the potential of being used as a triage of abnormal cytology LSIL [43].

Beginning with 2010, Samarawardana et al. have demonstrated by statistical analysis that the sensitivity (Se) and specificity (Sp) of p16^{INK4a} for the detection of underlying CIN ≥ 2+ are 81.7% and 83.3%, respectively ($p = 0.81$). They underline that the Se and Sp of HR-HPV are lower than those of p16^{INK4a}, albeit statistically significant: 78.1% and 50.9%, respectively ($p < 0.01$) [42].

There are many research studies recommending the usage of p16^{INK4a} as a supplemental triage biomarker for ASC-US and LSIL cytologies, which have already been assigned as "high-risk" after HR-HPV detection [49, 50].

Large studies approached the comparison between the sensitivity and specificity of immunocytomarker p16 ^{INK4a} /Ki67dual stain versus HPV test in order to reveal if one of these tests is statistically more powerful to detect high-grade histopathological lesions ≥CIN2+. So, PALMS study is a bulky study which has enrolled 27,349 women from five European countries. All women aged 18 and older were tested by conventional cytology and p16/Ki67 dual test, while women aged 30 or older were tested by HPV DNA. The comparison between Se of p16^{INK4a} / Ki67 dual stain cytology versus Pap's test with regard to the detection of high-grade cervical intraepithelial neoplasia (HGCIN) has shown higher values for p16^{INK4a} /Ki67 test (86.7 vs 68.5%). As regards the Sp of the tests, it was comparable (95.2 vs 95.4%). By comparing Se and Sp of HPV DNA test versus p16^{INK4a} /Ki67 dual stain, the study remarks that HPV DNA test has a higher Se to detect CIN2+, 93.3 versus 84.7%, but a low drop in specificity, 93.0 versus 96%. On the other hand, the dual test p16/Ki67 sets the idea that the test offers the same high sensitivity and specificity to identify HGCIN (see **Table 1**). The conclusions of researchers published on August 2015 within the Specialist Forum concerning PALMS study underline that the immunoexpression of dual-stained p16/Ki67 biomarkers is a novel approach to scrutinize efficiently for HGCIN and to achieve the same specificity conferred by Pap's test.

Detection of HGCIN	p16/Ki67		Pap's test	
	Se	Sp	Se	Sp
p16/Ki67 dual test versus Pap's test	86.7%	95.2%	68.5%	95.4%
Detection of HGCIN	p16/Ki67		HPV DNA test	
	Se	Sp	Se	Sp
$p16^{INK4a}$ /Ki67 vs. HPV DNA	84.7%	96%	93.3%	93.00%

$p16^{INK4a}$/Ki67 = dual test CINTech Plus; Se = sensitivity; Sp = specificity; HGCIN = high-grade cervical intraepithelial neoplasia.

Table 1. Cellular markers able to detect HGCIN sensitivity and specificity—results of PALMS study.

Similar attention is given to the cervical cancer screening of vaccinated women. In this regard, the trial known as Compass Trial is being conducted today in Australia. This trial enrolled 121,000 HPV-vaccinated women who are analyzed from the point of view of cervical screening programs using HPV test versus cytology tests [52].

Methods	Unites States	Europe	Australia
HPV vaccine	NSP		NSP
HPV DNA testing	NSP primary test	GR-triage	NSP primary test
Co-test PAP	NSP		NO NSP
Pap's test	Conjunction to HPV DNA testing	NSP	
P16	GR—Triage	GR—Triage	GR—Triage
P16/Ki67	GR—Triage	GR—Triage	GR—Triage
E6/E7 mRNA	GR—Triage	GR—Triage	GR—Triage

NSP = National Screening Programme; GR—Triage = Guideline Recommendations—Triage; NO = negative.

Table 2. Cervical cancer screening programmes and guideline recommendations—update.

In line with the recent discoveries made by researches and the large studies mentioned above, the guidelines approved in the United States recommend HPV vaccination, HPV primary screening and co-testing with Pap's test, with major benefits in terms of sorting abnormally low cytologies and extending the screening interval. The ATHENA study prescribes the circumstances for applying the HPV test: triage of ASC-US in women over 21 years of age, HPV test with reflex Pap's cytology in women between 25 and 65 years, and HPV test with

HPV 16/18 genotyping for primary screening in women older than 25. As to the accepted screening interval, this is 3–5 years for women negative at both intraepithelial malign cervical lesions (NIEML) and HPV infection, and 12 months in cases with HPV-positive test, but cytology-negative for NIEML, followed up by classic advices when the tests are constantly changed. Positive test for HPV 16/18 genotyping push the screening directly to colposcopy due to the presence of an absolute risk for CIN3+ progression. The interval for screening is prolonged to 5 years when women are negative at co-testing. Access to this screening program is given only to women with healthcare insurance [53]. The present guideline recommendations and cervical cancer screening programs existing nowadays are summarized in **Table 2**.

In Europe, there are many differences as regards the modality of carrying out the screening of cervical cancer, because health policies and financial resources differ among Europe's demographic regions. The most commonly used national screening program is mainly Pap's test; however, it is complemented by other new markers and biotechnologies prescribed by physicians with the goal of increasing diagnosis accuracy.

The Australian National Screening Program recommends only the screening using HPV test, and encompasses ages between 25 and 74 (applicable if women were screened in the past). The program includes both vaccinated and unvaccinated women. If the HPV test is positive, the follow-up program will be in line with cervical screening pathway [52].

5. Conclusions

The detection of carcinogenetic HPV DNA, and especially of HPV 16/18 genotyping, stands for approved tests to be used as primary screening and for triage of equivocal cytology equally on vaccinated and unvaccinated women.

Recognition of E6/E7 mRNA is largely applied in adjunct to primary HPV screening to select cases with HPV integrated in the host cell. The result of E6/E7 mRNA is able to achieve the triage of equivocal or mildly abnormal cytology.

Uncovering of HPV protein by cytology and histology immunostaining underlines the accuracy of diagnosis and can be used together with primary HPV screening or for the triage of equivocal or mildly abnormal cytology.

The success that was achieved in researches across the world showed that the identification of immnuocytomarkers inside the same cervical cell—dual stain $p16^{INK4a}$ and Ki67—warns more accurately about the possibility of progression to cervical cancer.

Correctly performed and interpreted, the results of approved tests for cervical screening programs allow to obtain an extended interval screening between 2 and 5 years, with a larger number of advantages in terms of diagnosis accuracy and healthcare costs.

Author details

Ruxandra Stanculescu

Address all correspondence to: ruxandra_v_stanculescu@yahoo.com

Obstetrics and Gynaecology Department, "Carol Davila" University of Medicine, "St. Pantelimon"Clinical Emergency Hospital Bucharest, Romania

References

[1] Ferlay J, Soerjomataram I, Ervik M, Dikshit R, Eser S, Mathers C, Rebelo M, Parkin DM, Forman D, Bray F. GLOBOCAN 2012 v1.1, Cancer Incidence and Mortality Worldwide: IARC Cancer Base No. 11 2014. http://globocan.iarc.fr

[2] Bray F, Loos AH, McCarron P, Weiderpass E, Arbyn M, Møller H, Hakama M, Parkin DM. Trends in cervical squamous cell carcinoma incidence in 13 European countries: changing risk and the effects of screening. Cancer Epidemiol Biomarkers Prev. 2005;14(3):677–686.

[3] Wang SS, Sherman ME, Hildesheim A, Lacey JV, Devesa S. Cervical adenocarcinoma and squamous cell carcinoma incidence trends among white women and black women in the United States for 1976–2000. Cancer 2004;100(5):1035–1044; DOI: 10.1002/cncr.20064.

[4] Siebers AG, Klinkhamer PJ, Grefte JM, et al. Comparison of liquid-based cytology with conventional cytology for detection of cervical cancer precursors: a randomized controlled trial. JAMA 2009;302(16):1757–1764.

[5] Kulasingam SL, Hughes JP, Kiviat NB, et al. Evaluation of human papillomavirus testing in primary screening for cervical abnormalities: comparison of sensitivity, specificity, and frequency of referral. JAMA 2002;288(14):1749–1757.

[6] Sahasrabuddhe VV, Luhn P, Wentzensen N. Human papillomavirus and cervical cancer: biomarkers for improved prevention efforts. Future Microbiol 2011;6(9):1083–1098; 10.2217/fmb.11.87. doi: 10.2217/fmb.11.87.

[7] Abreu ALP, Souza RP,Gimenes F, Consolaro MEL. A review of methods for detect human Papillomavirus infection. Virol J 2012;9:262. doi: 10.1186/1743-422X-9-262

[8] Villa LL, Denny L. Methods for detection of HPV infection and its clinical utility. Int J Gyn Obst 2006;94(Suppl.1):71–80.

[9] Hwang SJ, Shroyer KR. Biomarkers of cervical dysplasia and carcinoma. J Oncol 2012 2012;507286.

[10] Brown AJ, Trimble CL. New technologies for cervical cancer screening. Best Pract Res Clin Obstet Gynaecol 2012;26(2):233–242. doi: 10.1016/j.bpobgyn.2011.11.001

[11] Doorbar J. Papillomavirus life cycle organization and biomarker selection. Dis Markers 2007;23(4):297–313.

[12] Cattani P, Zannoni GF, Ricci C, et al. Clinical performance of human papillomavirus E6 and E7 mRNA testing for high-grade lesions of the cervix. J Clin Microbiol 2009;47(12):3895–3901.

[13] Yoshida T, Sano T, Kanuma T, et al. Quantitative real- time polymerase chain reaction analysis of the type distribution, viral load, and physical status of human papillomavirus in liquid-based cytology samples from cervical lesions. Int J Gynecol Cancer 2008;18:121–127.

[14] Iaaks CD, Truter EJ, Khan S. Correlative analysis of CinteC p16 and detection of HPV DNA by PCR in cervical abnormalities. Med Technol SA 2011;25(2):23–27.

[15] Klaes R, Friedrich T, Spitkovsky D, et al. Overexpression of p16ink4a as a specific marker for dysplastic and neoplastic epithelial cells of the cervix uteri. Int J Cancer 2001;92(2):276–284.

[16] Zeng WJ, Li Y, Fei HL, et al. The value of p16ink4a expression by fluorescence *in situ* hybridization in triage for high risk HPV positive in cervical cancer screening. Gynecol Oncol 2011;120(1):84–88.

[17] Tsoumpou I, Arbyn M, Kyrgiou M, et al. p16(INK4a) immunostaining in cytological and histological specimens from the uterine cervix: a systematic review and meta-analysis. Cancer Treat Rev 2009;35(3):210–220.

[18] Wentzensen N, Bergeron C, Cas F, et al. Evaluation of a nuclear score for $p16^{INK4a}$ stained cervical squamous cells in liquid-based cytology samples. Cancer Cytopathol 2005;105:461–467.

[19] Waldstrøm M, Christensen R K, Ørnskov D. Evaluation of $p16^{INK4a}$/Ki-67 dual stain in comparison with an mRNA human papillomavirus test on liquid-based cytology samples with low-grade squamous intraepithelial lesion. Cancer Cytopathol. 2013; 121(3):136–145.

[20] Schmidt D, Bergeron C, Denton KJ, Ridder R, for the European CINtec. P16/ki-67 dual-stain cytology in the triage of ASCUS and LSIL Papanicolaou cytology. Results from the European equivocal or mildly abnormal Papanicolaou cytology study. Cancer Cytopathol. 2011;119:158–166.

[21] Shroyer KR, Homer P, Heinz D, Singh M. Validation of a novel immunocytochemical assay for topoisomerase II-a and minichromosome maintenance protein 2 expression in cervical cytology. Cancer (Cancer Cytopathol) 2006;108:324–330. DOI 10.1002/cncr. 22171

[22] Wentzensen N, Sherman ME, Schiffman M, Wang SS. Utility of methylation markers in cervical cancer early detection: appraisal of the state-of-the-science. Gynecol Oncol 2009;112(2):293–299.

[23] Turan T, Kalantari M, Calleja-Macias IE, et al. Methylation of the human papillomavirus-18 L1 gene: a biomarker of neoplastic progression? Virology 2006;349(1):175–183.

[24] Heselmeyer-Haddad K, Sommerfeld K, White NM, et al. Genomic amplification of the human telomerase gene (TERC) in pap smears predicts the development of cervical cancer. Am J Pathol 2005;166(4):1229–1238.

[25] Cuzick J, Arbyn M, Sankaranarayanan R, et al. Overview of human papillomavirus-based and other novel options for cervical cancer screening in developed and developing countries. Vaccine 2008;26(Suppl. 10):K29–41. doi: 10.1016/j.vaccine.2008.06.019 PMID: 18847555

[26] Cong X, Cox DD, Cantor SB. Bayesian meta-analysis of Papanicolaou smear accuracy. Gynecol Oncol 2007;107(Suppl 1):S133–S137.

[27] Arbyn M, Bergeron C, Klinkhamer P, et al. Liquid compared with conventional cervical cytology: a systematic review and meta-analysis. Obstet Gynecol 2008;111:167–177. doi: 10.1097/01.AOG.0000296488.85807.b3

[28] Whitlock EP, Vesco KK, Ederet M et al. Liquid-based cytology and human papillomavirus testing to screen for cervical cancer: a systematic review for the U.S. Preventive Services Task Force. Annals Int Med (Online) 2011. 155(10):687–697.

[29] Dillner J, Rebolj M, Birembaut P, et al. Long term predictive values of cytology and human papillomavirus testing in cervical cancer screening: joint European cohort study. BMJ 2008;337:A1754.

[30] Stoler MH, Schiffman M. Interobserver variability of cervical cytologic and histologic interpretations: realistic estimates from the ASCUS-LSIL Triage Study. 2001;285:1500–1505.

[31] MacDonald CF. Assessing secondary prevention methods for cervical cancer: costs and benefits in managed care. Am J Manag Care. 2008;14(6 Suppl 1):S185–S192.

[32] Arbyn M, Buntinx F, Van Ranst M, Paraskevaidis E, Martin-Hirsch P, Dillner J. Virologic versus cytologic triage of women with equivocal Pap smears: a meta-analysis of the accuracy to detect high-grade intraepithelial neoplasia. J Natl Cancer Inst 2004;96(4):280–293.

[33] Arbyn M, Paraskevaidis E, Martin-Hirsch P, Prendiville W, Dillner J. Clinical utility of HPV-DNA detection: triage of minor cervical lesions, follow-up of women treated for high-grade CIN: an update of pooled evidence. Gynecol Oncol. 2005;99(3 Suppl 1):S7–S11.

[34] Hwang SJ, Shroyer KR. Biomarkers of cervical dysplasia and carcinoma. J Oncol 2012;2012:507286. doi: 10.1155/2012/507286

[35] Bartholomew DA, Luff RD, Quigley NB, Curtis M, Olson MC. Analytical performance of Cervista HPV 16/18 genotyping test for cervical cytology samples. J Clin Virol 2011;51:38–43.

[36] Johnson LR, Starkey CR, Palmer J, et al. A comparasion of two methods to determine the presence of high-risk HPV cervical infections. Am J Clin Pathol 2008;130:401–408.

[37] Wentzensen N. Triage of HPV-positive women in cervical cancer screening. Lancet Oncol 2013;14:107–109.

[38] Cuschieri K, Wentzensen N. Human papillomavirus mRNA and p16 detection as biomarkers for the improved diagnosis of cervical neoplasia. Cancer Epidemiol Biomarkers Prev 2008;17(10):2536–2545.

[39] Wentzensen N, Fetterman B, Tokugawa D, Schiffman M, Castle PE, Wood SN, Stiemerling E. Interobserver reproducibility and accuracy of p16/Ki-67 dual-stain cytology in cervical cancer screening. Cancer Cytopathol 2014;122(12):914–920. DOI: 10.1002/cncy.21473

[40] Wentzensen N, Fetterman B, Castle PE, et al. p16/Ki-67 dual stain cytology for detection of cervical precancer in HPV-positive women. JNCI J Natl Cancer Inst 2015;107(12):djv257. doi: 10.1093/jnci/djv257

[41] Bergeron C, Ordi J, Schmidt D, Trunk MJ, Keller T, Ridder R. Conjunctive p16INK4a testing significantly increases accuracy in diagnosing high-grade cervical intraepithelial neoplasia. Am J Clin Pathol 2010;133(3):395–406.

[42] Samarawardana P, Dehn DL, Singh M, et al. $p16^{INK4a}$ is superior to high-risk human papillomavirus testing in cervical cytology for the prediction of underlying high-grade dysplasia. Cancer Cytopathol 2010;118(3):146–156.

[43] Denton KJ, Bergeron C, Klement P, Trunk MJ, Keller T, Ridder R. The sensitivity and specificity of p16INK4a cytology vs HPV testing for detecting high-grade cervical disease in the triage of ASC-US and LSIL Pap cytology results. Am J Clin Pathol 2010;134(1):12–21.

[44] Castle PE, Stoler MH, Wright TC Jr. et al. Performance of carcinogenetic human papillomavirus (HPV) testing and HPV16 or HPV18 genotyping for cervical cancer screening of women aged 25 years and older: a subanalysis of the ATHENA study. Lancet Oncol 2011;12(9):880–890.

[45] Samarawardana P, Singh M, Shroyer KR. Dual stain immunohistochemical localization of p16INK4A and ki-67: a synergistic approach to identify clinically significant cervical mucosal lesions. Immunohistochem Mol Morphol 2011;19(6):514–518.

[46] Donà MG, Vocaturo A, Giuliani M, Ronchetti L, Rollo F, Pescarmona E, Carosi M, Vocaturo G, Benevolo M. p16/Ki-67 dual staining in cervico-vaginal cytology: correla-

tion with histology, human papillomavirus detection and genotyping in women undergoing colposcopy. Gynecol Oncol 2012;126(2):198–202.

[47] Roelens J, Reuschenbach M, Doeberitz M; Wentzensen N, Bergeron C, Arbyn M, p16ink4a Immunocytochemistry Versus Human Papillomavirus Testing for Triage of Women With Minor Cytologic Abnormalities, Cancer Cytopathology. 2012 October 25; 120 (5): 294–307

[48] Holladay B, Logan S, Arnold J, Knesel B, Smith GD. A comparison of the clinical utility of p16^{INK4a} immunolocalization with the presence of human papillomavirus by hybrid capture 2 for the detection of cervical dysplasia/neoplasia. Cancer Cytopathol 2006;108(6):451–461.

[49] Wentzensen N, Bergeron C, Cas F, Vinokurova S, Doeberitz M K; Triage of women with ASCUS and LSIL cytology, Cancer Cytopathology, 2007 February 25;111(1):58–66.

[50] Nasioutziki M, Daniilidis A, Dinas K, Kyrgiou M, Valasoulis G, Loufopoulos PD, et al.; The evaluation of p16INK4a immunoexpression/immunostaining and human papillomavirus DNA test in cervical liquid-based cytological samples. Int J Gynecol Cancer, 2011;21(1):79–85.

[51] Gustinucci D, Passamonti B, Cesarini E, Butera D, Palmieri E A, Buletti S, et al.; Role Of p16ink4a Cytology Testing as an Adjunct to Enhace the Diagnostic Specificity And Accuracy in Human Palillomavirus- Positive Women within an Organized Cervical Cancer Screening Program; Acta Cytologica 2012;56(5):506–514

[52]] Canfell K The Australian Exemple: an integrated approach to HPV vaccination and cervical screening Newletter on Human Papillomavirus- HPV Today 2015; 38:25–30 www.HPVTODAY.COM

[53] Benard V,Saraiya M. HPV Testing in the United States Perspectives from Systems Providers and Women Newletter on Human Papillomavirus- HPV Today 2015;38:25–30 www.HPVTODAY.COM

5

Human Papillomavirus in Head and Neck Cancer

Makbule Tambas, Musa Altun and Deniz Tural

Abstract

Throughout the last three decades, there has been a notable shift in the epidemiology of head and neck cancer (HNC) worldwide. A rapidly spreading subtype of HNCs is caused by human papillomavirus (HPV) infection. HPV-related cancers are now considered to constitute 30–65% of all HNC cases and 50–80% of oropharyngeal cancers. HPV-positive oropharyngeal cancers have a unique demographic profile and tumor biology characteristics. HPV-associated patients predominantly consist of younger men with better performance status and fewer comorbid diseases. They have better dentition, higher numbers of oral sex partners, and use less amount of tobacco or alcohol, higher amount of marijuana compared with HPV-negative patients. In addition, patients with HPV-positive tumors have a 60–80% reduced mortality rates, a finding that was confirmed by multiple trials and led to several ongoing deintensification studies. This chapter describes epidemiologic features of HPV-positive HNC, risk factors for HPV infection and HPV-associated oropharyngeal cancer, HPV detection methods, mechanisms of carcinogenesis and improved treatment response, and the impact of HPV status on clinical outcome as well as deintensification approaches and potential of vaccination.

Keywords: head and neck cancer, human papillomavirus, epidemiology, carcinogenesis, treatment

1. Introduction

Head and neck cancer (HNC) involves a wide field of tumors that originate from the skull base to the clavicles including the orbits, paranasal sinuses, nasopharynx, oropharynx, hypopharynx, oral cavity, and larynx. Worldwide, the incidence of HNC accounts for more than half a million each year, 5% of all cancer cases, with being the fifth most common cancer in the world [1, 2]. The distribution of HNC varies around world, such that it is 3–4% of all cancer diagnosed in North America and the Europe, whereas HNC consists of 30% of all cancer cases in men in India [3]. Yet, around 300,000 people die from HNC that can be seen in the global picture of the disease [4].

The well-known risk factors for HNC comprise tobacco, alcohol, poor oral health, human papillomavirus (HPV) infection (for oropharyngeal cancer), and Epstein-Barr virus (EBV) infection (for nasopharyngeal carcinoma) [5, 6]. Traditionally, HNC was related to tobacco use and alcohol exposure, and the synergistic increased risk with the combination of them [7]. HNCs are most common among 50–60 year-old individuals who are heavy smokers and alcohol users with lower socioeconomic status [8]. Additionally, the squamous cell carcinoma constitutes more than 90% of histological subtype of HNC [1].

2. Epidemiology

2.1. Changing trends in epidemiology of HPV-associated HNCs

Throughout the last three decades, there has been a notable shift in the epidemiology of HNC worldwide. The decrease in tobacco consumption has resulted in an entire reduction in the incidence of HNC during the past 30 years [9]. Since smoking maintains as the primary risk factor for the oral cavity, larynx, and hypopharynx, this declining trend is marked for these sites. However, up to 25% of all HNCs recently diagnosed are not related to tobacco use. A rapidly spreading subtype of HNCs is caused by HPV infection [10].

First suggested in 1983 by Syrjanen, HPV was reported as an initiative factor of HNC owing to its oncogenic potential, the parallel clinical characteristics in oral and genital damages, epithelia similarities, and HPV affinity for epithelial cells [11]. The evidence for a significant correlation was insufficient, until recently. In the 2000s, several reports, mainly from Sweden, established that a remarkable ratio of tonsillar cancers included HPV DNA. The increases by 2.8- and 2.9-fold were detected in the incidence of tonsillar cancer and ratio (23–68%) of HPV-positive tonsillar cancer between 1970 and 2002, in Sweden, in 2006 [12]. Immediately after this, in 2007, an arising HPV epidemic correlating with oropharyngeal SCC was reported in the United States [13]. The striking increases up to sevenfold in both HPV-positive tonsillar and base of tongue were demonstrated during the periods of 1970–2007 and 1998–2006 in 2009 and 2010 from Sweden, respectively [14, 15]. Following Dalianis group definition of "epidemic of viral-induced carcinoma," due to observation that most of the tonsillar carcinomas were HPV-associated in 2009 [14], a retrospective analysis of clinical trial material detected that HPV-related oropharyngeal cancer rate was 64% in the USA [16]. Similar retrospective analyses on oropharyngeal tumor samples revealed an increase in HPV incidence from 23, 28 to 57% from 1970s, 1980s to 1990s, respectively. Also, a constant trend in the increase was detected for recent term (68, 77, 93% incidence rates during 2000–2002, 2003–2005, 2006–2007, respectively [14]. Similarly, HPV association rate in oropharyngeal cases was increased from 16% to 73%, from 1984–1989 to 2000–2004 in the United States [17]. Furthermore, during the same periods, reports delivering similar striking rises in both oropharyngeal and HPV-positive oropharyngeal cancers have accumulated from several Western countries [3, 12–15, 17–23].

The oropharynx is distinctively sensitive to HPV, and as high as 70% of oropharyngeal cancers in the USA are HPV-related oropharyngeal squamous cell carcinomas [24]. The past 30-year Surveillance, Epidemiology, and End Results (SEER) population-based data were analyzed by Chaturvedi et al, and they evaluated the incidence trends of HPV-related and -unrelated HNC. They demonstrated a significant decline (1.85% annual reduction) in the incidence of HNC in HPV-unrelated fields (hypopharynx, oral cavity, larynx) and a remarkable rise (0.8% annual increase) in the incidence of HNC in HPV-associated oropharyngeal regions during the same period [9]. In addition, the incidence of hypopharyngeal, oral cavity, and laryngeal carcinomas notably reduced due to smoking and alcohol consumption declining in many countries [25]. On the contrary, the oropharyngeal carcinoma incidence has been reported to be increased in many countries including the UK [26], Canada [27], Australia [28], Norway [29], Denmark [30], and the Netherlands [20] over the last two decades, besides Sweden [12] and the USA [9]. HPV-related cancers are now considered to constitute 30–65% of all HNC cases and 50–80% of oropharyngeal cancers [9, 16]. HPV-positive HNC, which has distinctive epidemiologic and prognostic features [5–14] has become an expanding public health issue, is expected to be the main factor for HNC development in the forthcoming period [17].

Currently, the highest HPV-positive HNC incidence rates have been reported in Sweden and the USA. The genital HPV infection prevalence, sexual habits, and smoking and alcohol use may affect the population-specific HPV-positive HNC incidences. The focus of HPV-related malignancies has been shifted from anogenital cancers developing predominantly in women to oropharyngeal cancers developing mainly in men due to the fact that men were reported to have >70% HPV-positive oropharyngeal cancer cases [9, 12, 15, 16, 20–22]. By 2020, the number of HPV-mediated oropharyngeal patients per year is reflected to outnumber HPV-related cervical cancer cases in the USA [17]. The HPV-mediated oropharyngeal cancer has become an epidemic of our era [31].

2.2. HPV positivity in non-oropharyngeal sites of HNC

HPV detection rates were currently reported to be between 12.6% and 90.9% in oropharyngeal carcinoma [32]. One-quarter to one-half of unknown primaries originates from oropharyngeal region [33, 34] and the HPV presence in cervical lymph node metastases is a strong marker of oropharyngeal subsite for unknown primary regions [33, 35]. Although the association between oropharyngeal carcinoma (predominantly soft palate, the tonsils, base of tongue) and HPV is well known, the role of HPV in other head and neck subsites etiology is not well established. The presence of HPV DNA was not demonstrated in laryngeal, nasopharyngeal, hypopharyngeal, and oral cavity cancers in older studies, whereas recently published studies using more advanced methodologies and analyzed HPV gene expression products (e.g., p16) reported that HPV existed in non-oropharyngeal sites in small proportions which explains the increased incidence of oropharyngeal carcinoma compared with other HNCs [1, 36–38].

The prevalence of HPV-mediated HNCs was found as 25.9% in a systematic review of 60 published studies using PCR-based methods while it was higher in oropharyngeal carcinoma (35.6%) than both oral (23.5%) and laryngeal (24.0%) carcinoma. HPV-16 and the second most common high-risk type HPV-18 were detected in 86.7% and only 2.8% of the HPV-positive oropharyngeal carcinoma [39]. In addition, in a meta-analysis of 39 publications with 3649 HNC patients which investigated HPV in European population, the prevalence of HPV was found to be 40.0%, while it was most dominant in tonsillar cancer (66.4%) and lowest in pharyngeal (15.3%) and tongue (25.7%) cancers [36].

Unlike oropharyngeal cancers, HPV etiologic role in other HNC sites remains unclear. Concerning other head and neck subsites, HPV may play a role in the supraglottic larynx cancer [40], which might constitute the high-risk HPV infection rate established in laryngeal cancer, since its marginal field is adjacent with the oropharynx [28, 29, 41, 42]. Overall, contemporary studies using gold standard methods (type-specific HPV E6/E7 mRNA) from the United States detected the presence of HPV in less than 5% of non-oropharyngeal HNCs [17, 43]. Nevertheless, the estimate for the HPV infection-mediated non-oropharyngeal HNCs varies widely in the literature. While the estimated prevalence of HPV is 24% in the larynx, 31% in the nasopharynx, oral cavity 6–20%, and 21% in the sinonasal tract [44, 45], the studies mainly from the USA based on *in situ* hybridization (ISH) assays and E6/E7 mRNA detection suggest that the HPV association was found in 3% of oral cavity, 7% of larynx, and 0% of hypopharynx cancers [43]. Many factors including the border of anatomic classification of head and neck subsites and HPV detection methods contribute to this instability. The identification of certain markers of HPV-induced carcinogenesis and the correct rule out of the oropharynx as tumor origin site are substantial forthcoming issues in HPV-related non-oropharyngeal HNC estimation [43]. In addition, another topic which remains to be clarified is whether HPV tumor status in non-oropharyngeal sites may be implicated as a strong independent prognostic indicator such as in oropharyngeal cancers [16, 46–48].

2.3. The characteristics of HPV-positive HNC cancer patients

The demographic and risk features of HPV-positive and HPV-negative HNC patients differ remarkably. First, HPV(+) patients are younger than HPV(−) ones [49]. The HPV-related cancers develop in those aged 40–55 [50] who are 4–10 years younger than HPV-negative patients [16, 51]. This age difference might explain the increase in oropharyngeal cancer incidence in younger individuals in developed countries [17, 52]. Given that HPV-associated patients are younger at diagnosis, they have better performance status [16, 47, 50] with fewer comorbid diseases [16, 51, 53].

Second, although HNC is generally more common in men than women, a notably larger rate of HPV-positive oropharyngeal cancer is diagnosed in men than HPV-negative ones [17]. This is convenient with the data that oral HPV16 infection is five times more common in men compared with women in the USA [54].

Third, HPV-HNC has been found to develop more frequently in white than black patients. HPV-positivity rate is 29–34% in whites compared to only 0–4% in blacks [55, 56], while HPV-positive versus -negative rumors occurring in whites are 92–97% and 75–78%, respectively [16, 46, 55]. Thus, in contrast to blacks, the incidence of oropharyngeal cancer has increased in whites which is probably caused by higher HPV-HNC rates in whites compared with blacks in the USA [57]. Furthermore, the socioeconomic status differs in HPV-positive patients from

HPV-negative ones. HPV-positive patients have higher income and are more educated with higher rates of being married [51, 54].

The HPV-positive HNC patients have better dentition, higher numbers of oral sex partners, and use less amount of tobacco or alcohol, higher amount of marijuana compared with HPV-negative patients. In addition, these risk factors have a powerful dose effect, revealing the distinguishing risk profile for HPV-positive patients [17]. Furthermore, these patients without environmental risk factors have persistent infection with high-risk HPVs [17].

3. Risk factors for HPV infection and HPV(+) oropharyngeal cancers

HPV-16 which is detected in about 90% of the HPV(+) oropharyngeal cancers is the most common among several high-risk HPV types. Currently, HPV-16 is the only HPV type which is accepted as cancer inducing in the HNC [58, 59]. In addition, there are other high-risk HPV types with a less significant function and different manner than HPV-16 [37]. Among these, HPV-58, HPV-35, HPV-33, and HPV- 45 were detected in 10–15% of HPV(+) oropharyngeal cancer [38, 60, 61]. At present, HPV 16 constitutes 15- to 230-fold increased risk for oropharyngeal cancer [50, 62]. HPV has been confirmed to induce and promote the development of oropharyngeal cancer [63].

With the identification of HPV as a powerful and independent risk factor for HNC, data are accumulating concerning the oral HPV infection epidemiology. The prevalence of oral HPV infection has been estimated as 7% in population-based studies in the United States and significantly correlated with male gender, older age, current smoking, and various sexual habits (e.g., the number of oral sexual partners during lifetime) [54]. HPV infection which may be contaminated by any type of sexual contact has become the most frequent disease that transmits sexually in the world [64]. The estimated number of individuals who are currently infected and expected to be infected each year is 20 million and 6.2 million in the United States alone [65]. Even though the orally infected rate among the population aged between 14 and 69 (10% of men, 4% of women) is 7%, the cancer-causing HPV subtypes consist of only 1% of these infections [54].

HPV-infected persons are unaware of the infection, since there are no correlated signs or symptoms. No effective treatment has been developed for active HPV infection, currently. Fortunately, the virus will be cleared in most of the infected persons within 2 years. It remains unknown how to identify those in whom the infection will become chronic and progress to HPV-HNC in time. Since the most of carcinogenesis occurs deep in the crypts of the tonsils where simple "Pap smear equivalents" are inaccessible in contrast to anus or cervix, an efficient screening test for early detection of HPV-related oropharyngeal cancer does not exist, yet [31].

Marijuana smoking has been shown to be an independent risk factor for HPV-mediated HNC, while the duration, intensity, and total years of marijuana use increase the risk. Marijuana use is suggested to cause oropharyngeal cancer development since the cannabinoids bind to the

CB2 receptor of immune modulatory cells found in the tonsillar tissue which results in reduced immune response, lower resistance to viral infections, and antitumor functions [66].

It has been shown that HPV is less frequent in ex-, current-smokers, and tobacco chewers than nonsmokers and nonchewers [67]. Interestingly, in contrast to HPV(−) HNC, HPV(+) HNC decreases with increasing lifetime tobacco consumption [50]. On the one hand, rates of past and current tobacco use in HPV-oropharyngeal squamous cell carcinoma (OSCC) are reported to be 65% as opposed to 74% in HPV-negative OSCCs [6]. On the other hand, oral HPV infection presence is separately correlated with current smoking, but not lifetime smoking history [54]. Similarly, heavy alcohol consumption is less common in HPV(+) HNC patients compared with HPV-negative HNC ones [50]. Although heavy alcohol use (>21 drinks per week) is related to increased incidence of both HPV(+) and HPV(−) HNC, it is not correlated with oral HPV infection with the adjustment for sexual habits [54]. The complex role of alcohol remains to be identified.

Other significant factors in the increasing incidence of HPV infection and HPV(+) HNC are the changes in sexual behaviors, early sex debut, and number of oral-vaginal partners [68]. In addition, oral-oral contact and HPV transmission at birth may also lead to oral HPV infection [69, 70]. HPV transmits mainly through sexual contact directly with vaginal or anal intercourse, oral sex, or any mucosal contact. Also, oral HPV infection is more correlated with a genital HPV infection status, compared with oral sex activity in young males, suggesting autoinoculation as a potential HPV transmission route [71]. The first sexual encounter at younger ages, increasing number of sexual partners as well as more oral sex are reported by Americans [72, 73]. Additionally, the lifetime prevalence of oral sex was reported to be increased from 50% in 1970 to 90% in 2006 in a French study [73]. Furthermore, HPV exposure increases the HNC development risk, and HPV-16 seropositivity leads to cancer development 9 years earlier [74].

4. Diagnosis and histopathology

4.1. Clinical and pathologic presentation

An asymptomatic neck mass is the presentation of the disease in up to 90% of HPV(+) oropharyngeal cancer patients [75]. The neck nodes are generally in cystic structure which results in nondiagnostic aspiration materials. The diagnosis may be delayed due to no suspicious history because of being a nonsmoker, insufficient examination, and non-diagnostic aspirates of cystic lymph nodes. Ultrasound-guided fine-needle aspirates taken from cystic neck nodes may increase the chance of early diagnosis [76]. The utility of HPV detection in theses aspirates using p16 immunohistochemistry (IHC) and ISH has been shown [77]. In cases of unknown primary, a palatine and/or lingual tonsillectomy is superior to random biopsies.

HPV(+) oropharyngeal carcinoma exhibits a nonkeratinizing, basaloid, well-differentiated histology with diffuse nuclear and cytoplasmic p16 staining [66]. The HPV-positive tumor pathologic properties differ from HPV-negative ones showing lobular growth, having infiltrating lymphocytes, but not surface dysplasia or keratinization [66]. In addition, HPV-positive tumors present frequently with smaller primary tumors but advanced nodal metastasis [46, 50]. Despite being not pathognomonic, major histopathological features of HPV-mediated tumors are the presence of classic koilocytes, perinuclear cytoplasmic halos, nuclear dysplasia with the addition of presence of dyskeratosis, atypical immature metaplasia, macrocytes, and binucleation as minor properties [78].

4.2. HPV detection tests/methods

The detection of cyclin-dependent kinase inhibitor 2A (p16Ink4A or p16) by IHC is recognized as a standard test for HPV positivity in a tumor in many clinics and during clinical trial enrollment. The HPV-16 E7 protein downregulates Rb and frees E2F, its regulatory partner which upregulates p16. IHC detection of p16 is a fast, cheap, and easily available method and is the standard method for HPV status assessment in clinics [79].With a false-negative rate of 4%, p16 IHC is a reliable marker in HPV infection, given that strong nuclear and cytoplasmic staining is extremely predictive for HPV(+) HNC [80]. By contrast, in cases with intermediate p16 expression levels, ISH or reverse transcription-polymerase chain reaction (RT-PCR) is required [80]. The inability of PCR-based assays to distinguish integrated DNA from episomal viral DNA decreases the test specificity remarkably in contrast to ISH in which sensitivity is lower compared to PCR [81]. Furthermore, the RNA ISH E6/E7 microRNA probes enable the direct scanning of viral transcripts which means accurate HPV detection [82]. It may be used as a HPV confirmation test in p16-positive samples, due to the fact that p16 is also overexpressed in non-virally induced situations. Given the different survival rates of the p16(+)/HPV(−) subgroups, considering personalized approaches, these patients should be evaluated as a distinct subcategory that is why using both ISH and p16 is recommended for HPV assessment [83]. In a recent study, which used both three methods, the sensitivity of p16 was detected as 100%, whereas its specificity was 74% in oral cancer and 93% in oropharyngeal cancer [84]. Cancer Care Ontario recommends routine HPV test in oropharyngeal cancer, in metastatic cervical nodes from an unknown head and neck primary and the use of p16 IHC as an initial test for its high sensitivity in patients with HNC [31].

Antibodies against HPV in the serum can be used to measure the cumulative exposure to HPV infection [85]. HPV16 E6 or E7 antibodies were detected in 65% of HPV(+) oropharyngeal cancer patients which indicates that they are useful tools as HPV markers in the unavailability of appropriate cytologic or histologic materials [67]. The detection of HPV antibodies in saliva instead of serum may lead to common false negative results, since antibodies in oral sampling are fewer compared with those in serum [85].

Currently, several methods including The Roche linear array HPV genotyping test, the Hybrid Capture 2, and a PCR bead-based multiplex method present for HPV typing [86–88]. Nevertheless, since E6 and E7 mRNA by RT-PCR demonstrate functional HPV expression, it is widely accepted as the gold standard [89]. The correlation between the steps of HPV infection to cell, detection targets, and methods is shown in **Table 1**.

Step	HPV infection	Detection target	Suitable methods
1	HPV endocytosis HPV episome HPV DNA integration	DNA detection	PCR ISH
2	E6 mRNA E7 mRNA	RNA detection	PCR ISH
3	Protein E6 Protein E7	Oncoprotein detection	Monoclonal antibodies
4	Rb:E2F P16	P16 overexpression detection	Monoclonal antibodies

Table 1. Correlation between the steps of HPV infection to cell, detection targets and methods.

5. Carcinogenesis

Currently, HPVs consist of over 81 different subtypes of HPVs classified on the basis of their L1 protein, separated based on cutaneous and mucosal site tropism, and divided in low-, and high-risk viruses according to correlation with cancers [90]. The high-risk HPV types may be classified as follows: highest risk types (HPV 16, 18, 31, 45), other high-risk types (HPV 33, 35, 39, 51, 52, 56, 58, 59), and probably high-risk types (HPV 26, 53, 66, 68, 73, 82). Oncogenic HPV types 16, 18, 31, 33, and 35 are related to HPV(+) HNC, while HPV-16 is most frequently found in oropharyngeal cancer [91, 92]. Majority of the cases of HPV(+) HNC arise from the oropharyngeal region due to epithelial injury predisposition of its location and lack of protective keratin layer that leads to easy virus exposure of the basal cells [93].

HPVs are circular, non-enveloped, epitheliotrophic, double-stranded DNA viruses belonging to family *Papovaviridae* with an approximately 8000 base pair-sized viral genome carrying early open-reading frame (ORF), late ORF, and noncoding control region between these two regions with histones within a 52–55-nm virion [94]. HPV genome encodes two structural capsid proteins (L1 and L2), two regulatory proteins (E1, E2), three oncoproteins (E5, E6, E7) [94]. The early region encodes the regulatory proteins, E1-E2, E4-E7, which are responsible for gene regulation, replication, and pathogenesis, while the late region encodes the two structural proteins, L1, L2, which form the viral capsid and have no known role in carcinogenesis but are substantial immune response targets to HPV infection. The E4 protein is thought to ease viral particle release into the surroundings and be responsible for G2 arrest in HPV-infected cells [95, 96].

The best-known relation between high-risk HPVs and cancer is established for the uterine cervix. However, HPV is also correlated with vaginal, vulvar, anal, and penile cancers, and especially since 2007, it has also been demonstrated to be a risk factor for oropharyngeal cancer [15, 95, 96]. HPV-16 and HPV-18 remain the main mediating factors in most HPV-related cancers. For instance, they are associated with 70% of cases with cervical cancer [94]. Approximately 50% of penile cancers include HPV DNA, predominantly HPV-16 [93], while HPV-16 accounts for more than 90% of HPV(+) oropharyngeal cancers [74].

The palatine and lingual tonsils are predominant targets of HPV among all other potential sites of HNC. The basal cells are infected by HPV in the stratified squamous epithelium. The reticulated lymphoepithelium of tonsillar crypts expresses programmed death ligand 1 (PD-L1), which suppresses response of T-cells against HPV, and leads to an "immune-privileged" region for viral infection initiation and adaptation to immune resistance [97]. Virus enters through microinjuries in the epithelium, although the receptor and mechanism of this entry remain unknown. Prior to virus entry to the cell by endocytosis, heparin sulfate is considered to mediate the virus particle attachment to the cell [98]. HPV infection of epithelial cells causes different types of viral protein expression and production of 20 to 100 and thousands of viral DNA per cell in the basal layer and superficial layers, respectively [98]. While majority of other virus infections result in the production of progeny from the same target cell, the HPV-infected cells undergo mitosis and continue differentiation [99]. Thus, basal cells are not the only proliferating cells in the infected epithelium since infected suprabasal cells have active cell cycle and differentiation [100].

The three HPV oncoproteins E5, E6, and E7 promote uncontrolled cellular proliferation to lead viral amplification, initiate, and contribute to progression of cancer through the same mechanism and induce genomic instability [101–103]. As in cervical cancer, E6 and E7 oncoproteins are mainly responsible for the malignant transformation and progression in HNCs [101, 102]. Since silencing the E6 and E7 oncogene expression in HPV16(+) human oropharyngeal squamous cell lines led to p53 and Rb tumor suppressor activation and apoptosis induction, these two oncoproteins are thought to be required for maintaining malignant processes [104].

High-risk HPV E7 oncoproteins play a critical role in initiating DNA synthesis by binding and inactivating the Rb and its related pocket proteins p107 and p130 which are tumor suppressor genes by targeting them for degradation [98]. Rb, the most well-known pocket protein family member functions to prevent excessive cell growth by inhibiting cell cycle progression [105]. The Rb inactivation by E7 causes E2F transcription factor overexpression with the cell cycle gene upregulation, leading to the cell transition from G1 to S phase [106]. The inactivation of pRb increases levels of p16/CDKN2A which is an inhibitor of cdk4/cyclin D and cdk6/cyclin D and promotes aberrant cell proliferation [107]. Thus, increased levels of p16/CDKN2A expression correspond as a diagnostic biomarker for transcriptionally active HPV infection and virus-mediated deregulation of cell cycle [108]. E7 oncoproteins also have ability to affect gene transcription by influencing histone acetylation in regulatory regions via either histone acetyl transferases or histone deacetylases [109].

E7-mediated proliferation results in the activation of p53-dependent growth inhibition and apoptosis. To counteract this, HPV E6 causes p53 degradation which leads to apoptosis inhibition and uncontrolled cellular growth as a consequence [101]. E6 transcript produces a 19-kDa protein that binds with a ubiquitin protein ligase (E6AP) that will result in p53 tumor suppressor protein ubiquitination (posttranslational modification) and proteosomal degradation [101]. The p53 regulates the cell cycle by controlling the transition from G1 to the S phase at checkpoint by inducing cyclin inhibitor (p16, p21, and p27) expression [110]. Hence, E6 oncoprotein deregulates cell cycle checkpoints both at G1/S and G2/M in the case of cellular stress such as DNA damage which results in genomic instability. Moreover, E6 protein has the ability to downregulate p53 function either by direct binding or by interacting with the histone acetyltransferases (ADA3) and histone acetyltransferase binding proteins (p300 and CREB) [111, 112]. In addition, it can associate with *ras* and E7 for *in vitro* cell transformation [113]. Furthermore, E6 oncoprotein can activate cellular telomerase by upregulating human telomerase hTERT which leads to cellular immortalization [114]. E6 targets not only p53, but also Bak and Myc proteins which regulate apoptosis [115].

Additionally, the E5 protein works together with E6 and E7 to induce proliferation in infected cells and is considered to have a more minor role in host cell transformation. It also blocks apoptosis in the late process of HPV-induced carcinogenesis [103].

Several studies report that both E6 and E7 bind multiple complementary cooperators that perform oncogenic impacts other than p53 and pRb degradation. Despite the robust growth inducing functions of these HPV oncoproteins, extra oncogenic events are required for malignant development. Although high-risk E6 and E7 cause genomic instability [116], the mutation rate in HPV(+) tumors seem to be lower than in HPV(−) ones [59, 117]. E6 and E7 oncoproteins may lead to chromosomal segregation errors and aneuploidy development during mitosis [118]. Due to the E7 induction of CDK2 activation, multiple immature centrioles are formed which results in several centrosome synthesis rounds [119]. Eventually, E6 and E7 cause these cells with aberrant mitoses to proliferate by inhibiting G2-M checkpoint control and apoptosis [120].

It has been demonstrated that HPV-mediated carcinogenesis causes significantly fewer genomic changes than HPV-independent ones. Particularly, HPV(+) HNC is associated with less mutated p53, higher EGFR expression, and more chromosomal aberrations (3p, 9p, and 17p) [63, 121–123]. It has been confirmed by whole-exome sequencing of HNC that HPV(+) HNC has a distinct genetic entity from HPV(−) HNC which has more mutations compared with HPV(+) ones, independent of smoking [59, 117]. While HPV(+) tumors have no p53 mutation, p53 mutation rate was 78% in HPV(−) cancers [59]. These data indicate that HPV-mediated oncogenesis is correlated with cellular dysregulation to a lesser degree which may be the underlying explanation of better treatment response. HPV(+) tumor differs from HPV(−) HNC not only biologically, but also clinically. They tend to present at earlier T stage with extensive nodal involvement. Despite the fact that distant metastasis may constitute a major problem in HPV(+) tumors, their prognosis is better, especially in locally advanced diseases [124].

6. Mechanisms of improved response to treatment

The prognostic advantage of HPV positivity may be explained to some extent by the patient population features affected with younger age, higher performance status, fewer comorbid diseases, and less tobacco and alcohol exposure. However, after adjustment to these conditions in multivariate analyses, the improved survival of HPV(+) patients still maintains [16, 46].

Actually, these factors only account for approximately 9% of the survival difference between patients with HPV(+) and HPV(−) tumors, which means that the survival difference seems to be largely resulted by HPV status [16, 125]. It is clear that the higher response rate of HPV(+) tumor to therapy is caused by a basic biological difference between HPV(+) and HPV(−) HNCs. It is accepted that intrinsic factors of each individual tumor (e.g., mutations, HPV status) may modulate the microenvironment of tumors [126]. These alterations have the ability to influence immune response, stromal structure, and tumor vasculature [126]. Not only experimental studies but also several clinical studies have demonstrated that patients with HPV/p16(+) tumors had a much better prognosis compared with HPV/p16(−) ones [16].

It has been suggested that the immune system plays a significant role in rejection process of HPV(+) tumors because of viral protein expressions that reveal T-cell responses performing a long-term immunosurveillance. Accumulating evidence over the years appears to reinforce this hypothesis. Spanos et al. [127] showed superior tumor control in HPV(+) cell lines implanted into immunocompetent mice compared with immunocompromised mice [127]. HPV-specific circulating HPV16 E7-specific CD8+ T cells and IFNγ-producing T cells have been defined in patients with HPV(+) HNC [128]. A greater alteration from naive to effector and memory T cells has been shown in patients with HPV(+) compared with both healthy donors and patients with HPV(−) tumors which indicates higher tumor response in HPV(+) patients [129]. In addition, it has been reported that the programmed death-1 (PD-1) positive T-cell presence was associated with improved survival in HPV(+) HNC patients [130]. Moreover, circulating anti-HPV16 antibodies which are suggested to associate with clinical outcome have been detected in HPV(+) HNC patients [92]. Furthermore, radiation may induce expression loss of CD47 which is an important transmembrane cell surface marker in self-identification in HPV(+) cell lines that explains the interaction between the immune system and radiotherapy [131].

Even though radiosensitivity is mainly based on the cell ability to detect DNA damage and repair it, tumor oxygenation status may also be a factor for radiotherapy response [132]. In this context, in the Danish Head and Neck Cancer Group (DAHANCA)-5 study, the ratio of patients with high plasma osteopontin (a marker of hypoxia) levels was greater in HPV(−) tumors than in HPV(+) ones, indicating more hypoxia in HPV(−) group [133]. On the contrary, neither IHC staining for carbonic anhydrase IX (upregulated in hypoxic conditions) nor pO2 level of tumor was found to associate with HPV status of tumor in another study [134].

In two prospective trials investigating the impact of hypoxic modification (using nimorazole or tirapazamine) in HNC, the use of hypoxic cell radiosensitizer provided a trend toward better locoregional control in HPV(−) tumors but had no significant benefit in HPV(+) tumors [53, 135]. Surprisingly, HPV/p16-positive tumors appeared to be insensible to hypoxic modifier and revealed no benefit from nimorazole after which was suggested that HPV/p16(+) HNCs are less hypoxic than HPV(−) ones, and this might contribute to the better prognosis [135]. However, in studies evaluating the hypoxia with imaging markers including (18)F-fluoroazomycin arabinoside positron emission tomography/computed tomography (FAZA PET/CT)), dynamic contrast enhanced-MRI (DCE-MRI), and proton magnetic resonance spectroscopy ((1)H-MRS), no correlation between HPV positivity and intratumoral hypoxia was detected [136, 137]. Additionally, recent *in vitro* evidence comparing radiation response of HPV/p16(+) and (−) cell lines under hypoxia showed no difference regarding gene regulation patterns, while oxygen enhancement ratio (OER) of HPV/p16(+) cells was found similar to HPV/p16(−) ones [138].

Finally, it has been hypothesized that viral oncoproteins play a substantial role in improved treatment sensitivity. It has been shown that low levels of residual wild-type p53 in HPV(+) cells may be activated by radiation, resulting in increased cell death [139]. Recently, Rieckman et al. [140] demonstrated decreased survival fraction, increased double strand breaks levels, and extensive G2 arrest pointing to compromised DNA repair capacity in HPV/p16(+) cell lines compared with HPV(−) cell lines after irradiation [140].

7. Clinical considerations

7.1. Impact of HPV on prognosis (clinical studies)

The changing epidemiology of HPV-positive oropharyngeal cancer formed a new patient population in the clinic that consists of individuals at younger ages without a heavy alcohol or smoking history and with more advanced neck diseases [141]. The natural history of HPV-positive HNC began to be written with many retrospective studies published in the late 1990s to early 2000s. In a study of 42 patients, HPV(+) tonsil cancer revealed higher survival rates compared with HPV(−) ones [142]. In addition, in a German study including 208 HNC sample patients with HPV(+) samples had better survival despite more adverse pathological results [143]. Furthermore, in a Swedish study with 60 patients, HPV(+) oropharyngeal cancer patients were found to have higher 5-year OS rates (53.5% vs. 31.5%) and reduced recurrence risk irrespective of gender, age, or disease stage [144]. Gillison et al. retrospectively analyzed 252 HNC patients in 2000, and patients with HPV(+) HNC from all sites had a 40% reduction in death risk ($p = 0.07$) and a 59% reduction in disease-related death risk ($p = 0.02$) after adjustment for age, nodal status, and alcohol consumption [63]. Finally, a meta-analysis of 37 studies analyzing HPV and HNC reported that HPV(+) oropharyngeal cancer patients had a 28% reduced death risk and a 49% lower disease-failure risk compared with HPV(−) ones in 2007 [145].

In the Danish DAHANCA-5 phase III clinical trial, samples from 156 patients of whom 74 were oropharyngeal cancer patients were collected prospectively. Of oropharyngeal cancer samples, 24 were p16(+) and had a locoregional control benefit (OR, 5.1) compared with those with p16(−) samples [146]. In a phase II prospective trial of 42 oropharyngeal cancer patients of whom pretreatment biopsy HPV-positivity rate was 67%, HPV titer was correlated with improved induction chemotherapy response ($p = 0.001$), chemoradiation response ($p = 0.005$), overall survival ($p = 0.007$), and disease-specific survival (DSS) ($p = 0.008$) [147]. Similarly, in the Trans-Tasman Radiation Oncology Group (TROG), 20.02 trial which retrospectively reviewed for HPV and p16 status, a higher 2-year overall survival rate (91% vs. 74%; HR, 0.36; $p = 0.004$) and failure-free survival (87% vs. 72%; HR, 0.39; $p = 0.003$) were detected in 57% of 185 oropharyngeal cancer patients with p16 positivity compared with HPV(−) patients [53].

Several studies have demonstrated the favorable effect of HPV positivity in oropharyngeal cancer patients [46, 53, 148]. First, in 2008, the Eastern Cooperative Oncology Group (ECOG) 2399 trial which was a phase II prospective study including stages III and IV, M0, oropharynx and larynx cancer patients treated with paclitaxel/carboplatin induction chemotherapy followed by concurrent paclitaxel and radiotherapy showed that patients with HPV(+) oropharyngeal cancer (HPV detection method was p16 IHC) had a 61% lower death risk (HR, 0.39; $p = 0.06$) and a 62% lower progression risk (HR, 0.38; $p = 0.09$) than patients with HPV(−) ones, after adjustments for age, ECOG performance status, and disease stage [46]. Following this, Ang et al. [16] reported the largest retrospective examination of Radiation Therapy Oncology Group (RTOG) 0129 study about HPV effect on survival in oropharyngeal cancer where HPV positivity was tested by ISH. The 3-year overall survival rates were 82.4% and 57.1% in the HPV(+) and HPV(−) subgroups, respectively, while the 3-year progression-free survival rates were similarly better in HPV(+) subgroup compared with HPV(−) ones (73.7% vs. 43.4%). In addition, HPV(+) patients had a 58% lower death risk (HR, 0.42; $p < 0.001$) and a 51% lower progression risk (HR, 0.49; $p < 0.001$). Furthermore, patients were classified into risk-of-death categories (low, moderate, high) based on a recursive partitioning analysis according to HPV status, tumor burden, and tobacco use. The low-risk group included patients with HPV(+) cancer with the exception of smokers with advanced nodal metastasis, while smoker patients with HPV(+) tumors and advanced nodal metastasis or nonsmoker patients HPV(−) tumors of stage T2 or T3 were considered to be at intermediate risk. On the contrary, nonsmoker patients with HPV(−) T4 tumors or smoker patients with HPV(−) tumors consisted of high-risk group while 3-year survival rates of low-, moderate-, and high-risk patients were 93%, 70.8%, and 46.2%, respectively. Importantly, smoking had a negative factor on prognosis, regardless of HPV status [16]. Similarly, in the retrospective analysis of TAX 324 trial, which investigated triple-agent versus double-agent induction chemotherapy confirmed the better prognosis of HPV(+) patients, 5-year overall survival rates were significantly higher in HPV(+) group compared with HPV(−) (82% vs. 35%, $p < 0.0001$). The HPV status was tested using E6/E7 PCR methods in this study [47].

The retrospective subanalysis of 190 patients with oropharyngeal cancer in the RTOG 9003 study, a 4-arm, phase III trial which compared different RT protocols, p16 positivity was found to correlate with T1 stage, better performance status, absence of anemia, and less tobacco consumption. Independently from assigned treatment, the p16(+) oropharyngeal cancer group had better 5-year overall and progression-free survival, lower 5-year locoregional failure but similar 5-year distant metastasis rates compared with p16(−) ones [149]. Additionally, a recently published retrospective analysis of RTOG 0129 and RTOG 0522 revealed that HPV(+)oropharyngeal cancer patients had better overall survival even after disease progression compared with HPV(−) group. Moreover, salvage surgery was detected to provide significantly improved prognosis [150]. Another recent retrospective subanalysis of the phase III trial, IMCL-9815 Bonner trial [53, 54], which evaluated the impact of the role of cetuximab addition to radiotherapy in patients with locally advanced HNC, based on HPV status determined by p16 IHC, p16 positivity was confirmed as a powerful prognostic determinant for oropharyngeal cancer patients [151].

Likewise, surgical reports further confirmed the favorable effect of p16 positivity in oropharyngeal cancer. Rich et al. [148] reported that in a cohort of 84 stage III or IV oropharyngeal cancers, patients who received transoral laser microsurgery (TLM) ± adjuvant therapy, p16 positivity was significantly associated with higher 5-year overall survival (90% vs. 25%, $p <$ 0.0001) and disease-specific survival (DSS) rates (94% vs. 50%, $p = 0.0078$) [148]. Furthermore, two recent meta-analysis of clinical trial data of oropharyngeal cancer patients demonstrated hazard ratios for better overall survival of 0.49 and 0.47 correlated with HPV positivity [125, 152]. Overall, patients with HPV(+) tumors have a 60–80% reduced mortality rates, a finding that was confirmed by multiple trials.

The HPV(+) tumors had some unique features. The TAX324 trial analysis showed that HPV(+) patients had T1 or T2 tumors more commonly (49% vs. 20%) and better ECOG performance status (ECOG 0: 77% vs.49%) [47] which was in parallel with the results TROG 02.02 and ECOG 2399 trials [46, 53]. In addition, it has been shown that cystic lymph node metastases were associated with HPV(+) tonsil cancer in a surgical series of neck dissection [153]. Furthermore, Princess Margaret Hospital data of N2-3 HNC patients ($n = 493$) detected that HPV(+) lymph nodes ($n = 257$) were larger (2.9 vs. 2.5 cm), more commonly in cystic structure (38% vs. 6%), regressed more frequently after treatment (36% vs. 41%), and more likely to be eliminated after 36 weeks (90% vs. 0%) compared with HPV(–) ones [154].

7.2. The role of HPV in recurrent/metastatic HNC

The characteristics of metastatic disease in HPV(+) patients differ from HPV(–) ones in terms of sites and time, since metastases is more likely to develop at sites other than lungs and may occur after 2 years following the initial treatment. Locally advanced diseases (T4 and N3-N2C) are the risk factors for metastasis development in HPV(+) disease [16]. Princess Margaret Hospital reviewed the distant metastasis rates in 457 HPV(+) and 167 HPV(–) oropharyngeal cancer cases and found that metastasis rates were similar at 3 years. HPV(+) tumors were more likely to develop metastases after a long interval, such that metastases occurred within 2 years in 24 of 25 HPV(–) cases, while metastasis development were detected 3 years post treatment in 13% of HPV(+) cases. In addition, dissemination pattern was more common in HPV(+) patients (33% vs. 0%). Nevertheless, post-metastases 2-year survival was significantly better in HPV(+) group compared with HPV(–) group (11% vs. 4%, $p = 0.02$) [155]. These findings were confirmed by additional recent retrospective reports showing similar unique metastatic spread patterns [53, 156–158].

Recently, the impact of HPV in recurrent-metastatic HNC was evaluated in large trials. In the phase III EXTREME randomized trial which assessed the benefit of cetuximab addition to platinum + 5-fluorouracil (5-FU) in patients with recurrent-metastatic HNC as first-line therapy, paired tissue samples were analyzed for p16 expression by IHC using a 70% expression cutoff value and HPV via oligonucleotide hybridization test [159]. The p16 and HPV positivity was correlated with higher survival rates compared with p16 and HPV negativity in both cetuximab and control groups [159]. Since the predictive analyses indicated that cetuximab addition to chemotherapy improved survival rates independently from p16 or HPV status, these biomarkers did not have any significance in treatment efficacy prediction. By contrast, in the phase III SPECTRUM randomized trial which assessed the benefit of panitumumab addition to chemotherapy instead of cetuximab in recurrent-metastatic HNC, a nonsignificant difference between HPV(+) and HPV(−) groups was demonstrated. Furthermore, the benefit of panitumumab was not detected in p16(+) group in contrast to p16(−) group [159].

The pooled analysis of patients with recurrent-metastatic HNC from E1395, a phase III trial comparing platinum + 5-fluorouracil with cisplatin + paclitaxel and E3301, a phase II trial evaluating irinotecan + docetaxel demonstrated that patients with HPV(+)/p16(+) disease had better overall survival than HPV(−)/p16(−) ones [160]. Taken together, these three studies indicate the positive impact of HPV positivity on improved survival. The efficiency of anti-EGFR antibodies on survival of HPV(+) and HPV(−) patients remains to be clarified. Hence, further studies including only oropharyngeal cancer patients are required in recurrent-metastatic setting since the impact of HPV positivity at other sides of HNC is not fully known.

7.3. Prognostic factors

Combined with being a nonsmoker, HPV DNA/RNA presence and p16 overexpression are strong prognostic markers [16]. Smoking, the most important risk factor for HNC overall, affects negative survival and response to treatment [161]. In addition, tobacco exposure has been shown to be a significant independent factor for prognosis in patients with HPV(+) oropharyngeal cancer, as it predicted progression and death risk in a dose-dependent pattern. Independently from HPV status and other factors, each pack-year of smoking increases the progression and death risk and the risk of second primary cancers of by 1% and 1.5%, respectively. Furthermore, the risk of death doubles if patients do not quit smoking during radiotherapy [161]. Based on the data of RTOG 0129 trial, a risk stratification for oropharyngeal cancer patients was developed using HPV status, history of smoking (>10 pack-years), and disease stage [16].

Other factors which are correlated with poor prognosis are local extension, disease stage at presentation, cervical node involvement, and rich vascular and lymphatic network [162]. Tumor thickness greater than 5 mm is significantly correlated with occult lymph node metastasis which is suggested to be a stronger determiner of prognosis than TNM staging by some authors. It has been shown that tumor differentiation, angiogenesis, extracapsular extension, and perineural invasion had significant role in prognosis determination [162]. Regarding treatment associated factors, cervical node dissection and disease free margins are important [162], since local relapse rates are 64–84% in patients with positive surgical margins [163].

Concerning the molecular markers, aberrations in chromosomes 3, 9, 11, 13, and 17 and tumor suppressor genes (p53 and pRb) are significant for prognosis [162]. In addition, cytokeratin 8/18 has been shown to be an independent factor correlated with poor prognosis [162, 163]. Furthermore, the absent/low expression of MHC class I, CD44, or CD98 has strong prognostic value for HPV(+) oropharyngeal cancer patients such that MHC class I staining absence defines 3-year disease-free and overall survival with 95–100% probability [164–166]. Moreover, higher

CD8+ tumor infiltrating lymphocyte (TIL) counts is also a prognostic marker for patients with HPV(+) oropharyngeal cancer [167].

HPV16 E6 and E7 in serum were demonstrated to be the most predictive factor in determining the HNC prognosis among the several biomarkers. E6/E7 seropositivity was associated with improved survival, whereas their seronegativity was correlated with poor prognosis irrespective of the DNA or p16 status [168]. Another suggested prognostic factor for survival is pretreatment tumor HPV copy number; higher tumor HPV copy number was correlated with better induction chemotherapy (p = 0.001) and chemoradiotherapy (p = 0.005) response, disease-specific (p = 0.004) and overall survival and (p = 0.008) after adjustment for other significant factors [147]. Similarly, higher viral load was shown to be correlated with improved recurrence-free (p = 0.0037) and overall (p = 0.028) survival in tonsil cancer patients [169]. Furthermore, the presence of both HPV16 and p16 indicated significantly improved prognosis compared with either p16 or HPV16 alone [170].

7.4. Deintensification of treatment in HPV(+) oropharyngeal cancer

Three principal routes have been drawn in treatment deintensification: (1) EGFR inhibitor use (mostly Cetuximab) instead of cisplatin, concurrently with radiotherapy; (2) radiotherapy dose reduction with concurrent chemotherapy (based on induction chemotherapy response); and (3) minimally invasive transoral surgery use followed by reduced adjuvant treatment according to the histopathological properties of the excised tumor.

Since responses to treatment alter even between HPV(+) oropharyngeal cancer patients, defining appropriate patient subgroup is essential. It must be emphasized that all patients with HPV(+) oropharyngeal cancer are not suitable candidates for deintensification approaches. The clinical trial cohorts' analysis indicates some evidence. Some of them suggest that lifetime tobacco use history of >10 pack-years in HPV(+) patients with advanced regional nodal metastasis (N2b, N3) as well as smoking during radiotherapy decreases survival time (3-year overall survival rate of 70.8%) [16, 161]. The Italian study which reported that intermediate-risk patients are not convenient for deintensification trials confirmed these findings [171]. Furthermore, O'Sullivan et al. [27] demonstrated that the 3-year distant control rates of HPV(+) oropharyngeal cancer with advanced T stage (T4) or nodal (N3) was 72% and 78%, respectively [124]. Hence, late recurrences and relapses as distant metastasis are not rare in HPV(+) oropharyngeal cancer. These data indicate the presence of a limit of the biologic advantage provided by HPV positivity and may be helpful in determining patient subgroup that requires chemotherapy use in order to treat early micrometastasis. Both amount of smoking and locoregionally advanced disease have implications in designing deintensification trials for HPV(+) oropharyngeal cancer patients.

Many clinical trials have been planned to evaluate the efficiency of treatment deintensification in HNC patients and recently they have been reviewed by Masterson et al. [152] in detail. Enrolling patients into these trials to define optimum treatment of HPV(+) oropharyngeal cancer is encouraged. Nevertheless, besides as a clinical trial, there is not sufficient data for the treatment reduction or modification according to HPV positivity until we receive the results from these deintensification studies.

7.5. Prevention-vaccination

There are two prophylactic HPV vaccines available commercially; Gardasil® (Merck & Co., Whitehouse Station, NJ, USA) and Cervarix® (GlaxoSmithKline Biologicals, Rixensart, Belgium). The virus-like proteins (VLPs) are used to create HPV major capsid protein L1 neutralizing antibodies. Gardasil is a quadrivalent L1 VLP recombinant vaccine protecting against HPV6, -11, -16, and -18, while Gardasil 9 provides protection against five additional HPV genotypes 16, 18, 31, 33, 45, 52, and 58. In contrast, Cervarix is a bivalent L1 VLP recombinant vaccine against HPV-16 and -18. Both HPV vaccines are highly effective in anogenital HPV infection prevention and consequent anal and cervical cancer development.

Despite the fact that the prophylactic value of vaccination for oropharyngeal cancer has not been proven in randomized trials yet, both the Cervarix and Gardasil vaccines are expected to prevent oropharyngeal HPV16 and -18 infections and consequent oropharyngeal cancer, since HPV16 is the most common type detected in oropharyngeal cancer [172]. The vaccination efficiency was estimated as 93.3% in 7466 women who were aged 18–25 years and randomized to HPV16/18 (Cervarix) vaccine versus hepatitis A vaccine as control for oral HPV 16/18 prevalence evaluation 4 years after vaccination [173]. In addition, cross-sectional study of US population as part of the National Health and Nutrition Examination Survey (NHANES) oral HPV infection prevalence was reduced significantly in 290 vaccinated women compared with 1985 unvaccinated women (0% vs. 0.5%) [54].

Author details

Makbule Tambas[1*], Musa Altun[2] and Deniz Tural[3]

*Address all correspondence to: makbule_tambas@hotmail.com

1 Department of Radiation Oncology, Okmeydani Training and Research Hospital, Istanbul, Turkey

2 Department of Radiation Oncology, Istanbul Faculty of Medicine, Istanbul University, Istanbul, Turkey

3 Department of Medical Oncology, Bakirkoy Dr. Sadi Konuk Education and Research Hospital, Istanbul, Turkey

References

[1] Torre LA, Bray F, Siegel RL, Ferlay J, Lortet-Tieulent J, Jemal A. Global cancer statistics, 2012. CA: A Cancer Journal for Clinicians. 2015;65(2):87–108. Epub 2015/02/06.10.3322/caac.21262

[2] Jemal A, Bray F, Center MM, Ferlay J, Ward E, Forman D. Global cancer statistics. CA: A Cancer Journal for Clinicians. 2011;61(2):69–90. Epub 2011/02/08.10.3322/caac.20107

[3] Ramshankar V, Krishnamurthy A. Human papilloma virus in head and neck cancers-role and relevance in clinical management. Indian Journal of Surgical Oncology. 2013;4(1):59–66. Epub 2014/01/16.10.1007/s13193-012-0196-5

[4] Mehanna H, Paleri V, West CM, Nutting C. Head and neck cancer – part 1: epidemiology, presentation, and prevention. BMJ. 2010;341:c4684. Epub 2010/09/22.10.1136/bmj.c4684

[5] Hashibe M, Brennan P, Chuang SC, Boccia S, Castellsague X, Chen C, et al. Interaction between tobacco and alcohol use and the risk of head and neck cancer: pooled analysis in the International Head and Neck Cancer Epidemiology Consortium. Cancer Epidemiology, Biomarkers & Prevention. 2009;18(2):541–50. Epub 2009/02/05.10.1158/1055-9965.EPI-08-0347

[6] Guha N, Boffetta P, Wunsch Filho V, Eluf Neto J, Shangina O, Zaridze D, et al. Oral health and risk of squamous cell carcinoma of the head and neck and esophagus: results of two multicentric case-control studies. American Journal of Epidemiology. 2007;166(10):1159–73. Epub 2007/09/01.10.1093/aje/kwm193

[7] Mashberg A, Boffetta P, Winkelman R, Garfinkel L. Tobacco smoking, alcohol drinking, and cancer of the oral cavity and oropharynx among U.S. veterans. Cancer. 1993;72(4):1369–75. Epub 1993/08/15.

[8] Johnson S, McDonald JT, Corsten M, Rourke R. Socio-economic status and head and neck cancer incidence in Canada: a case-control study. Oral Oncology. 2010;46(3):200–3. Epub 2010/02/09.10.1016/j.oraloncology.2009.12.004

[9] Chaturvedi AK, Engels EA, Anderson WF, Gillison ML. Incidence trends for human papillomavirus-related and unrelated oral squamous cell carcinomas in the United States. Journal of Clinical Oncology: Official Journal of the American Society of Clinical Oncology. 2008;26(4):612–9. Epub 2008/02/01.10.1200/JCO.2007.14.1713

[10] de Martel C, Ferlay J, Franceschi S, Vignat J, Bray F, Forman D, et al. Global burden of cancers attributable to infections in 2008: a review and synthetic analysis. The Lancet Oncology. 2012;13(6):607–15. Epub 2012/05/12.10.1016/S1470-2045(12)70137-7

[11] Martin-Hernan F, Sanchez-Hernandez JG, Cano J, Campo J, del Romero J. Oral cancer, HPV infection and evidence of sexual transmission. Medicina Oral, Patologia Oral y Cirugia Bucal. 2013;18(3):e439–44. Epub 2013/03/26.

[12] Hammarstedt L, Lindquist D, Dahlstrand H, Romanitan M, Dahlgren LO, Joneberg J, et al. Human papillomavirus as a risk factor for the increase in incidence of tonsillar cancer. International Journal of Cancer. 2006;119(11):2620–3. Epub 2006/09/23.10.1002/ijc.22177

[13] Sturgis EM, Cinciripini PM. Trends in head and neck cancer incidence in relation to smoking prevalence: an emerging epidemic of human papillomavirus-associated cancers? Cancer. 2007;110(7):1429–35. Epub 2007/08/29.10.1002/cncr.22963

[14] Nasman A, Attner P, Hammarstedt L, Du J, Eriksson M, Giraud G, et al. Incidence of human papillomavirus (HPV) positive tonsillar carcinoma in Stockholm, Sweden: an epidemic of viral-induced carcinoma? International Journal of Cancer. 2009;125(2):362–6. Epub 2009/03/31.10.1002/ijc.24339

[15] Attner P, Du J, Nasman A, Hammarstedt L, Ramqvist T, Lindholm J, et al. The role of human papillomavirus in the increased incidence of base of tongue cancer. International Journal of Cancer. 2010;126(12):2879–84. Epub 2009/10/27.10.1002/ijc.24994

[16] Ang KK, Harris J, Wheeler R, Weber R, Rosenthal DI, Nguyen-Tan PF, et al. Human papillomavirus and survival of patients with oropharyngeal cancer. The New England Journal of Medicine. 2010;363(1):24–35. Epub 2010/06/10.10.1056/NEJMoa0912217

[17] Chaturvedi AK, Engels EA, Pfeiffer RM, Hernandez BY, Xiao W, Kim E, et al. Human papillomavirus and rising oropharyngeal cancer incidence in the United States. Journal of Clinical Oncology: Official Journal of the American Society of Clinical Oncology. 2011;29(32):4294–301. Epub 2011/10/05.10.1200/JCO.2011.36.4596

[18] Conway DI, Stockton DL, Warnakulasuriya KA, Ogden G, Macpherson LM. Incidence of oral and oropharyngeal cancer in United Kingdom (1990–1999) – recent trends and regional variation. Oral Oncology. 2006;42(6):586–92. Epub 2006/02/14.10.1016/j.oraloncology.2005.10.018

[19] Hammarstedt L, Dahlstrand H, Lindquist D, Onelov L, Ryott M, Luo J, et al. The incidence of tonsillar cancer in Sweden is increasing. Acta Oto-Laryngologica. 2007;127(9):988–92. Epub 2007/08/23.10.1080/00016480601110170

[20] Braakhuis BJ, Visser O, Leemans CR. Oral and oropharyngeal cancer in the Netherlands between 1989 and 2006: Increasing incidence, but not in young adults. Oral Oncology. 2009;45(9):e85–9. Epub 2009/05/22.10.1016/j.oraloncology.2009.03.010

[21] Marur S, D'Souza G, Westra WH, Forastiere AA. HPV-associated head and neck cancer: a virus-related cancer epidemic. The Lancet Oncology. 2010;11(8):781–9. Epub 2010/05/11.10.1016/S1470-2045(10)70017-6

[22] Ramqvist T, Dalianis T. Oropharyngeal cancer epidemic and human papillomavirus. Emerging Infectious Diseases. 2010;16(11):1671–7. Epub 2010/10/30.10.3201/eid1611.100452

[23] Ramqvist T, Dalianis T. An epidemic of oropharyngeal squamous cell carcinoma (OSCC) due to human papillomavirus (HPV) infection and aspects of treatment and prevention. Anticancer Research. 2011;31(5):1515–9. Epub 2011/05/28.

[24] Ryerson AB, Peters ES, Coughlin SS, Chen VW, Gillison ML, Reichman ME, et al. Burden of potentially human papillomavirus-associated cancers of the oropharynx and

oral cavity in the US, 1998-2003. Cancer. 2008;113(10 Suppl.):2901–9. Epub 2008/11/05.10.1002/cncr.23745

[25] Carvalho AL, Nishimoto IN, Califano JA, Kowalski LP. Trends in incidence and prognosis for head and neck cancer in the United States: a site-specific analysis of the SEER database. International Journal of Cancer. 2005;114(5):806–16. Epub 2004/12/21.10.1002/ijc.20740

[26] Reddy VM, Cundall-Curry D, Bridger MW. Trends in the incidence rates of tonsil and base of tongue cancer in England, 1985-2006. Annals of the Royal College of Surgeons of England. 2010;92(8):655–9. Epub 2010/07/10.10.1308/003588410X12699663904871

[27] Auluck A, Hislop G, Bajdik C, Poh C, Zhang L, Rosin M. Trends in oropharyngeal and oral cavity cancer incidence of human papillomavirus (HPV)-related and HPV-unrelated sites in a multicultural population: the British Columbia experience. Cancer. 2010;116(11):2635–44. Epub 2010/03/26.10.1002/cncr.25087

[28] Hong AM, Grulich AE, Jones D, Lee CS, Garland SM, Dobbins TA, et al. Squamous cell carcinoma of the oropharynx in Australian males induced by human papillomavirus vaccine targets. Vaccine. 2010;28(19):3269–72. Epub 2010/03/17.10.1016/j.vaccine.2010.02.098

[29] Mork J, Moller B, Dahl T, Bray F. Time trends in pharyngeal cancer incidence in Norway 1981-2005: a subsite analysis based on a reabstraction and recoding of registered cases. Cancer Causes & Control. 2010;21(9):1397–405. Epub 2010/05/01.10.1007/s10552-010-9567-9

[30] Blomberg M, Nielsen A, Munk C, Kjaer SK. Trends in head and neck cancer incidence in Denmark, 1978-2007: focus on human papillomavirus associated sites. International Journal of Cancer. 2011;129(3):733–41. Epub 2010/09/30.10.1002/ijc.25699

[31] Lewis A, Kang R, Levine A, Maghami E. The new face of head and neck cancer: the HPV epidemic. Oncology (Williston Park). 2015;29(9):616–26. Epub 2015/09/20.

[32] Mammas IN, Sourvinos G, Zaravinos A, Spandidos DA. Vaccination against human papilloma virus (HPV): epidemiological evidence of HPV in non-genital cancers. Pathology Oncology Research. 2011;17(1):103–19. Epub 2010/07/20.10.1007/s12253-010-9288-0

[33] El-Mofty SK, Zhang MQ, Davila RM. Histologic identification of human papillomavirus (HPV)-related squamous cell carcinoma in cervical lymph nodes: a reliable predictor of the site of an occult head and neck primary carcinoma. Head and Neck Pathology. 2008;2(3):163–8. Epub 2008/09/01.10.1007/s12105-008-0066-1

[34] Vent J, Haidle B, Wedemeyer I, Huebbers C, Siefer O, Semrau R, et al. p16 expression in carcinoma of unknown primary: diagnostic indicator and prognostic marker. Head & Neck. 2013;35(11):1521–6. Epub 2013/01/25.10.1002/hed.23190

[35] Begum S, Gillison ML, Nicol TL, Westra WH. Detection of human papillomavirus-16 in fine-needle aspirates to determine tumor origin in patients with metastatic squamous

cell carcinoma of the head and neck. Clinical Cancer Research: An Official Journal of the American Association for Cancer Research. 2007;13(4):1186–91. Epub 2007/02/24.10.1158/1078-0432.CCR-06-1690

[36] Abogunrin S, Di Tanna GL, Keeping S, Carroll S, Iheanacho I. Prevalence of human papillomavirus in head and neck cancers in European populations: a meta-analysis. BMC Cancer. 2014;14:968. Epub 2014/12/18.10.1186/1471-2407-14-968

[37] Venuti A, Badaracco G, Rizzo C, Mafera B, Rahimi S, Vigili M. Presence of HPV in head and neck tumours: high prevalence in tonsillar localization. Journal of Experimental & Clinical Cancer Research. 2004;23(4):561–6. Epub 2005/03/04.

[38] Koskinen WJ, Chen RW, Leivo I, Makitie A, Back L, Kontio R, et al. Prevalence and physical status of human papillomavirus in squamous cell carcinomas of the head and neck. International Journal of Cancer. 2003;107(3):401–6. Epub 2003/09/25.10.1002/ijc.11381

[39] Stephen JK, Divine G, Chen KM, Chitale D, Havard S, Worsham MJ. Significance of p16 in site-specific HPV positive and HPV negative head and neck squamous cell carcinoma. Cancer and Clinical Oncology. 2013;2(1):51–61. Epub 2013/08/13.10.5539/cco.v2n1p51

[40] Bussu F, Sali M, Gallus R, Vellone VG, Zannoni GF, Autorino R, et al. HPV infection in squamous cell carcinomas arising from different mucosal sites of the head and neck region. Is p16 immunohistochemistry a reliable surrogate marker? British Journal of Cancer. 2013;108(5):1157–62. Epub 2013/02/14.10.1038/bjc.2013.55

[41] Almadori G, Cadoni G, Cattani P, Posteraro P, Scarano E, Ottaviani F, et al. Detection of human papillomavirus DNA in laryngeal squamous cell carcinoma by polymerase chain reaction. European Journal of Cancer. 1996;32A(5):783–8. Epub 1996/05/01.

[42] Almadori G, Galli J, Cadoni G, Bussu F, Maurizi M. Human papillomavirus infection and cyclin D1 gene amplification in laryngeal squamous cell carcinoma: biologic function and clinical significance. Head & Neck. 2002;24(6):597–604. Epub 2002/07/12.10.1002/hed.10097

[43] Combes JD, Franceschi S. Role of human papillomavirus in non-oropharyngeal head and neck cancers. Oral Oncology. 2014;50(5):370–9. Epub 2013/12/18.10.1016/j.oraloncology.2013.11.004

[44] Isayeva T, Li Y, Maswahu D, Brandwein-Gensler M. Human papillomavirus in non-oropharyngeal head and neck cancers: a systematic literature review. Head and Neck Pathology. 2012;6(Suppl. 1):S104–20. Epub 2012/07/13.10.1007/s12105-012-0368-1

[45] Lingen MW, Xiao W, Schmitt A, Jiang B, Pickard R, Kreinbrink P, et al. Low etiologic fraction for high-risk human papillomavirus in oral cavity squamous cell carcinomas. Oral Oncology. 2013;49(1):1–8. Epub 2012/07/31.10.1016/j.oraloncology.2012.07.002

[46] Fakhry C, Westra WH, Li S, Cmelak A, Ridge JA, Pinto H, et al. Improved survival of patients with human papillomavirus-positive head and neck squamous cell carcinoma

in a prospective clinical trial. Journal of the National Cancer Institute. 2008;100(4):261–9. Epub 2008/02/14.10.1093/jnci/djn011

[47] Posner MR, Lorch JH, Goloubeva O, Tan M, Schumaker LM, Sarlis NJ, et al. Survival and human papillomavirus in oropharynx cancer in TAX 324: a subset analysis from an international phase III trial. Annals of Oncology: Official Journal of the European Society for Medical Oncology/ESMO. 2011;22(5):1071–7. Epub 2011/02/15.10.1093/annonc/mdr006

[48] Lassen P, Eriksen JG, Krogdahl A, Therkildsen MH, Ulhoi BP, Overgaard M, et al. The influence of HPV-associated p16-expression on accelerated fractionated radiotherapy in head and neck cancer: evaluation of the randomised DAHANCA 6 & 7 trial. Radiotherapy and Oncology: Journal of the European Society for Therapeutic Radiology and Oncology. 2011;100(1):49–55. Epub 2011/03/25.10.1016/j.radonc.2011.02.010

[49] Lajer CB, von Buchwald C. The role of human papillomavirus in head and neck cancer. APMIS: Acta Pathologica, Microbiologica, et Immunologica Scandinavica. 2010;118(6–7):510–9. Epub 2010/06/18.10.1111/j.1600-0463.2010.02624.x

[50] Gillison ML, D'Souza G, Westra W, Sugar E, Xiao W, Begum S, et al. Distinct risk factor profiles for human papillomavirus type 16-positive and human papillomavirus type 16-negative head and neck cancers. Journal of the National Cancer Institute. 2008;100(6):407–20. Epub 2008/03/13.10.1093/jnci/djn025

[51] Schwartz SR, Yueh B, McDougall JK, Daling JR, Schwartz SM. Human papillomavirus infection and survival in oral squamous cell cancer: a population-based study. Otolaryngology – Head and Neck Surgery: Official Journal of American Academy of Otolaryngology – Head and Neck Surgery. 2001;125(1):1–9. Epub 2001/07/18.10.1067/mhn.2001.116979

[52] Shiboski CH, Schmidt BL, Jordan RC. Tongue and tonsil carcinoma: increasing trends in the U.S. population ages 20-44 years. Cancer. 2005;103(9):1843–9. Epub 2005/03/18.10.1002/cncr.20998

[53] Rischin D, Young RJ, Fisher R, Fox SB, Le QT, Peters LJ, et al. Prognostic significance of p16INK4A and human papillomavirus in patients with oropharyngeal cancer treated on TROG 02.02 phase III trial. Journal of Clinical Oncology: Official Journal of the American Society of Clinical Oncology. 2010;28(27):4142–8. Epub 2010/08/11.10.1200/JCO.2010.29.2904

[54] Gillison ML, Broutian T, Pickard RK, Tong ZY, Xiao W, Kahle L, et al. Prevalence of oral HPV infection in the United States, 2009-2010. JAMA. 2012;307(7):693–703. Epub 2012/01/28.10.1001/jama.2012.101

[55] Settle K, Posner MR, Schumaker LM, Tan M, Suntharalingam M, Goloubeva O, et al. Racial survival disparity in head and neck cancer results from low prevalence of human papillomavirus infection in black oropharyngeal cancer patients. Cancer Prevention Research (Phila). 2009;2(9):776–81. Epub 2009/07/31.10.1158/1940-6207.CAPR-09-0149

[56] Weinberger PM, Merkley MA, Khichi SS, Lee JR, Psyrri A, Jackson LL, et al. Human papillomavirus-active head and neck cancer and ethnic health disparities. The Laryngoscope. 2010;120(8):1531–7. Epub 2010/06/22.10.1002/lary.20984

[57] Jemal A, Simard EP, Dorell C, Noone AM, Markowitz LE, Kohler B, et al. Annual Report to the Nation on the Status of Cancer, 1975-2009, featuring the burden and trends in human papillomavirus (HPV)-associated cancers and HPV vaccination coverage levels. Journal of the National Cancer Institute. 2013;105(3):175–201. Epub 2013/01/09.10.1093/jnci/djs491

[58] Bouvard V, Baan R, Straif K, Grosse Y, Secretan B, El Ghissassi F, et al. A review of human carcinogens – part B: biological agents. The Lancet Oncology. 2009;10(4):321–2. Epub 2009/04/08.

[59] Stransky N, Egloff AM, Tward AD, Kostic AD, Cibulskis K, Sivachenko A, et al. The mutational landscape of head and neck squamous cell carcinoma. Science. 2011;333(6046):1157–60. Epub 2011/07/30.10.1126/science.1208130

[60] Glombitza F, Guntinas-Lichius O, Petersen I. HPV status in head and neck tumors. Pathology, Research and Practice. 2010;206(4):229–34. Epub 2010/02/09.10.1016/j.prp.2009.11.007

[61] Deng Z, Hasegawa M, Yamashita Y, Matayoshi S, Kiyuna A, Agena S, et al. Prognostic value of human papillomavirus and squamous cell carcinoma antigen in head and neck squamous cell carcinoma. Cancer Science. 2012;103(12):2127–34. Epub 2012/09/04.10.1111/cas.12009

[62] D'Souza G, Gross ND, Pai SI, Haddad R, Anderson KS, Rajan S, et al. Oral human papillomavirus (HPV) infection in HPV-positive patients with oropharyngeal cancer and their partners. Journal of Clinical Oncology: Official Journal of the American Society of Clinical Oncology. 2014;32(23):2408–15. Epub 2014/04/30.10.1200/JCO.2014.55.1341

[63] Gillison ML, Koch WM, Capone RB, Spafford M, Westra WH, Wu L, et al. Evidence for a causal association between human papillomavirus and a subset of head and neck cancers. Journal of the National Cancer Institute. 2000;92(9):709–20. Epub 2000/05/04.

[64] Jay N, Moscicki AB. Human papillomavirus infections in women with HIV disease: prevalence, risk, and management. The AIDS Reader. 2000;10(11):659–68. Epub 2001/02/24.

[65] Cates W, Jr. Estimates of the incidence and prevalence of sexually transmitted diseases in the United States. American Social Health Association Panel. Sexually Transmitted Diseases. 1999;26(4 Suppl.):S2–7. Epub 1999/05/05.

[66] Westra WH. The changing face of head and neck cancer in the 21st century: the impact of HPV on the epidemiology and pathology of oral cancer. Head and Neck Pathology. 2009;3(1):78–81. Epub 2009/03/01.10.1007/s12105-009-0100-y

[67] Herrero R, Castellsague X, Pawlita M, Lissowska J, Kee F, Balaram P, et al. Human papillomavirus and oral cancer: the International Agency for Research on Cancer multicenter study. Journal of the National Cancer Institute. 2003;95(23):1772–83. Epub 2003/12/05.

[68] Anaya-Saavedra G, Ramirez-Amador V, Irigoyen-Camacho ME, Garcia-Cuellar CM, Guido-Jimenez M, Mendez-Martinez R, et al. High association of human papillomavirus infection with oral cancer: a case-control study. Archives of Medical Research. 2008;39(2):189–97. Epub 2008/01/01.10.1016/j.arcmed.2007.08.003

[69] D'Souza G, Agrawal Y, Halpern J, Bodison S, Gillison ML. Oral sexual behaviors associated with prevalent oral human papillomavirus infection. The Journal of Infectious Diseases. 2009;199(9):1263–9. Epub 2009/03/27.10.1086/597755

[70] Syrjanen S, Puranen M. Human papillomavirus infections in children: the potential role of maternal transmission. Critical Reviews in Oral Biology and Medicine: An Official Publication of the American Association of Oral Biologists. 2000;11(2):259–74. Epub 2002/05/11.

[71] D'Souza G, Kreimer AR, Viscidi R, Pawlita M, Fakhry C, Koch WM, et al. Case-control study of human papillomavirus and oropharyngeal cancer. The New England Journal of Medicine. 2007;356(19):1944–56. Epub 2007/05/15.10.1056/NEJMoa065497

[72] Turner CF, Danella RD, Rogers SM. Sexual behavior in the United States 1930-1990: trends and methodological problems. Sexually Transmitted Diseases. 1995;22(3):173–90. Epub 1995/05/01.

[73] Bajos N, Bozon M, Beltzer N, Laborde C, Andro A, Ferrand M, et al. Changes in sexual behaviours: from secular trends to public health policies. AIDS. 2010;24(8):1185–91. Epub 2010/03/20.10.1097/QAD.0b013e328336ad52

[74] Gillison ML, Koch WM, Shah KV. Human papillomavirus in head and neck squamous cell carcinoma: are some head and neck cancers a sexually transmitted disease? Current Opinion in Oncology. 1999;11(3):191–9. Epub 1999/05/18.

[75] Garden AS, Kies MS, Morrison WH, Weber RS, Frank SJ, Glisson BS, et al. Outcomes and patterns of care of patients with locally advanced oropharyngeal carcinoma treated in the early 21st century. Radiation Oncology. 2013;8:21. Epub 2013/01/31.10.1186/1748-717X-8-21

[76] Atula TS, Varpula MJ, Kurki TJ, Klemi PJ, Grenman R. Assessment of cervical lymph node status in head and neck cancer patients: palpation, computed tomography and low field magnetic resonance imaging compared with ultrasound-guided fine-needle aspiration cytology. European Journal of Radiology. 1997;25(2):152–61. Epub 1997/09/01.

[77] Compton AM, Moore-Medlin T, Herman-Ferdinandez L, Clark C, Caldito GC, Wang XI, et al. Human papillomavirus in metastatic lymph nodes from unknown primary head and neck squamous cell carcinoma. Otolaryngology – Head and Neck Surgery:

Official Journal of American Academy of Otolaryngology – Head and Neck Surgery. 2011;145(1):51–7. Epub 2011/04/16.10.1177/0194599811400385

[78] Nishat R, Behura SS, Ramachandra S, Kumar H, Bandyopadhyay A. Human papilloma virus (HPV) induced head & neck squamous cell carcinoma: a comprehensive retrospect. Journal of Clinical and Diagnostic Research. 2015;9(6):ZE01–4. Epub 2015/08/13.10.7860/JCDR/2015/13948.6056

[79] Fischer CA, Kampmann M, Zlobec I, Green E, Tornillo L, Lugli A, et al. p16 expression in oropharyngeal cancer: its impact on staging and prognosis compared with the conventional clinical staging parameters. Annals of Oncology: Official Journal of the European Society for Medical Oncology/ESMO. 2010;21(10):1961–6. Epub 2010/04/29.10.1093/annonc/mdq210

[80] Lewis JS, Jr. p16 Immunohistochemistry as a standalone test for risk stratification in oropharyngeal squamous cell carcinoma. Head and Neck Pathology. 2012;6(Suppl. 1):S75–82. Epub 2012/07/13.10.1007/s12105-012-0369-0

[81] Westra WH. Detection of human papillomavirus (HPV) in clinical samples: evolving methods and strategies for the accurate determination of HPV status of head and neck carcinomas. Oral Oncology. 2014;50(9):771–9. Epub 2014/06/17.10.1016/j.oraloncology.2014.05.004

[82] Shi W, Kato H, Perez-Ordonez B, Pintilie M, Huang S, Hui A, et al. Comparative prognostic value of HPV16 E6 mRNA compared with *in situ* hybridization for human oropharyngeal squamous carcinoma. Journal of Clinical Oncology: Official Journal of the American Society of Clinical Oncology. 2009;27(36):6213–21. Epub 2009/11/04.10.1200/JCO.2009.23.1670

[83] Perrone F, Gloghini A, Cortelazzi B, Bossi P, Licitra L, Pilotti S. Isolating p16-positive/HPV-negative oropharyngeal cancer: an effort worth making. The American Journal of Surgical Pathology. 2011;35(5):774–7; author reply 7–8. Epub 2011/03/26.10.1097/PAS.0b013e3182116a45

[84] Pannone G, Rodolico V, Santoro A, Lo Muzio L, Franco R, Botti G, et al. Evaluation of a combined triple method to detect causative HPV in oral and oropharyngeal squamous cell carcinomas: p16 immunohistochemistry, consensus PCR HPV-DNA, and *in situ* hybridization. Infectious Agents and Cancer. 2012;7:4. Epub 2012/03/02.10.1186/1750-9378-7-4

[85] Cameron JE, Snowhite IV, Chaturvedi AK, Hagensee ME. Human papillomavirus-specific antibody status in oral fluids modestly reflects serum status in human immunodeficiency virus-positive individuals. Clinical and Diagnostic Laboratory Immunology. 2003;10(3):431–8. Epub 2003/05/10.

[86] Clavel C, Masure M, Bory JP, Putaud I, Mangeonjean C, Lorenzato M, et al. Hybrid capture II-based human papillomavirus detection, a sensitive test to detect in routine

high-grade cervical lesions: a preliminary study on 1518 women. British Journal of Cancer. 1999;80(9):1306–11. Epub 1999/07/29.10.1038/sj.bjc.6690523

[87] Gravitt PE, Peyton CL, Apple RJ, Wheeler CM. Genotyping of 27 human papillomavirus types by using L1 consensus PCR products by a single-hybridization, reverse line blot detection method. Journal of Clinical Microbiology. 1998;36(10):3020–7. Epub 1998/09/17.

[88] Schmitt M, Bravo IG, Snijders PJ, Gissmann L, Pawlita M, Waterboer T. Bead-based multiplex genotyping of human papillomaviruses. Journal of Clinical Microbiology. 2006;44(2):504–12. Epub 2006/02/04.10.1128/JCM.44.2.504-512.2006

[89] Lindquist D, Romanitan M, Hammarstedt L, Nasman A, Dahlstrand H, Lindholm J, et al. Human papillomavirus is a favourable prognostic factor in tonsillar cancer and its oncogenic role is supported by the expression of E6 and E7. Molecular Oncology. 2007;1(3):350–5. Epub 2007/12/01.10.1016/j.molonc.2007.08.005

[90] Doorbar J, Quint W, Banks L, Bravo IG, Stoler M, Broker TR, et al. The biology and life-cycle of human papillomaviruses. Vaccine. 2012;30(Suppl. 5):F55–70. Epub 2012/12/05.10.1016/j.vaccine.2012.06.083

[91] Munoz N, Bosch FX, de Sanjose S, Herrero R, Castellsague X, Shah KV, et al. Epidemiologic classification of human papillomavirus types associated with cervical cancer. The New England Journal of Medicine. 2003;348(6):518–27. Epub 2003/02/07.10.1056/NEJMoa021641

[92] Kreimer AR, Clifford GM, Boyle P, Franceschi S. Human papillomavirus types in head and neck squamous cell carcinomas worldwide: a systematic review. Cancer Epidemiology, Biomarkers & Prevention. 2005;14(2):467–75. Epub 2005/03/01.10.1158/1055-9965.EPI-04-0551

[93] Ringstrom E, Peters E, Hasegawa M, Posner M, Liu M, Kelsey KT. Human papillomavirus type 16 and squamous cell carcinoma of the head and neck. Clinical Cancer Research: An Official Journal of the American Association for Cancer Research. 2002;8(10):3187–92. Epub 2002/10/11.

[94] McLaughlin-Drubin ME, Munger K. Oncogenic activities of human papillomaviruses. Virus Research. 2009;143(2):195–208. Epub 2009/06/23.10.1016/j.virusres.2009.06.008

[95] Tertipis N, Villabona L, Nordfors C, Nasman A, Ramqvist T, Vlastos A, et al. HLA-A*02 in relation to outcome in human papillomavirus positive tonsillar and base of tongue cancer. Anticancer Research. 2014;34(5):2369–75. Epub 2014/04/30.

[96] Nordfors C, Grun N, Tertipis N, Ahrlund-Richter A, Haeggblom L, Sivars L, et al. CD8+ and CD4+ tumour infiltrating lymphocytes in relation to human papillomavirus status and clinical outcome in tonsillar and base of tongue squamous cell carcinoma. European Journal of Cancer. 2013;49(11):2522–30. Epub 2013/04/11.10.1016/j.ejca.2013.03.019

[97] Lyford-Pike S, Peng S, Young GD, Taube JM, Westra WH, Akpeng B, et al. Evidence for a role of the PD-1:PD-L1 pathway in immune resistance of HPV-associated head

and neck squamous cell carcinoma. Cancer Research. 2013;73(6):1733–41. Epub 2013/01/05.10.1158/0008-5472.CAN-12-2384

[98] Doorbar J. The papillomavirus life cycle. Journal of Clinical Virology: The Official Publication of the Pan American Society for Clinical Virology. 2005;32(Suppl. 1):S7–15. Epub 2005/03/09.10.1016/j.jcv.2004.12.006

[99] Chow LT, Broker TR, Steinberg BM. The natural history of human papillomavirus infections of the mucosal epithelia. Acta Pathologica, Microbiologica, et Immunologica Scandinavica. 2010;118(6–7):422–49. Epub 2010/06/18.10.1111/j.1600-0463.2010.02625.x

[100] Cheng S, Schmidt-Grimminger DC, Murant T, Broker TR, Chow LT. Differentiation-dependent up-regulation of the human papillomavirus E7 gene reactivates cellular DNA replication in suprabasal differentiated keratinocytes. Genes & Development. 1995;9(19):2335–49. Epub 1995/10/01.

[101] Scheffner M, Werness BA, Huibregtse JM, Levine AJ, Howley PM. The E6 oncoprotein encoded by human papillomavirus types 16 and 18 promotes the degradation of p53. Cell. 1990;63(6):1129–36. Epub 1990/12/21.

[102] Munger K, Werness BA, Dyson N, Phelps WC, Harlow E, Howley PM. Complex formation of human papillomavirus E7 proteins with the retinoblastoma tumor suppressor gene product. The EMBO Journal. 1989;8(13):4099–105. Epub 1989/12/20.

[103] DiMaio D, Mattoon D. Mechanisms of cell transformation by papillomavirus E5 proteins. Oncogene. 2001;20(54):7866–73. Epub 2001/12/26.10.1038/sj.onc.1204915

[104] Rampias T, Sasaki C, Weinberger P, Psyrri A. E6 and e7 gene silencing and transformed phenotype of human papillomavirus 16-positive oropharyngeal cancer cells. Journal of the National Cancer Institute. 2009;101(6):412–23. Epub 2009/03/12.10.1093/jnci/djp017

[105] Indovina P, Marcelli E, Casini N, Rizzo V, Giordano A. Emerging roles of RB family: new defense mechanisms against tumor progression. Journal of Cellular Physiology. 2013;228(3):525–35. Epub 2012/08/14.10.1002/jcp.24170

[106] Strati K, Lambert PF. Role of Rb-dependent and Rb-independent functions of papillomavirus E7 oncogene in head and neck cancer. Cancer Research. 2007;67(24):11585–93. Epub 2007/12/20.10.1158/0008-5472.CAN-07-3007

[107] Khleif SN, DeGregori J, Yee CL, Otterson GA, Kaye FJ, Nevins JR, et al. Inhibition of cyclin D-CDK4/CDK6 activity is associated with an E2F-mediated induction of cyclin kinase inhibitor activity. Proceedings of the National Academy of Sciences of the United States of America. 1996;93(9):4350–4. Epub 1996/04/30.

[108] Klaes R, Friedrich T, Spitkovsky D, Ridder R, Rudy W, Petry U, et al. Overexpression of p16(INK4A) as a specific marker for dysplastic and neoplastic epithelial cells of the cervix uteri. International Journal of Cancer. 2001;92(2):276–84. Epub 2001/04/06.

[109] Brehm A, Nielsen SJ, Miska EA, McCance DJ, Reid JL, Bannister AJ, et al. The E7 oncoprotein associates with Mi2 and histone deacetylase activity to promote cell growth. The EMBO Journal. 1999;18(9):2449–58. Epub 1999/05/06.10.1093/emboj/18.9.2449

[110] Kessis TD, Slebos RJ, Nelson WG, Kastan MB, Plunkett BS, Han SM, et al. Human papillomavirus 16 E6 expression disrupts the p53-mediated cellular response to DNA damage. Proceedings of the National Academy of Sciences of the United States of America. 1993;90(9):3988–92. Epub 1993/05/01.

[111] Patel D, Huang SM, Baglia LA, McCance DJ. The E6 protein of human papillomavirus type 16 binds to and inhibits co-activation by CBP and p300. The EMBO Journal. 1999;18(18):5061–72. Epub 1999/09/16.10.1093/emboj/18.18.5061

[112] Kumar A, Zhao Y, Meng G, Zeng M, Srinivasan S, Delmolino LM, et al. Human papillomavirus oncoprotein E6 inactivates the transcriptional coactivator human ADA3. Molecular and Cellular Biology. 2002;22(16):5801–12. Epub 2002/07/26.

[113] Yamada T, Yamashita T, Nishikawa T, Fujimoto S, Fujinaga K. Biologic activity of human papillomavirus type 16 E6/E7 cDNA clones isolated from SiHa cervical carcinoma cell line. Virus Genes. 1995;10(1):15–25. Epub 1995/01/01.

[114] James MA, Lee JH, Klingelhutz AJ. HPV16-E6 associated hTERT promoter acetylation is E6AP dependent, increased in later passage cells and enhanced by loss of p300. International Journal of Cancer. 2006;119(8):1878–85. Epub 2006/05/19.10.1002/ijc.22064

[115] Pillai MR, Nair MK. Development of a condemned mucosa syndrome and pathogenesis of human papillomavirus-associated upper aerodigestive tract and uterine cervical tumors. Experimental and Molecular Pathology. 2000;69(3):233–41. Epub 2000/12/15.10.1006/exmp.2000.2335

[116] Fan X, Liu Y, Heilman SA, Chen JJ. Human papillomavirus E7 induces rereplication in response to DNA damage. Journal of Virology. 2013;87(2):1200–10. Epub 2012/11/16.10.1128/JVI.02038-12

[117] Agrawal N, Frederick MJ, Pickering CR, Bettegowda C, Chang K, Li RJ, et al. Exome sequencing of head and neck squamous cell carcinoma reveals inactivating mutations in NOTCH1. Science. 2011;333(6046):1154–7. Epub 2011/07/30.10.1126/science.1206923

[118] Duensing S, Lee LY, Duensing A, Basile J, Piboonniyom S, Gonzalez S, et al. The human papillomavirus type 16 E6 and E7 oncoproteins cooperate to induce mitotic defects and genomic instability by uncoupling centrosome duplication from the cell division cycle. Proceedings of the National Academy of Sciences of the United States of America. 2000;97(18):10002–7. Epub 2000/08/16.10.1073/pnas.170093297

[119] Duensing A, Liu Y, Tseng M, Malumbres M, Barbacid M, Duensing S. Cyclin-dependent kinase 2 is dispensable for normal centrosome duplication but required for

oncogene-induced centrosome overduplication. Oncogene. 2006;25(20):2943–9. Epub 2005/12/07.10.1038/sj.onc.1209310

[120] Finzer P, Aguilar-Lemarroy A, Rosl F. The role of human papillomavirus oncoproteins E6 and E7 in apoptosis. Cancer Letters. 2002;188(1–2):15–24. Epub 2002/10/31.

[121] Kumar B, Cordell KG, Lee JS, Worden FP, Prince ME, Tran HH, et al. EGFR, p16, HPV Titer, Bcl-xL and p53, sex, and smoking as indicators of response to therapy and survival in oropharyngeal cancer. Journal of Clinical Oncology: Official Journal of the American Society of Clinical Oncology. 2008;26(19):3128–37. Epub 2008/05/14.10.1200/JCO.2007.12.7662

[122] Licitra L, Perrone F, Bossi P, Suardi S, Mariani L, Artusi R, et al. High-risk human papillomavirus affects prognosis in patients with surgically treated oropharyngeal squamous cell carcinoma. Journal of Clinical Oncology: Official Journal of the American Society of Clinical Oncology. 2006;24(36):5630–6. Epub 2006/12/21.10.1200/JCO.2005.04.6136

[123] Braakhuis BJ, Snijders PJ, Keune WJ, Meijer CJ, Ruijter-Schippers HJ, Leemans CR, et al. Genetic patterns in head and neck cancers that contain or lack transcriptionally active human papillomavirus. Journal of the National Cancer Institute. 2004;96(13):998–1006. Epub 2004/07/09.

[124] O'Sullivan B, Huang SH, Siu LL, Waldron J, Zhao H, Perez-Ordonez B, et al. Deintensification candidate subgroups in human papillomavirus-related oropharyngeal cancer according to minimal risk of distant metastasis. Journal of Clinical Oncology: Official Journal of the American Society of Clinical Oncology. 2013;31(5):543–50. Epub 2013/01/09.10.1200/JCO.2012.44.0164

[125] O'Rorke MA, Ellison MV, Murray LJ, Moran M, James J, Anderson LA. Human papillomavirus related head and neck cancer survival: a systematic review and meta-analysis. Oral Oncology. 2012;48(12):1191–201. Epub 2012/07/31.10.1016/j.oraloncology.2012.06.019

[126] Hanahan D, Weinberg RA. Hallmarks of cancer: the next generation. Cell. 2011;144(5):646–74. Epub 2011/03/08.10.1016/j.cell.2011.02.013

[127] Spanos WC, Nowicki P, Lee DW, Hoover A, Hostager B, Gupta A, et al. Immune response during therapy with cisplatin or radiation for human papillomavirus-related head and neck cancer. Archives of Otolaryngology – Head & Neck Surgery. 2009;135(11):1137–46. Epub 2009/11/18.10.1001/archoto.2009.159

[128] Heusinkveld M, Goedemans R, Briet RJ, Gelderblom H, Nortier JW, Gorter A, et al. Systemic and local human papillomavirus 16-specific T-cell immunity in patients with head and neck cancer. International Journal of Cancer. 2012;131(2):E74–85. Epub 2011/10/25.10.1002/ijc.26497

[129] Turksma AW, Bontkes HJ, van den Heuvel H, de Gruijl TD, von Blomberg BM, Braakhuis BJ, et al. Effector memory T-cell frequencies in relation to tumour stage,

location and HPV status in HNSCC patients. Oral Diseases. 2013;19(6):577–84. Epub 2012/11/28.10.1111/odi.12037

[130] Badoual C, Hans S, Merillon N, Van Ryswick C, Ravel P, Benhamouda N, et al. PD-1-expressing tumor-infiltrating T cells are a favorable prognostic biomarker in HPV-associated head and neck cancer. Cancer Research. 2013;73(1):128–38. Epub 2012/11/09.10.1158/0008-5472.CAN-12-2606

[131] Vermeer DW, Spanos WC, Vermeer PD, Bruns AM, Lee KM, Lee JH. Radiation-induced loss of cell surface CD47 enhances immune-mediated clearance of human papillomavirus-positive cancer. International Journal of Cancer. 2013;133(1):120–9. Epub 2013/01/08.10.1002/ijc.28015

[132] Yoshimura M, Itasaka S, Harada H, Hiraoka M. Microenvironment and radiation therapy. BioMed Research International. 2013;2013:685308. Epub 2013/03/20.10.1155/2013/685308

[133] Overgaard J, Eriksen JG, Nordsmark M, Alsner J, Horsman MR. Plasma osteopontin, hypoxia, and response to the hypoxia sensitiser nimorazole in radiotherapy of head and neck cancer: results from the DAHANCA 5 randomised double-blind placebo-controlled trial. The Lancet Oncology. 2005;6(10):757–64. Epub 2005/10/04.10.1016/S1470-2045(05)70292-8

[134] Kong CS, Narasimhan B, Cao H, Kwok S, Erickson JP, Koong A, et al. The relationship between human papillomavirus status and other molecular prognostic markers in head and neck squamous cell carcinomas. International Journal of Radiation Oncology, Biology, Physics. 2009;74(2):553–61. Epub 2009/05/12.10.1016/j.ijrobp.2009.02.015

[135] Lassen P, Eriksen JG, Hamilton-Dutoit S, Tramm T, Alsner J, Overgaard J. HPV-associated p16-expression and response to hypoxic modification of radiotherapy in head and neck cancer. Radiotherapy and Oncology: Journal of the European Society for Therapeutic Radiology and Oncology. 2010;94(1):30–5. Epub 2009/11/17.10.1016/j.radonc.2009.10.008

[136] Mortensen LS, Johansen J, Kallehauge J, Primdahl H, Busk M, Lassen P, et al. FAZA PET/CT hypoxia imaging in patients with squamous cell carcinoma of the head and neck treated with radiotherapy: results from the DAHANCA 24 trial. Radiotherapy and Oncology: Journal of the European Society for Therapeutic Radiology and Oncology. 2012;105(1):14–20. Epub 2012/10/23.10.1016/j.radonc.2012.09.015

[137] Jansen JF, Carlson DL, Lu Y, Stambuk HE, Moreira AL, Singh B, et al. Correlation of a priori DCE-MRI and (1)H-MRS data with molecular markers in neck nodal metastases: Initial analysis. Oral Oncology. 2012;48(8):717–22. Epub 2012/03/01.10.1016/j.oraloncology.2012.02.001

[138] Sorensen BS, Busk M, Olthof N, Speel EJ, Horsman MR, Alsner J, et al. Radiosensitivity and effect of hypoxia in HPV positive head and neck cancer cells. Radiotherapy and

Oncology: Journal of the European Society for Therapeutic Radiology and Oncology. 2013;108(3):500–5. Epub 2013/08/21.10.1016/j.radonc.2013.06.011

[139] Kimple RJ, Smith MA, Blitzer GC, Torres AD, Martin JA, Yang RZ, et al. Enhanced radiation sensitivity in HPV-positive head and neck cancer. Cancer Research. 2013;73(15):4791–800. Epub 2013/06/12.10.1158/0008-5472.CAN-13-0587

[140] Rieckmann T, Tribius S, Grob TJ, Meyer F, Busch CJ, Petersen C, et al. HNSCC cell lines positive for HPV and p16 possess higher cellular radiosensitivity due to an impaired DSB repair capacity. Radiotherapy and Oncology: Journal of the European Society for Therapeutic Radiology and Oncology. 2013;107(2):242–6. Epub 2013/04/23.10.1016/j.radonc.2013.03.013

[141] Goon PK, Stanley MA, Ebmeyer J, Steinstrasser L, Upile T, Jerjes W, et al. HPV & head and neck cancer: a descriptive update. Head & Neck Oncology. 2009;1:36. Epub 2009/10/16.10.1186/1758-3284-1-36

[142] Portugal LG, Goldenberg JD, Wenig BL, Ferrer KT, Nodzenski E, Sabnani JB, et al. Human papillomavirus expression and p53 gene mutations in squamous cell carcinoma. Archives of Otolaryngology – Head & Neck Surgery. 1997;123(11):1230–4. Epub 1997/11/21.

[143] Andl T, Kahn T, Pfuhl A, Nicola T, Erber R, Conradt C, et al. Etiological involvement of oncogenic human papillomavirus in tonsillar squamous cell carcinomas lacking retinoblastoma cell cycle control. Cancer Research. 1998;58(1):5–13. Epub 1998/01/13.

[144] Mellin H, Friesland S, Lewensohn R, Dalianis T, Munck-Wikland E. Human papillomavirus (HPV) DNA in tonsillar cancer: clinical correlates, risk of relapse, and survival. International Journal of Cancer. 2000;89(3):300–4. Epub 2000/06/22.

[145] Ragin CC, Taioli E. Survival of squamous cell carcinoma of the head and neck in relation to human papillomavirus infection: review and meta-analysis. International Journal of Cancer. 2007;121(8):1813–20. Epub 2007/06/05.10.1002/ijc.22851

[146] Lassen P, Eriksen JG, Hamilton-Dutoit S, Tramm T, Alsner J, Overgaard J. Effect of HPV-associated p16INK4A expression on response to radiotherapy and survival in squamous cell carcinoma of the head and neck. Journal of Clinical Oncology: Official Journal of the American Society of Clinical Oncology. 2009;27(12):1992–8. Epub 2009/03/18.10.1200/JCO.2008.20.2853

[147] Worden FP, Kumar B, Lee JS, Wolf GT, Cordell KG, Taylor JM, et al. Chemoselection as a strategy for organ preservation in advanced oropharynx cancer: response and survival positively associated with HPV16 copy number. Journal of Clinical Oncology: Official Journal of the American Society of Clinical Oncology. 2008;26(19):3138–46. Epub 2008/05/14.10.1200/JCO.2007.12.7597

[148] Rich JT, Milov S, Lewis JS, Jr., Thorstad WL, Adkins DR, Haughey BH. Transoral laser microsurgery (TLM) +/- adjuvant therapy for advanced stage oropharyngeal cancer:

outcomes and prognostic factors. The Laryngoscope. 2009;119(9):1709–19. Epub 2009/07/03.10.1002/lary.20552

[149] Gillison ML, Zhang Q, Ang K, Fu KK, Hammond ME, Jordan R, Trotti A, Spencer S, Rotman M, Chung CH. Analysis of the effect of p16 and tobacco packyears (p-y) on overall (OS) and progression-free survival (PFS) for patients with oropharynx cancer (OPC) in Radiation Therapy Oncology Group (RTOG) protocol 9003. Journal of Clinical Oncology: Official Journal of the American Society of Clinical Oncology. 2010;28:abstract 5510.

[150] Fakhry C, Zhang Q, Nguyen-Tan PF, Rosenthal D, El-Naggar A, Garden AS, et al. Human papillomavirus and overall survival after progression of oropharyngeal squamous cell carcinoma. Journal of Clinical Oncology: Official Journal of the American Society of Clinical Oncology. 2014;32(30):3365–73. Epub 2014/06/25.10.1200/JCO.2014.55.1937

[151] Rosenthal DI, Harari P, Giralt J, Bell D, Raben D, Liu J, Schulten J, Ang KK, Bonner JA. Impact of p16 status on the results of the phase III cetuximab (cet)/radiotherapy (RT). Journal of Clinical Oncology: Official Journal of the American Society of Clinical Oncology. 2014;32:abstract 6001.

[152] Masterson L, Moualed D, Liu ZW, Howard JE, Dwivedi RC, Tysome JR, et al. De-escalation treatment protocols for human papillomavirus-associated oropharyngeal squamous cell carcinoma: a systematic review and meta-analysis of current clinical trials. European Journal of Cancer. 2014;50(15):2636–48. Epub 2014/08/06.10.1016/j.ejca.2014.07.001

[153] Goldenberg D, Begum S, Westra WH, Khan Z, Sciubba J, Pai SI, et al. Cystic lymph node metastasis in patients with head and neck cancer: an HPV-associated phenomenon. Head & Neck. 2008;30(7):898–903. Epub 2008/04/03.10.1002/hed.20796

[154] Huang SH, O'Sullivan B, Xu W, Zhao H, Chen DD, Ringash J, et al. Temporal nodal regression and regional control after primary radiation therapy for N2-N3 head-and-neck cancer stratified by HPV status. International Journal of Radiation Oncology, Biology, Physics. 2013;87(5):1078–85. Epub 2013/11/12.10.1016/j.ijrobp.2013.08.049

[155] Huang SH, Perez-Ordonez B, Weinreb I, Hope A, Massey C, Waldron JN, et al. Natural course of distant metastases following radiotherapy or chemoradiotherapy in HPV-related oropharyngeal cancer. Oral Oncology. 2013;49(1):79–85. Epub 2012/08/25.10.1016/j.oraloncology.2012.07.015

[156] Huang SH, Perez-Ordonez B, Liu FF, Waldron J, Ringash J, Irish J, et al. Atypical clinical behavior of p16-confirmed HPV-related oropharyngeal squamous cell carcinoma treated with radical radiotherapy. International Journal of Radiation Oncology, Biology, Physics. 2012;82(1):276–83. Epub 2010/10/19.10.1016/j.ijrobp.2010.08.031

[157] O'Sullivan B, Huang SH, Perez-Ordonez B, Massey C, Siu LL, Weinreb I, et al. Outcomes of HPV-related oropharyngeal cancer patients treated by radiotherapy alone

using altered fractionation. Radiotherapy and Oncology: Journal of the European Society for Therapeutic Radiology and Oncology. 2012;103(1):49–56. Epub 2012/03/14.10.1016/j.radonc.2012.02.009

[158] McBride SM, Busse PM, Clark JR, Wirth LJ, Ancukiewicz M, Chan AW. Long-term survival after distant metastasis in patients with oropharyngeal cancer. Oral Oncology. 2014;50(3):208–12. Epub 2014/01/07.10.1016/j.oraloncology.2013.10.020

[159] Vermorken JB, Psyrri A, Mesia R, Peyrade F, Beier F, de Blas B, et al. Impact of tumor HPV status on outcome in patients with recurrent and/or metastatic squamous cell carcinoma of the head and neck receiving chemotherapy with or without cetuximab: retrospective analysis of the phase III EXTREME trial. Annals of Oncology: Official Journal of the European Society for Medical Oncology/ESMO. 2014;25(4):801–7. Epub 2014/03/01.10.1093/annonc/mdt574

[160] Mehra R. Analysis of HPV and ERCC1 in recurrent or metastatic squamous cell carcinoma of the head and neck (R/M SCCHN). Journal of Clinical Oncology: Official Journal of the American Society of Clinical Oncology. 2013;31:abstract 6006.

[161] Gillison ML, Zhang Q, Jordan R, Xiao W, Westra WH, Trotti A, et al. Tobacco smoking and increased risk of death and progression for patients with p16-positive and p16-negative oropharyngeal cancer. Journal of Clinical Oncology: Official Journal of the American Society of Clinical Oncology. 2012;30(17):2102–11. Epub 2012/05/09.10.1200/JCO.2011.38.4099

[162] Massano J, Regateiro FS, Januario G, Ferreira A. Oral squamous cell carcinoma: review of prognostic and predictive factors. Oral Surgery, Oral Medicine, Oral Pathology, Oral Radiology, and Endodontics. 2006;102(1):67–76. Epub 2006/07/13.10.1016/j.tripleo.2005.07.038

[163] Jadhav KB, Gupta N. Clinicopathological prognostic implicators of oral squamous cell carcinoma: need to understand and revise. North American Journal of Medical Sciences. 2013;5(12):671–9. Epub 2014/01/10.10.4103/1947-2714.123239

[164] Nasman A, Andersson E, Nordfors C, Grun N, Johansson H, Munck-Wikland E, et al. MHC class I expression in HPV positive and negative tonsillar squamous cell carcinoma in correlation to clinical outcome. International Journal of Cancer. 2013;132(1):72–81. Epub 2012/05/18.10.1002/ijc.27635

[165] Lindquist D, Ahrlund-Richter A, Tarjan M, Tot T, Dalianis T. Intense CD44 expression is a negative prognostic factor in tonsillar and base of tongue cancer. Anticancer Research. 2012;32(1):153–61. Epub 2012/01/04.

[166] Rietbergen MM, Martens-de Kemp SR, Bloemena E, Witte BI, Brink A, Baatenburg de Jong RJ, et al. Cancer stem cell enrichment marker CD98: a prognostic factor for survival in patients with human papillomavirus-positive oropharyngeal cancer. European Journal of Cancer. 2014;50(4):765–73. Epub 2013/12/10.10.1016/j.ejca.2013.11.010

[167] Nasman A, Romanitan M, Nordfors C, Grun N, Johansson H, Hammarstedt L, et al. Tumor infiltrating CD8+ and Foxp3+ lymphocytes correlate to clinical outcome and human papillomavirus (HPV) status in tonsillar cancer. PLoS One. 2012;7(6):e38711. Epub 2012/06/16.10.1371/journal.pone.0038711

[168] Liang C, Marsit CJ, McClean MD, Nelson HH, Christensen BC, Haddad RI, et al. Biomarkers of HPV in head and neck squamous cell carcinoma. Cancer Research. 2012;72(19):5004–13. Epub 2012/09/20.10.1158/0008-5472.CAN-11-3277

[169] Cohen MA, Basha SR, Reichenbach DK, Robertson E, Sewell DA. Increased viral load correlates with improved survival in HPV-16-associated tonsil carcinoma patients. Acta Oto-Laryngologica. 2008;128(5):583–9. Epub 2008/04/19.10.1080/00016480701558880

[170] Weinberger PM, Yu Z, Haffty BG, Kowalski D, Harigopal M, Brandsma J, et al. Molecular classification identifies a subset of human papillomavirus--associated oropharyngeal cancers with favorable prognosis. Journal of Clinical Oncology: Official Journal of the American Society of Clinical Oncology. 2006;24(5):736–47. Epub 2006/01/13.10.1200/JCO.2004.00.3335

[171] Bossi P, Orlandi E, Miceli R, Perrone F, Guzzo M, Mariani L, et al. Treatment-related outcome of oropharyngeal cancer patients differentiated by HPV dictated risk profile: a tertiary cancer centre series analysis. Annals of Oncology: Official Journal of the European Society for Medical Oncology/ESMO. 2014;25(3):694–9. Epub 2014/02/11.10.1093/annonc/mdu004

[172] Dempsey AF, Patel DA. HPV vaccine acceptance, utilization and expected impacts in the U.S.: Where are we now? Human Vaccines. 2010;6(9):715–720. Epub 2010/09/22.10.4161/hv.6.9.12730

[173] Herrero R, Quint W, Hildesheim A, Gonzalez P, Struijk L, Katki HA, et al. Reduced prevalence of oral human papillomavirus (HPV) 4 years after bivalent HPV vaccination in a randomized clinical trial in Costa Rica. PLoS One. 2013;8(7):e68329. Epub 2013/07/23.10.1371/journal.pone.0068329

6

Cervical Cancer Screening at a Crossroads: Learnings from the Past Driving Change for the Future

Laurence M. Vaughan, Brian R. Faherty,
Erin C. Gutierrez, James M. Harris,
William A. Nussbaumer and Ryan J. Schwab

Abstract

Cervical cancer screening has been one of the most impactful human interventions in medical history, saving the lives of countless thousands of women since the introduction of organized cytology screening programs. Today, we stand at a crossroads in the fight against cervical cancer, with several countries actively engaged in introducing primary human papillomavirus (HPV) testing and vaccination as more effective means of prevention. This chapter discusses the history of organized screening and how this led to HPV test methods to detect cervical cancer. We go on to examine the technologies used to screen for high-risk HPV types and how they affect clinical performance. We examine the evidence for primary HPV screening and review recent self-collection initiatives to reach underserved women, including the use of urine as novel sample type. In addition, we critically examine the evolution of HPV test methods and make the case for the use of extended genotyping as an improved risk stratification tool for guiding clinical management. Finally, we look to the future of cervical cancer screening and consider options for future management programs.

Keywords: genotyping, HPV screening tests/strategies, Pap, risk stratification, self-sampling

1. Introduction

Cervical cancer screening has advanced considerably since the introduction of the Pap smear in the 1960s: organized cytology screening programs have successfully reduced the burden of disease associated with human papillomavirus (HPV) and sensitive new molecular methods have been developed to detect the virus. Perhaps more importantly, safe and efficacious HPV vaccines are now widely available and offer the prospect of greatly reducing the incidence of cervical cancer if sufficient numbers of the target population can be vaccinated. Vaccines offer the best hope for developing countries, which lack the resources to implement an effective screening program. Despite the introduction of vaccination, there is still a need for improved screening modalities as both screening and vaccination will necessarily coexist for some decades to come. It is against this backdrop that we briefly review the history of the Pap smear and the development of organized cytology screening programs and then go on to discuss the development of molecular methods. We discuss the pros and cons of the different molecular assay design approaches and review the case for primary HPV screening. Despite the effective tools at our disposal, reaching underserved women remains the biggest challenge to controlling cervical disease. However, new self-sampling methods offer the prospect of an effective outreach program to reach women most in need. Finally, we discuss the benefits of extended genotyping and how this might influence future screening algorithms. We conclude that the biggest hurdle to preventing and detecting cervical disease may lie in our inability to adapt to change and effectively implement new strategies. This history of cervical cancer screening suggests that the pace of change is slow but we must respond more quickly to the global threat posed by cervical cancer and make efficient use of the tools at our disposal.

2. The history of organized screening programs

George Nicholas Papanicolaou is almost single-handedly credited with developing cervical cancer screening. He was encouraged to leave his native Greece by the renowned geneticist, Thomas Hunt Morgan, who helped him gain a position in the Department of Pathology and Bacteriology at New York Hospital as an assistant, and later at the Department of Anatomy at Cornell Medical School. Dr. Papanicolaou began to study vaginal secretions in women, beginning with a case study of his wife, Mary [1]. Later work led to the observation of cancer cells while studying smears of women in the New York Hospital, which led him to propose that a systematic study of smears could lead to early cancer detection. His "New Cancer Diagnosis" theory was initially very poorly received by his peers [2]. It was not until over 10 years later that a successful collaboration with Herbert Traut (1894–1963), a renowned gynecologist and pathologist at Cornell University, resulted in a more widely received manuscript "The diagnostic value of vaginal smears in carcinoma of the uterus." This work was presented to the New York Gynecological Society in 1941 and published in the prestigious *American Journal of Obstetrics and Gynecology* [3]. In 1947, Dr. Papanicolaou and the head of the Anatomy Department, Dr. Joseph Hinsey, began focusing on training other physicians on the new technique. This led to a gradual adoption of the screening method, and by 1960 it was being adopted across the United States. However, it was not until just before Papanicolaou's death that the impact of his discovery was becoming apparent and he finally began to get the recognition he deserved. Today, he is remembered as "the father of exfoliative cytology" and cervical cytology stands as one of the most successful clinical interventions of the twentieth century. Organized cervical cancer screening has led to an over two-fold reduction in the incidence of cervical cancer in the United States in the period 1975–2012. This success in the United States has been replicated in other countries with organized screening programs such as the United Kingdom, which has seen a similar reduction in mortality from 1985 to 2012. However, over the last decade it has become evident that cytology screening may have reached the limits of its effectiveness in terms of reducing the incidence rate, with both the US and UK trend lines reaching a plateau (**Figure 1**).

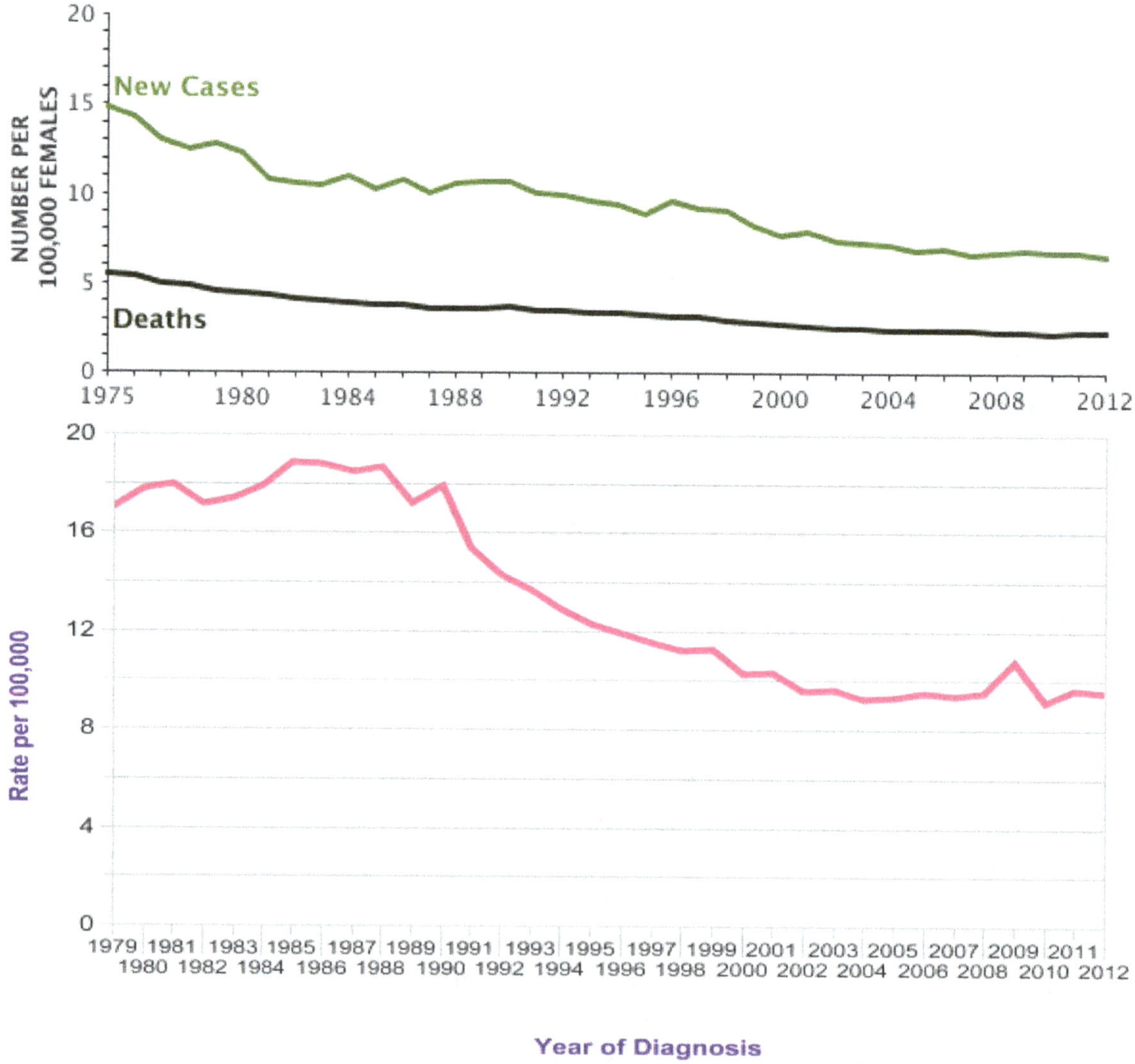

Figure 1. (A) US age-standardized incidence and mortality rates per 100,000 women (1975–2012). Source: http://seer.cancer.gov/statfacts/html/cervix.html (accessed January 2016). (B) United Kingdom age-standardized incidence rates per 100,000 women (1979–2012). Source: Cancer Research UK, http://www.cancerresearchuk.org/health-professional/cancer-statistics/statistics-by-cancer-type/cervical cancer/incidence#heading-Two (accessed January 2016).

3. The development of molecular screening tools

The development of molecular biology techniques in the late 1970s and early 1980s paved the way for the discovery that the HPV was both necessary and responsible for cervical disease. zur Hausen played a pivotal role in establishing the link between papillomaviruses and cervical cancer [4]. As interest intensified, novel HPV types began to be isolated from genital warts (HPV6 [5–7] and laryngeal papillomas (HPV11) [8]). The detection of additional type-specific viral sequences followed: [9, 10], HPV16 [11], HPV18 [12–14], and high-risk types HPV31 and HPV45, which were first described by Lorincz et al. [15] in the United States [16]. These discoveries laid the foundation for the development of cervical cancer diagnostic tests and the development of the first HPV cancer vaccines. Harald zur Hausen went on to win the Nobel Prize in Physiology or Medicine in 2008 for this work on the association of papillomaviruses with human cancers.

While the work of Harald zur Hausen and others set the stage for modern cervical cancer diagnostics, it took another wave of development to advance HPV detection to the point that it could be widely adopted in the clinical laboratory. The early work led to rapid development of basic laboratory tests to detect various HPV types. However, the techniques employed involved the use of ^{32}P-labeled probes that were hybridized using Southern blotting or slot blot methods, which meant they were labor intensive. These early methods (ViraPap and ViraType) were commercialized by Life Technologies Inc. and later sold to the Digene Corporation but they did not achieve widespread adoption, primarily because they did not detect all oncogenic HPV types and also lacked sensitivity. This period also saw the development of *in situ* hybridization (ISH) techniques by Enzo Diagnostics and Life Technologies Inc., and additional methods were later automated by Ventana Medical Systems (now a Roche Company), the Dako Corporation, and others [17]. These tests also suffered from lack of sensitivity [18] and were ultimately not adopted as screening tools. However, ISH methods may prove to be useful in assisting in the diagnosis of Cervical Intraepithelial Neoplasia cases (CIN) [19].

4. The *digene*hybrid capture 2 assay

The Digene Corporation (now part of QIAGEN) under the scientific leadership of another early HPV molecular pioneer, Dr. Attila Lorincz [15, 16], developed the modern market for HPV cervical cancer screening. Lorincz et al. developed a technology called hybrid capture that fused traditional immunoassay techniques with the newer nucleic acid isolation technology [20]. The core principle leveraged the fact that DNA–RNA hybrids have a distinct shape different than a DNA helix that is detectable using antibodies. By generating *in vitro* RNA transcripts of each of the target HPV types and pooling them into a single probe cocktail, the method was capable of detecting as many as 13 high-risk HPV types at once. The capture antibody is bound to a solid surface that binds cognate target hybrids which in turn are then detected using a secondary antibody coupled with alkaline phosphatase using a chemiluminescent substrate. The first generation hybrid capture assay utilized two mixtures of single-stranded RNA probes: one for low-risk HPV types 6, 11, 42, 43, and 44, and one for high-risk

HPV types 16, 18, 31, 33, 35, 45, 51, 52, and 56. The analytic sensitivity of the first generation test was estimated at 50,000 copies of HPV16 DNA [21, 22], and this was not found to be sensitive enough versus polymerase chain reaction (PCR) and histology [23]. Digene researchers then launched a second generation assay (Hybrid Capture 2) whose analytical sensitivity was increased to 1000 HPV DNA copies by the reformulation of hybridization reagents and by the addition of new probes for four high-risk HPV types, 39, 58, 59, and 68. This assay was launched in Europe in 1998 and was subsequently approved by the US Food and Drug Administration (FDA) in 2003, for the triage of Atypical Squamous Cells of Undetermined Significance (ASC-US) cytology patients and as an adjunctive test with cytology for cervical cancer screening [23]. The assay went on to achieve worldwide acceptance and became the *de facto* clinical standard for all subsequent assay development. It has the largest body of clinical evidence supporting its use, and it has been used in numerous clinical trials across the globe [24, 25].

5. PCR- and other amplification-based technologies

The development of PCR technology [26, 27] meant that small quantities of DNA or RNA could now be amplified and detected either directly in endpoint PCR [28] or through the use of accumulating fluorescence that could be monitored continuously in real-time (RT) PCR [29–31]. As with most new techniques, refinements and improvements overcame some of the early difficulties such as assay robustness and the potential for contamination/false positives [32, 33]. The use of PCR to detect HPVs mirrored that of other methods, with HPV initially being detected using gel analysis of PCR products [34] and subsequently using real-time methods [35, 36]. Type-specific primer amplification methods eventually gave way to consensus PCR approaches where multiple HPV types could be detected in one reaction [37]. Most PCR approaches targeted the L1 gene region, and included the MY09–MY11 (MY09/MY11) and GP51–GP61 (GP51/GP61) primer systems. The MY primers were later redesigned to improve performance (PGMY09/PGMY11 [38]) as were the GP primers, to GP5+/GP6+, which were subsequently widely adopted [39, 40]. PCR-based tests are intrinsically more analytically sensitive than Hybrid Capture 2 technology, detecting as little as 10–100 copies of target. However, the Hybrid Capture 2 assay established that approximately 1 pg/ml or 5000 copies of HPV16 target DNA per reaction equated to an actionable clinical result (CIN2+ histology) [41]. Therefore, assays that are clinically more sensitive than this would have poor specificity, referring low level infections unnecessarily to follow colposcopy and possible biopsy or treatment. This has been the subject of discussion in cervical cancer screening since the introduction of highly sensitive molecular methods. Key opinion leaders have cautioned against the use of analytically validated assays whose clinical performance has not been well established in large longitudinal studies, emphasizing the need to strike the proper balance between sensitivity and specificity [42]. In one case, even an FDA approved test was considered clinically unacceptable due to its high HPV positivity [43]. The issue is compounded by the fact that even large reference laboratories and smaller commercial companies cannot afford to fund large studies with a minimum of 3-year follow up of enrolled patients. This led a group of international HPV experts to propose acceptance criteria for HPV tests that wish to be used in primary HPV screening [44]. These criteria, commonly known as "Meijer Criteria" after the lead author, were founded on the principle that "candidate high-risk HPV tests to be used for screening should reach an optimal balance between clinical sensitivity and specificity for detection of high-grade CIN and cervical cancer to minimize redundant or excessive follow-up procedures for high-risk HPV positive women without cervical lesions" and set forth the following guidelines for an acceptable HPV screening test:

1. The sensitivity of the candidate test for ≥CIN2 should be at least 90% of the sensitivity of the HC2 (i.e., relative sensitivity of at least 90%) as assessed by a noninferiority score test.

2. The specificity of the candidate test for ≥CIN2 should be at least 98% of the specificity of HC2.

3. The intralaboratory reproducibility in time and interlaboratory agreement should be determined by evaluation of at least 500 samples, 30% of which tested positive in a reference laboratory using a clinically validated assay. This should result in a percentage of agreement with a lower confidence bound not less than 87% (kappa value of at least 0.5 in this series of samples including 30% positives).

Meijer criteria have been well accepted as a critical litmus test in the absence of large-scale longitudinal trial data and have become a clinical benchmark for validation of tests, especially in the European Union. Despite the use of this leaner approach where the disease samples can be sourced retrospectively, only a small number of existing commercially available assays have actually met the criteria. A 2015 review of currently available commercial assays "identified 193 distinct commercial HPV tests" [45]. However, Arbyn et al. [46], also reported in the same year that only five commercially available tests fully met the Meijer criteria and could be considered suitable for use in primary HPV screening: PapilloCheck® HPV-Screening test; Abbott RealTime hrHPV test; cobas® 4800 HPV test; BD Onclarity™ HPV assay; HPV-Risk assay and the Aptima assay, targeting E6/E7 mRNA. The authors stated that the Cervista® assay should also be added to the list, despite one report of a lack of noninferiority for specificity (see also reference [104]). Three other assays met the sensitivity/specificity criteria but did not disclose accuracy and reproducibility data and were thus considered to partially meet the criteria (an in-house quantitative RT-PCR targeting E6/E7DNAsequences, a GP5+/GP6+ PCR with Luminex identification of high-risk types and a MALDITOF assay). The authors also concluded that the Aptima assay, while fully meeting the criteria, needed further longitudinal validation of its long-term negative predictive value (NPV) because it was an RNA-based assay and to date this had only been established for DNA assays [46].

E6 and E7 gene RNA-based assays have been extensively tested in cervical cancer screening. The impetus for using RNA- versus a DNA-based targets, is likely based on the observation that both the E6 and E7 genes encode oncogenes that are involved in the development of cancer and are upregulated as disease progresses [47]. E6 and E7 viral oncoproteins bind and modulate cellular gene products (p53 and pRb) that play a key role in cell cycle control and DNA repair. The resulting genomic instability caused by E6 and E7 oncoproteins is a necessary condition for cell transformation and immortalization [48, 49]. Thus, it is reasonable to postulate that an E6/E7 RNA target might offer an advantage over DNA in that it should be overexpressed in high- versus low-grade disease and that it might offer both a sensitivity and specificity advantage. There are two commercially based E6/E7 RNA assays: the Proofer Assay (Norchip, Klokkarstua, Norway) is a real-time multiplex nucleic acid sequence-based amplification assay(NASBA) for isothermal amplification and detection of E6/E7 mRNA from five high-risk oncogenic types, HPV16, 18, 31, 33, and 45, using molecular beacon probes, and the Aptima® HPV Assay (Hologic—GenProbe) that is a qualitative nucleic acid amplification test that detects HPV E6/E7 mRNA from 14 high-risk HPV types [50]. The Aptima assay uses target amplification using transcription-mediated amplification (TMA) [51] and detection of the amplification products (amplicon) by the hybridization protection assay (HPA) [52]. HPV mRNA is captured on magnetic particles and then amplified using TMA that is a transcription-based nucleic acid amplification method that utilizes two enzymes, Moloney Murine Leukemia Virus (MMLV) reverse transcriptase and T7 RNA polymerase. The reverse transcriptase is used to generate a DNA copy of the target mRNA sequence containing a promoter sequence for T7 RNA polymerase. T7 RNA polymerase produces multiple copies of RNA amplicon from the DNA copy template. Detection of the amplicon is achieved by HPA using single-stranded nucleic acid probes with chemiluminescent labels that are complementary to the amplicon. The labeled nucleic acid probes hybridize specifically to the amplicon. The selection reagent differentiates between hybridized and unhybridized probes by inactivating the label on the unhybridized probes. During the detection step, light emitted from the labeled RNA–DNA hybrids is measured as photon signals called relative light units (RLU) in a luminometer. Final assay results are interpreted based on the analyte signal-to-cutoff (S/CO) [53]. The Norchip Proofer assay has been shown to be substantially less sensitive but more specific when compared to other clinically validated assays, including Roche cobas and Hybrid Capture 2 [54–56]. Arbyn et al. [57] performed a meta-analysis of the performance of the Aptima HPV assay versus Hybrid Capture 2 and found that for both triage of ASC-US and Low-Grade Squamous Intraepithelial Lesion (LSIL), Aptima is as sensitive but more specific than HC2 for detecting cervical precancer. In head to head tests, Aptima had a substantially higher sensitivity than Proofer in both a screening and a referral population, but Proofer showed improved specificity [55, 56]. The Aptima test has broader clinical application and relevance because it detects all 14 high-risk types versus just five high-risk types in the Proofer assay. However, as noted above, it needs further confirmation of its long-term NPV over at least a 5-year period, as recommended by Arbyn et al. [46]. A recent report with a 3-year longitudinal follow up found that the NPV is similar to that of Hybrid Capture 2 and again that its specificity was significantly better (96.3% compared with HC2 specificity of 94.8%; $P < 0.001$ [58]. A comprehensive review of the clinical performance of the assay versus HC2 also concluded that the NPV was sufficient to justify a 3-year interval and that the specificity of the assay was consistently higher [59]. The increase in specificity is similar to that previously reported [57] and is relatively modest. It could also result from a slight clinical cut-point bias toward the specificity axis of the receiver operating characteristic (ROC) plot of sensitivity versus 1–specificity for this assay. Whatever the driver, it seems clear that there is no significant difference in sensitivity when comparing RNA- and DNA-based assays and the specificity differences are not as high as one might have predicted from the upregulation of E6/E7 RNA during oncogenesis. The latter may reflect that one does not see the full potential of upregulation when screening for less severe cellular abnormalities versus cancer. The answer may also lie in the observation that neither assay exclusively targets RNA: both assays have been reported to detect cognate DNA sequences present in endocervical specimens at levels where one might expect the DNA signal alone to be sufficient to record a positive clinical result [60, 61]. Thus, it is conceivable that this could render otherwise RNA-negative specimens positive, reducing the specificity of the assay.

6. How target regions impact assay performance

6.1. Which target region to choose?

HPV is double-stranded DNA virus whose circular genome is approximately 8000 base pairs long. It encodes eight open reading frames (ORFs) that are divided into early and late genes (**Figure 2**) involved in replication (i.e., E1 and E2) and packaging (i.e., L1 and L2) with the remaining genes (E6, E7, E5, and E4), playing roles in driving cell cycle entry, immune evasion, and virus release (reviewed in [49]). Papillomaviruses are ancient in origin, believed to have arisen in reptiles approximately 350 million years ago. They have evolved in their various host lineages (including humans) over the millennia and they have relatively stable genomes given their (redundant) double-stranded DNA structure. The rate of nucleotide substitution for HPV18 has been estimated at ~4.5×10^{-7} subs/site/year [62]. This means that assay developers can look across the entire genome for conserved target regions in which to design gene probes.

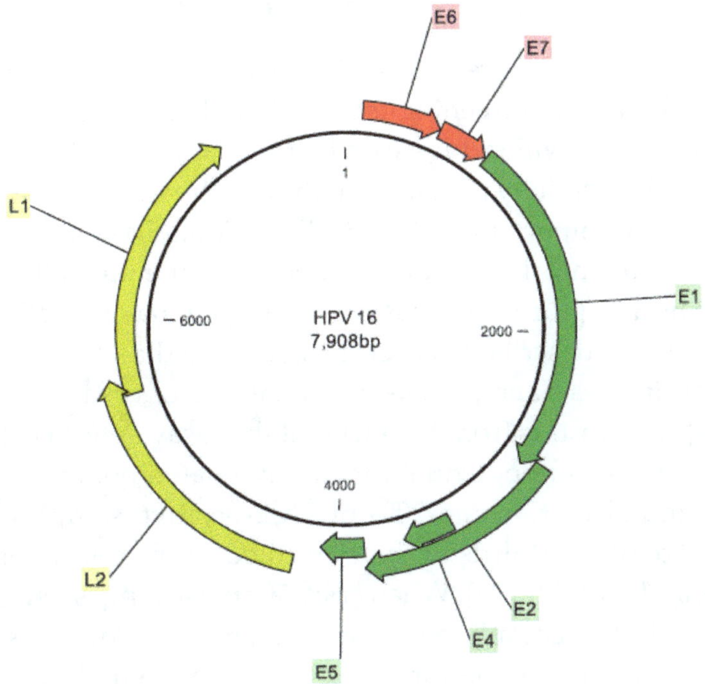

Figure 2. Physical map of the HPV16 genome.

Given the aforementioned large number of commercial assays available on the market, not surprisingly most ORFs have been targeted by one or more assays, including L1 [63], E1 [64], and E6/E7 [65, 66]. However, most commercial assays to date have been developed using the L1 gene as a target region [45, 63], including the Roche cobas assay that has received FDA approval [67].

The question one must then ask is: does it matter which region of the genome you use—are all genomic regions created equal? While a detailed phylogenetic and evolutionary analysis (beyond the scope of the current work) would be required to fully address this question, the following sections discuss some important topics with respect to target analyte performance in clinical diagnostics and how this can influences clinical results.

6.2. Cross-reactivity with nontarget HPV types

There is general agreement that only high-risk types cause cervical cancer and that low-risk types should not be screened for as a part of routine cervical cancer prevention [68]. Previously, there was consensus that 14 high-risk types caused the majority of cancers. However, more recently the evidence for HPV66 in cervical cancers was considered too weak to keep it in the group of 14 high-risk types and it was recommended to remove it [69]. However, all FDA tests approved to date detect HPV66 as part of their 14 high-risk panel (Roche cobas, Hologic-Genprobe Aptima, and Hologic Cervista) and the Hybrid Capture 2 assay detects it via cross-reactivity [70]. In addition, a number of possible/probably carcinogenic types (including HPV66) have been shown to have oncogenic potential and "are biologically active and affect the same cellular pathways as any of the fully recognized carcinogenic HR-HPV types" [71]. Thus, it is difficult to draw an absolute line between known carcinogenic types and those that have that potential but very infrequently result in cancers [69].

Whether you take the view that there are 14 high-risk types or 13 high-risk types (omitting HPV66), there is little doubt that screening for additional HPV types will not increase sensitivity for cancer detection and will reduce specificity. In addition, it may do harm to patients both psychologically and potentially physically if they are treated for lesions that will not result in cancer [68, 72]. Thus, it is important that clinically validated assays perform inclusivity and exclusivity studies to ensure that the assay detects only the intended HPV types for which they have claims. They Hybrid Capture 2 test has been shown to have excellent clinical sensitivity for CIN2+ endpoints and as described earlier, has been used as a clinical benchmark for the last decade. However, it does have a well-documented cross-reactivity with non-high-risk HPV types [70, 73, 74]. This results from the fact that the assay detects the entire HPV genome (**Figure 2**) and thus there is more potential for closely related nononcogenic sequences to be detected. One study found that "some 20% of HC2-positive samples did not contain the targeted HPV types. About two-thirds of them resulted from cross-hybridization, especially with HPV53, HPV66, and HPV70" [75]. When split sample testing is performed with HC2 and a second assay, one typically sees a larger proportion of HC2+/other assay–results which, if they are resolved by third-party genotyping or sequencing method, shows both low-risk and no HPV present results, confirming the negative result as truth with respect to high-risk HPV [66, 76]. In another recent study ($n = 6172$) comparing Roche cobas assay with Hybrid Capture

2, where discordants were resolved using the Roche Linear Array genotyping assay, the authors reported that "HC2+/COBAS– were less likely to contain hrHPV genotypes (12.3 versus 68.9%; $P < 0.0001$) and more likely to contain only lrHPV genotypes (52.8 versus 12.1%; $P < 0.0001$) than those HC2–/COBAS+" and they found "lower CIN2+ rates among women with HC2+/COBAS– results" [77].

The clinical impact of this cross-reactivity has not been widely discussed in the literature. Castle et al. used a more stringent dual reference assay method to determine the level of HC2 cross-reactivity and concluded that about 8% of all HPV positives were due to cross-reactivity with non-high-risk HPV types in the referred (ALTS Study) population. They concluded that cross-reactivity would likely be further reduced in a screening population where there is less overall infection. However, they cautioned that these non-high-risk HPV "cases of CIN2 might be treated by excisional procedures, which can cause iatrogenic morbidity and adversely affect reproductive outcomes" [70]. The previously cited study of Gillio-Tos et al. [75] concluded "If only the samples containing HC2-targeted types tested positive, the positive predictive value (PPV) would have increased from 7.0% (95% CI, 6.1–8.0%) to 8.4% (95% CI, 7.3–9.6%), although 4.9% (95% CI, 2.4–8.8%) of cervical intraepithelial neoplasia grade 2+ (CIN2+) cases would have been missed". Regarding the latter point, "missing" CIN2+ disease caused by non-high-risk HPV types should be the goal of future assays since it has an extremely low risk of resulting in cancer. In summary, there is an 8–20% false-positivity associated with the Hybrid Capture 2 assay that unfortunately is correlated with bona fide abnormal cytology and histology (CIN2+). However, it is important to recognize that since these abnormalities are *not* caused by high-risk HPV types, they have a very low cancer risk and should be managed accordingly. While this phenomenon is well documented, it tends to be largely ignored and considered noise in the overall clinical performance of an assay. It does however have implications for benchmarking studies and in our view should also be taken into account in any future revisions of the Meijer criteria, since it has a direct impact on the maximum sensitivity and specificity of any assay which only detects high-risk HPV.

6.3. L1 consensus-based versus gene-specific PCR approaches

All molecular assays require some sort of amplification technology in order for them to have the required sensitivity to detect small quantities of target nucleic acid. This can take the form of signal amplification such as that described for the Hybrid Capture 2 assay (where the signal rather than the target is amplified using a chemiluminescent substrate), or in the case of the Hologic Cervista assay, where signal amplification is achieved through the use of a unique isothermal Invader® chemistry that leverages a reusable universal flap and fluorescence energy transfer (FRET) to amplify the signal [78, 79] or it can use RNA amplification (Proofer and Aptima assays described earlier) or PCR that accounts for the majority of HPV assays on the market [45]. Traditional PCR methods where the amplicon is detected in a secondary process such as on an agarose gel or via hybridization on strips have gradually been replaced by real-time detection methods for clinical use, although the Roche Linear Array and InnoLIPA line blot assays have remained popular where researchers are interested in determining which genotypes are present in clinical samples or for discordant result analysis [76, 80, 81]. With PCR one can choose to selectively amplify each viral gene target individually (gene-specific PCR) or utilize a consensus (broad spectrum) primer approach. The latter typically uses degenerate primer sequences to detect conserved protein coding regions of multiple HPV types [82]. This has the advantage that multiple (e.g., all high-risk) HPV types can be detected in a single reaction but it means that you can only record a pooled type result, unless you use a secondary method such as a line blot or bead approach to subsequently identify the specific genotypes present [83–85]. Gene-specific detection approaches offer the possibility of direct individual genotype detection but require the use of multiple reactions [86] or the combining of one or more genotypes in different fluorescent channels using real-time PCR technology [66, 87]. **Table 1** lists the major approaches to HPV DNA detection and details some of their advantages and disadvantages. Head to head testing suggests that the top performing assays have broadly similar clinical sensitivity and specificity [55, 56, 88, 89] so clinical laboratories have a choice in the assay they use. The decision on which assay to adopt may be made based on the needs of a particular laboratory. However, it is instructive to consider the following assay characteristics when choosing an HPV test:

Assay name	HPV target region	Nucleic acid type	Consensus or gene-specific	High-risk type coverage	Advantages	Disadvantages	References
QIAGEN Hybrid Capture 2	Entire genome	DNA(signal amplification)	Not applicable	13	Single reaction Clinically validated CE marked/FDA approved	No genotyping or internal control. High level of nontarget cross-reactivity	[41, 70, 75]
PreTect HPV-Proofer	E6/E7	RNA	Gene-specific	5	High specificity CE marked	Low sensitivity Does not detect all cancer-causing types	[55, 56]
Hologic Aptima (screening)	E6/E7	RNA	Gene-specific	14	Single reaction Clinically validated CE marked/FDA approved Fully automated	No genotyping. Sample processing control only	[53, 90]
Hologic Aptima (genotyping)	E6/E7	RNA	Gene-specific	3—HPV16, HPV18+45	Single reaction Clinically validated CE marked/FDA approved Fully automated	Additional test required for limited genotyping Sample processing control only	[91]

Assay name	HPV target region	Nucleic acid type	Consensus or gene-specific	High-risk type coverage	Advantages	Disadvantages	References
Hologic Cervista (screening)	E6/E7/L1	DNA	Gene-specific	14	Single reaction Clinically validated. Internal control CE marked/FDA approved	No genotyping High positivity rate (clinical specificity has been questioned)	[43, 78]
Hologic Cervista (genotyping)	E6/E7/L1	DNA	Gene-specific	2—HPV16, HPV18	Single reaction Clinically validated. Internal control CE marked/FDA approved	Additional test required for limited genotyping Limited genotyping	[79]
Abbott Real-time high-risk HPV	L1	DNA	Consensus	14	Single reaction that includes HPV16/18 genotyping. Internal control Semiautomated, CE marked	Limited genotyping	[92, 93]
Greiner Papillocheck	E1	DNA	Consensus (genotypes resolved using array hybridization)	24—includes 14 high-risk Or 14 high-risk only	Full genotyping CE marked	Labor-intensive workflow requiring three separate rooms	[64, 94]
Sonic Laboratories (formerly RIATOL) E6/E7 real-time PCR test	E6/E7	DNA	Gene-specific	14 + 3 moderate risk types	Full genotyping Partially validated per Meijer criteria Semiautomated	17 individual PCR reactions plus controls required Laboratory developed test (LDT)	[86]
BD Onclarity HPV Assay	E6/E7	DNA	Gene-specific	14	Extended genotyping HPV16, 18, 45, 31, 51, 52 Clinically validated Fully automated CE marked	Three-well assay design reduces throughput	[66, 95, 96]
Cepheid Xpert® HPV	E6/E7	DNA	Gene-specific	14	Single reaction that includes HPV16/18+45 genotyping. Internal control	Limited genotyping capability, Meijer criteria not yet established	[87]

Assay name	HPV target region	Nucleic acid type	Consensus or gene-specific	High-risk type coverage	Advantages	Disadvantages	References
					CE marked		
Roche cobas assay	L1	DNA	Consensus	14	Single reaction that includes HPV16/ HPV18 genotyping. Internal control. Clinically validated CE marked and FDA approved(cotesting and primary screening) Semiautomated	Limited genotyping capability	[72, 97]

Table 1. HPV detection methods.

1. Is the assay and required equipment cost competitive?
2. What level of automation is involved—manual processing, semiautomated, or a fully integrated workflow?
3. What is the time to result and the hands on time of laboratory personnel to run the assay?
4. Is the assay part of a complete offering or does the user have to procure third party equipment or reagents to complement the workflow?
5. Does the assay target only high-risk HPV types?
6. Does the assay provide the required level of genotyping information to assist with informed patient management and risk stratification?
7. Has the assay demonstrated the required ability to accurately diagnose both single and mixed infections?
8. Has the clinical performance of the assay been demonstrated in the intended target population using the specified collection devices and preservative media (sensitivity/ specificity/longitudinal NPV and PPV)?
9. Have the required regulatory approvals and quality requirements for the product been fully met?
10. Has the clinical cutoff of the assay been tested in several different patient populations with different risk profiles to ensure that patients are neither being over-or underreferred for biopsy and treatment?

The first decision one may want to make is whether to choose an assay that targets RNA or DNA. Clinical performance is very similar so it may come down to a practical decision on workflow and laboratory suitability. At the current time, the long-term NPV of DNA-based assays is well established and enshrined in consensus guidelines whereas the evidence for

RNA assays is still accumulating [58, 59, 98]. DNA assays also have the advantage of improved target stability which imposes stricter adherence to laboratory cleaning methods to avoid degrading the more labile RNA targets [53]. As mentioned above, real-time PCR approaches now predominate in the market so one has the choice of either a consensus-based primer design or a gene-specific primer approach (**Table 1**). Consensus approaches yield a pooled high-risk result with HPV16/HPV18 genotype identification from a single well whereas gene-specific approaches can offer more extended genotyping information which can limit throughput. The clinical benefits of extended genotyping will be discussed later in this chapter but here we will focus on the analytical performance of the two assay design approaches.

6.4. The link between analytical and clinical assay performance

Good analytical assay performance is a requirement but not a guarantee of clinical assay performance. The viral load that correlates well with prediction of CIN2+ risk is approximately 5000 copies per reaction as established by the Hybrid Capture 2 test [41]. Thus, it is important to determine the clinical cutoff (a level of positivity in the assay that best correlates with histologically confirmed disease) for each individual assay using standard receiver operating characteristic plots of sensitivity versus 1–specificity so as to provide the highest possible sensitivity and an optimal specificity [55, 56, 88]. Assays that are analytically too sensitive will refer an unacceptably high number of women to colposcopy for possible biopsy and treatment [43]. **Table 2** describes some of the unique diagnostic challenges associated with cervical cancer screening that make this task a complicated one. This is reflected in the reports in the literature on viral load measurements, which are mixed at best. While HPV16 viral load has been shown to correlate with disease progression [99, 100], non-HPV16 types have been reported to show less correlation [101]. A recent well controlled study that focused exclusively on single infections found that HPV16/HPV18/HPV31/HPV45 viral load was correlated with abnormal cytology. This study is likely to have benefited by excluding the complication of mixed infections and the use of a high quality E6 gene-specific real-time PCR assay [102]. A positive correlation for these types (and HPV33) with disease severity was also confirmed in an independent study with histological endpoints [103]. These apparent discrepancies may be explained by analytical performance differences in the methods used to measure viral load. As mentioned above, most commercial assays use consensus L1 primers because of the ease of use offered by a single reaction that can detect 14 high-risk viruses. However, consensus primer designs exhibit poor detection of mixed infections due to HPV-type suppression or restriction, where the overabundance of one HPV type in a mixed infection can lead to failure to detect lower levels of a coinfecting virus. Van Doorn et al. were one of the first to demonstrate this phenomenon using spiking experiments where detectable levels of HPV18 were eliminated using an increasing concentration of a competing HPV16 target [104]. This result was later confirmed in cervical smear and biopsy specimens where the L1 SPF10 consensus primer assay was compared to a gene-specific E6 assay where significantly more genotypes ($P <$ 0.0001) were identified by the E6 assay, especially for HPV types 16, 35, 39, 45, 58, and 59 and the authors concluded "that broad-spectrum PCRs are hampered by type competition when multiple HPV genotypes are present in the same sample" [105]. Similar results have been reported by Mori et al. who found that "three consensus primers frequently caused incorrect genotyping in the selected clinical specimens containing HPV16 and one or two of HPV18, 31, 51, 52, and 58" and went on to conclude "that PCR with consensus primers is not suitable for genotyping HPV in specimens containing multiple HPV types" [106]. Given that approximately one-third or more of clinical specimens can harbor more than one HPV type [107], this should be considered carefully when designing vaccine monitoring or other studies requiring genotyping. This has recently been underlined by a *post-hoc* analysis of the PATRICIA vaccine trial where Struyf et al. found that an E6-based multiplex type-specific PCR and reverse hybridization assay showed improved sensitivity versus the L1-based SPF10 PCR-DNA enzyme immunoassay (DEIA)/line probe assay (LiPA25) used in the original trial, resulting in higher vaccine efficacy estimates for nonvaccine oncogenic HPV types [108]. The E6-assay was developed by Van Doorn et al. and had previously been shown to increase genotype detection by 14.3% [105]. Another negative impact of HPV-type suppression was reported by Cornall et al. who hypothesized that the sensitivity of consensus-based PCR approaches could be altered in highly vaccinated populations such as Australia. They confirmed their hypothesis using the Roche HPV linear array genotype assay by simulating samples containing 1000 copies of one or two high-risk HPV DNA genomes in the presence and the absence of 10,000 copies of the HPV16 genome. HPV16 alone did not affect detection of other high-risk genotypes; however, when HPV16 and an additional genotype were present, detection of HPV31, 33, 51, or 59 was impeded, indicating potential for misrepresentation of population-based prevalence of these genotypes and false evidence for type replacement following vaccination [109]. A next-generation sequencing (NGS) method also found that consensus MY09/MY11 primers had "lower sensitivity for some HPV types than LiPA, conceivably due to the poor sensitivity of the MY09/MY11-based primers"[110]. The results from the WHO LabNet genotyping panel broadly support these findings. The panel consists of approximately 43 DNA standardized DNA samples with single and mixed infections of the 14 high-risk HPV types (and low-risk types HPV6 and HPV11) and three cell line extraction controls. Candidate assays are considered proficient if they can detect 50 international units (IU) of HPV type 16 (HPV16) and HPV18 DNA and 500 genome equivalents (GE) for the other 14 HPV types. The 2010 panel results reported the data from 98 laboratories who submitted 132 datasets, only ~20% of which were deemed proficient for all HPV types. In addition, approximately 35% of the test panels had multiple false positive results and were considered nonproficient. Virtually all of the assays that submitted test results were L1 consensus-primer based [63]. The results from the 2014 panel from 119 participating global laboratories (146 datasets) were recently reported and the overall results showed an improvement, with 59% of the test results deemed 100% proficient and 20% nonproficient [111]. Nevertheless, there is little room for complacency when one considers that this implies that 40% of current assays do not accurately detect HPV types. In summary, assay design has a direct impact on clinical performance and the ability to accurately genotype both single and mixed infections will play an ever-increasing role, especially in a postvaccination era.

Diagnostic challenge	Impact	Mitigation	Current status	Comments
Most infections do no result in cancer	Cancer incidence can be as low as 5–8 per 100,000 women screened [112]	Organized screening programs need to reach as many women as possible	50% of cancers still occur in women who have not been screened	Need to continue to expand programs to reach underserved women (self-sampling)
Younger women are more likely to be infected with HPV	Screening of women < 25–30 may lead to overdiagnosis [113]	Current guidelines recommend not screening women <25 or <30	Primary screening approved in US for >25, with >30 more common for cotesting with cytology	Ongoing countrywide programs will shed more light on the correct age to start screening (which could be population specific)
Older women are more likely to develop cancer	Overtesting may cause unnecessary anxiety in younger patients	Adhere to expert guidelines and screen appropriately		
Analytical positive ≠ clinical positive [42]	Over- and underreferral possible	Establish appropriate clinical cutoff in target population	Meijer guidelines and FDA approval provide reassurance but in-country real-world validation is also informative	Need more research on the impact of cross-reactivity and molecular mimics as well as mixed infections
Results impacted by quality of specimen collection	Poorly collected or expressed samples increases unsatisfactory rate and can lead to false negative results if no cellular control present	Include cellular versus PCR processing control in the assay	Performance of different collection devices should be considered [114, 115]	Physicians and laboratory personnel need to adhere to recommended procedures for collection and processing of specimens
Large number of normal versus abnormal cells present in sample leads to sampling variation	Sampling errors can occur and lead to false negative results [116]	Assay needs to be robust to differences in pipetting volumes around recommended test volume	Most of the newer assays have a cellular processing control which helps mitigate this risk Semiautomated or fully automated methods improve reliability (**Table 1**)	Most manufacturers have adapted their methods for the two common liquid-based-cytology media on the market
Most endocervical samples are collected in preservative which lead to clumping of exfoliated cells		Samples need to be vortexed adequately and aliquots removed promptly prior to robust extraction and		

Diagnostic challenge	Impact	Mitigation	Current status	Comments
		homogenization of the specimen [67, 117]		
Samples can be inhibited with a variety of exogenous and endogenous interfering substances [118]	False negative or indeterminate results obtained	Product needs to undergo rigorous analytical validation with a variety of interfering substances	Most assays are robust to interfering substances	Less of an issue than sampling variation
Infections are dynamic and can produce a large dynamic range of viral titers	Infections may be regressing or proliferating leading to false results	Correlate with cytology or other biomarker results and repeat test as needed	Clinically validated assays have good correlation with disease endpoints. One assay reported predictive ability of viral load measurements taken sequentially [119]	Viral load measurements are difficult to perform and may not be clinically practical if sequential. Genotyping provides information on persistence which may aid in patient management
The same pathology can be cause by non-high-risk HPV or other "mimics"	Non-high-risk HPV pathology can lead to overtreatment	Assays should not detect nontarget HPV types. Histology results should be considered in the context of high-risk HPV results	Newer assays have no cross-reactivity to nontarget types. Pathology review and biomarker qualification improve diagnostic cytopathology accuracy	The belief that "gold standard" pathology is truth needs to be critically challenged [120]
Viral clearance may precede resolution of cellular abnormalities	Lingering pathology complicates patient management	Adhere to screening guidelines and retest as needed	p16 biomarker is increasingly being used to augment diagnosis and guidelines have been proposed [121]	Extended genotyping offers improved risk stratification which may aid in patient management [96]

Table 2. Diagnostic challenges associated with cervical cancer screening.

6.5. HPV integration-induced deletions: impact on screening programs?

It is now well established that the HPV viral genome can integrate into the host genome during disease progression. The ability to integrate varies by high-risk HPV type with approximately 70% of HPV16-associated cervical cancers containing integrated HPV16 sequences, rising to almost 100% for HPV18 [122, 123]. Next-generation sequencing methods are now shedding new light on this phenomenon and the emerging picture suggests the following:

1. Viral integration appears to be a random (nontargeted) event with disruption of a wide variety of host genes across the human genome [124–126].

2. Integration is associated with fragile sites in human DNA and is likely opportunistic, with the HPV virus taking advantage of exposed DNA to integrate into the host genome. Regions of microhomology between the viral and human sequences are enriched near integration sites suggesting that integration may be driven by the host DNA repair machinery [124, 125].

3. Viral sequences are frequently deleted during the integration process [124, 125].

4. Contrary to what was previously believed E6 and E7 oncogenes can also be deleted during integration. However, this occurs less frequently than in other viral genes such as L1, L2, E1, and E2 and there appears to be significant enrichment of (intact) viral gene E7 > E4 > E5 > E6 reads among the cervical tumor samples [124, 125, 127].(It is possible that this may simply due to the random nature of the integration process and reflect the fact that L1, L2, E1, and E2 are the largest ORFs in the HPV genome, **Figure 2**).

5. Viral integration appears to occur at a higher frequency than perhaps previously understood and can also be detected in Pap smears, one study reporting integration in 53% of cytology samples with histology grades CIN1–3 [124].

Thus, it appears that viral integration HPV integration is an unintended consequence of HPV replication and that following integration, the virus life cycle is aborted. Nevertheless, virus integration is a routine consequence of infection and the observation that it can occur earlier in the disease progression prompts the question whether it has a measureable effect on the ability of HPV assays to detect the virus. Several authors have expressed concern that L1-based assays can fail to detect late-stage cancers due to target deletion [128–130] and there is no doubt that L1-deleted cancers occur as evidenced by case studies [129, 131]. Several studies have reported that the E6/E7 assays have increased sensitivity for cancer versus L1-based assays [132–134]. Some have dismissed this as due to earlier methodological differences due to the difficulty of detecting longer L1 amplicons in formalin fixed paraffin embedded (FFPE) tissue. However, this is not supported by more recent literature where even using gold standard FFPE processing methods, one group reported only a 91% detection rate in cancer specimens with two different L1 primer assays [135]. Another recent study of cervical adenocarcinomas reported that PCR using a very sensitive L1-based SPF10-PCR resulted in 482 cases (67%) positive for HPV DNA, but that testing using type-specific E6 PCR added 53 HPV-positive cases (a 7% increase in detection). The study design also accounted for DNA adequacy in the samples [136]. Adenocarcinomas represent about 25% of all cervical cancers [137, 138] and are known to be prone to HPV DNA integration, so this increase in sensitivity for detection of adenocarcinomas could potentially translate to the detection of another 1–2% of total cancer cases (assuming an increase in just adenocarcinoma cases). Large-scale studies will be needed to address the question of whether or not the above reported difference in assay performance (due to increased maintenance of intact target regions postintegration) has a measureable impact on clinical sensitivity in cervical cancer screening. This warrants further study, especially given the reported ability of the virus to integrate in approximately 50% of cervical smears from patients with CIN [124]. Finally, the Roche cobas assay has recently been reported to have a 94% detection rate in the smears from women with histologically confirmed invasive cervical cancer [139].

7. The evolution of HPV screening

7.1. Cotesting with cytology versus primary HPV screening

It has been known for 10 years that HPV testing is substantially more sensitive in detecting CIN2+ than cytology (96.1 versus 53.0%) but less specific (90.7 versus 96.3%) [140]. In the intervening period, large randomized controlled trials (RCTs) have continued to reaffirm this point. Pileggi et al. [141] recently performed a meta-analysis of global RCTs which included trials from Italy (NTCC trials I+II [142, 143]), the UK (ARTISTIC Trial [144]), Finland [145], India [146], Canada [147], and the Netherlands (POBASCAM [148]). The analysis from this larger more comprehensive dataset showed a significantly higher detection of both CIN2+ and CIN3+ by HPV testing versus cytology and that the relative specificity of cytology was higher. However, in women greater than 30 years of age, the specificity was not statistically different ("almost overlapping"). In addition, the pooled relative PPV was not significantly lower for HPV compared with cytology. These results suggest that the difference in specificity is actually less than previously thought, at least in women over 30. A recent US *post-hoc* analysis of a large group of women from multiple practices reported that positive Pap + HPV (cotest) was more sensitive than either a positive HPV alone or Pap alone for detection of CIN3+ and suggested that HPV primary screening might miss cancers if not combined with the Pap [149]. However, the study design has come under criticism from an independent expert, because the short follow up time of 1 year biases results in favor of cytology and all women were not followed equally [150]. Thus, large global studies support the use of primary HPV testing as a means to improve cervical cancer detection and it explains why many countries are now in the process of implementing either pilot or countrywide programs to replace cytology and/or cotesting [151, 152]. In the United States, one HPV test has received FDA approval for primary screening in women >25 years of age [153] and interim guidelines for its use have been issued [113]. The reaction to this decision has been mixed with some arguing that cotesting detects more disease [154]. However, data continue to accumulate both in the United States and in Europe that supports the long-term NPV of a primary HPV negative result, thus permitting safe interval extension [155, 156]. A study comparing primary HPV versus cotesting versus primary cytology concluded that "primary HPV testing every 3 years might provide as much, if not more, reassurance against precancer and cancer, compared to primary Pap testing every 3 years and cotesting every 5 years"[156]. Thus, the choice of which screening paradigm to adopt will likely be influenced by the resources available together with the desired screening interval and risk tolerance of the medical community and the patients they serve. Despite the slow pace of change, it seems clear that HPV primary screening will gradually be adopted worldwide, especially in countries which do not have current cytology infrastructure. HPV testing is considerably more reproducible than cytology [157] and with the advent of automation, highly skilled personnel are no longer required to implement IVD-qualified tests. It should be noted, however, that primary HPV screening cannot be used in isolation to refer women to colposcopy. Biomarkers such as p16 [121] or cytology or HPV16/HPV18 genotyping need to be considered to increase specificity and reduce the number of unnecessary colposcopies [72, 153, 158].

7.2. Reaching underserved women: self-sampling methods

It is well established that the effectiveness of cervical cancer screening programs is limited by the number of women who do not participate—with 50% or more of disease being detected in women who have not been screened [159–162]. While there may be many reasons (cultural, socioeconomic, and religious) why women choose not to participate in screening programs available to them, it is clear that self-collection offers an effective outreach tool with which to increase participation. For example, in Finland the participation rate was <70% but was increased to 72.6–79.9% by sending reminder letters to nonattendees in 22 municipalities, and to 83.4% by sending self-collection kits to those who did not attend after receiving the initial invitation letter [163]. Similar finding on outreach were reported in Sweden where telephone invitations to long-term nonattendees increased the participation rate within the following 12 months to 18.0% versus 10.6% in a control group [164]. In Canada, reminder letters were compared head to head with sending a self-sampling kit and standard screening and women receiving the self-collected HPV kit were 3.7 times more likely to undergo screening compared with the standard of care [165]. Finally, a recent Danish outreach program where 5000 women were invited to "opt-in" and receive a self-collection kit resulted in the detection of nine cancers. This translates to yield of 1.8 per 1000, a dramatic enrichment for disease detection versus the Danish population rate, estimated at 12.9 per 100,000 women [166, 167]. Thus, self-sampling is emerging as a very important tool in national screening programs and one that continues to generate a high degree of interest [168]. Two principal self-collection methods that have been described in the literature: cervico-vaginal collection and urine collection.

7.2.1. Cervico-vaginal collection methods

A number of different cervico-vaginal methods have been described in the literature (reviewed in [169, 170]) and range from simple brush devices currently used by physicians to custom designed self-collection devices such as the Rovers® Evalyn® brush (Rovers Medical Devices BV, the Netherlands) and HerSwab™ (Eve Medical, Canada). Earlier literature reported mixed results versus physician collected endocervical samples in terms of sensitivity and specificity. However, more recent studies have confirmed that self-collected specimens can have the same sensitivity for CIN2+ as physician-collected specimens [171]. A recent meta-analysis concluded that signal amplification methods were not sensitive enough for self-collection use but that certain PCR methods had similar sensitivity to physician-collected samples [172]. This has been confirmed in a number of small studies using clinically validated HPV tests where sensitivities for CIN2+ were similar to physician-collected samples [173–176]. It is likely that both the quality of the instructions used and the sample workflow/assay play a role in the ability to accurately detect infections. Further large-scale studies are needed to further demonstrate the utility of these methods in screening populations.

7.2.2. HPV testing from urine

HPV testing from urine has been performed for over 20 years and similar to cervico-vaginal methods, early studies were somewhat discouraging with decreased sensitivity versus physician-collected endocervical samples being reported [177]. This was compounded by the demonstration that male urine samples were a poor sample type for HPV detection [178], which has been confirmed in more recent studies and likely reflects a true biological difference between men and women [179, 180]. The general interest in self-sampling and the introduction of HPV vaccines, which can benefit from noninvasive population-based monitoring, has resulted in a renewed interest in urine as an alternative sample type for cervical cancer screening [181]. There is now a growing body of evidence that urine, in particular first void urine, has a lot of potential for detecting HPV infections [182, 183]. The basic premise of HPV urine testing is founded on the hypothesis that "at the start of the void, urine gets contaminated by debris and impurities lining the urethra opening, including mucus and debris of exfoliated cells from the vagina, cervix and uterus" [181]. Recent research has also demonstrated that optimal sample workflows and sensitive detection methods improve clinical performance:

1. Urine contains substantial amounts of free-DNA and virus, so processing methods that utilize recovered cell pellets may underestimate the amount of virus present. Processing of neat urine is preferable [184, 185]. A recent study found similar performance using 0.5 ml of neat urine versus up to 80-fold concentrated cell pellets [186]. Another study found HPV DNA sequences in both urinary tract infection positive and negative patient urine using cesium chloride density gradient-purified virus particles, suggesting that intact virions are present [187].(Urine also contains transrenal DNA [short DNA fragments from the blood circulation that has passed the kidney barrier [188], but this is not believed to be the main source of HPV target DNA as evidenced by the observation that first void urine collected during menses is contaminated with blood and cells.)

2. Urine from HPV positive women appears to be consistently positive even when sampled multiple times from the same patient. However, first void urine samples are analytically more positive, especially if the initial catchment is in a smaller volume [181, 182, 186, 189].

3. Virus appears to be shed continuously from infected women and is simply flushed out of the vaginal canal during urination. Therefore, it is not advisable to clean the local area with alcohol wipes prior to collection in order to maximize recovery of cells, virus, and free-DNA [181].

4. Urine samples are labile at room temperature (due to the action of proteases and nucleases) so urine samples should be mixed promptly with an appropriate preservative such as EDTA to ensure sample integrity. Addition of the preservative to the urine cup or collection tube is optimal since degradation can occur immediately post-collection prior to the arrival of the sample in the testing laboratory [184, 188, 190–192].

5. An assay cellularity control targeting a human gene is recommended to ensure sample adequacy. Routine urine samples should be positive for human DNA and confirms that an adequate catchment has been obtained. Analytically sensitive molecular methods such

as real-time PCR should be used to ensure optimal results and clinical cutoff adjustments may be required versus endocervical specimens [193].

8. "Safety in numbers": time for extended genotyping in cervical cancer screening

The majority of (clinically validated) HPV screening tests have the ability to provide genotyping information on only two types, HPV16 and HPV18 [46]. There is now a growing body of evidence that extended genotyping (beyond types 16 and18) better stratifies a woman's risk for subsequent disease: A recent Danish study looked at the long-term absolute risk for CIN3+ in women following a baseline HPV genotyping result and found that HPV31 and HPV33 had the same or greater longitudinal risk as HPV18 over a 10-year period [194]; Schiffman et al. [195] confirmed this finding for HPV31 in a US cohort over a 15-year follow up period; Cuzick et al. [196] looked at the positive predictive value of genotyping in a referred UK population and found that HPV33 had a higher PPV than HPV16 (59.8 versus 57.8) and that HPV31 was higher than HPV18 (39.5 versus 29.3). Similar trends were reported in a much larger New Mexico study of 21,297 women of whom 77% had biopsies. Among women with CIN3+ (n = 1880), 14.9% were attributable to HPV31, 5.2% to HPV33 and 4.9% to HPV18, with HPV16 responsible for 54.1% [197]. Roche Linear Array genotyping analysis of patients from the ATHENA trial also support these findings: among 40,901 women aged ≥25 years HPV16 conferred the greatest absolute risk of ≥CIN3 both in women aged 25–29 and ≥30 years (14.2% and 15.1%, respectively) followed by HPV31 (8.0% and 7.9%), HPV52 (6.7% and 4.4%), and HPV18 (2.7% and 9.0%) [198].

While the majority of cancers are caused by HPV16 and HPV18, presumably due to the increased ability of these genotypes to persist and induce oncogenic changes, one must equally concede that HPV31, 33, 45, 52, and 58 are the next most potent carcinogens of the high-risk HPV types [199]. This is supported by the introduction of the nine-valent HPV vaccine, where the addition of these types is estimated to provide protection against an additional ~20% of cancers [200]. The clinical paradigm of equal management of equal risk [201] strongly suggests that knowledge of HPV31 and HPV33 infections has clinical value and can aid in patient management. In addition, the widespread introduction of the new nine-valent vaccine is expected to have a profound effect on the incidence of CIN3+ disease, further underlining the need for a more comprehensive genotype profile of pre- and postvaccinated women [202]. Finally, the use of gene-specific versus consensus PCR genotyping approaches can alleviate the issue of apparent type replacement in vaccinated women where HPV types such as HPV31 and HPV33 may appear to be increasing in prevalence but are simply being unmasked due to the reduced incidence of HPV16 and HPV18 in the postvaccination era [109].

Extended genotyping also offers a potential solution to key emerging issues in cervical cancer screening:

I. Accurate risk stratification—absolute risk calculations *a priori* are underestimated when two or more HPV types with different CIN3 risks are pooled together (e.g., the 10-year longitudinal study of Kahn et al. attributes a very low risk to pooled non-16/18 types [203] which has been consistently found *not* to be the case in subsequent studies where individual genotypes have been detected [194, 196–198]). Precise risk stratification is essential for consistent and informed patient management. This is especially true in cytology-negative HPV-positive women where genotyping can provide clinicians with a much more informed assessment of future risk versus a pooled HPV positive result.

II. On the other hand, extended genotyping allows one to group HPV types with similar risk, thereby simplifying patient management algorithms. Cuzick et al. [196] proposed a three tiered risk group approach to patient stratification based on the positive predictive value of different genotypes for CIN3+ disease in a referred population. Schiffman et al. recently published the largest longitudinal ASC-US population analysis to date (Persistence and Progression cohort with 13,890 women aged 21+with HC2 (QIAGEN)-positive ASC-US at enrollment and median follow-up of 3.0 years). The authors used the concept of equal management of equal risk approach and calculated the 3-year CIN3+ risk for all HC2-positive women with ASC-US (5.2%), using this as the "benchmark" risk for colposcopic referral. They concluded that the 3-year risk for developing CIN3+ associated with high-risk HPV types 35, 39, 51, 56, 59, 66, and 68 (2.7% for HPV51, 1.6% for HPV39/HPV68/HPV35, and 1.3% for HPV59/HPV56/HPV66) "might be low enough to recommend 1-year retesting, permitting viral clearance. This strategy would defer colposcopy for 40% of women with HPV-positive ASC-US, half of whom would be cotest-negative at 1-year return" [96].

Thus, extended genotyping offers the potential of improved risk stratification and simpler patient management, helping to improve patient outcomes with reduced intervention.

9. Future perspectives

While we have made great strides in both detecting and preventing cervical cancer over the last 20 years, it still represents a significant challenge in both developed and developing settings. In countries with a high disease burden such as Mexico, Ecuador, Samoa, and Colombia, it is the number one cancer in young women and the number two cancer in women of all ages, whereas in several areas in Africa and in Cambodia, it is primary cause of cancer and death [112]. With 50% of cancers occurring in underserved women, it is clear that the biggest remaining challenges are in implementation, not technology development. Self-collection methods offer new hope of reaching women who are currently not captured in traditional screening programs. Ongoing studies should shed further light on the ability of these methods to equal those used in the physician's office or at least provide a means to target these women for follow up in the medical system (analogous to current home pregnancy test kits). HPV vaccines have been shown to be safe and efficacious but here again the biggest hurdle is achieving the required vaccine coverage in the target population. It is hoped that the successful implementation models such as those in the UK and Australia will be adopted elsewhere to boost global vaccine coverage. It should also not go unmentioned that the other barrier to improved disease prevention and detection is resistance to change. While medicine can be understandably conservative, waiting for substantial bodies of evidence to accumulate prior to changing clinical management, we should also constantly challenge ourselves on this point, given the severity of the disease burden imposed by HPV. With the benefit of hindsight, one can justifiably argue that even the Pap smear itself took 30 years too long to be implemented, HPV primary screening could have been adopted 10 years ago based on the available evidence, and vaccine coverage is suffering today due to the emergence of vaccine opposition which is not supported by scientific evidence [204]. We should also continue to challenge the *status quo* on cervical cytology and histopathology—while they have an important role to play, their future role should be evaluated in the context of comprehensive screening strategies [205, 206]. There is an urgent need to eradicate cervical cancer for the sake of both the current generation of women and the men and women who follow them. At the same time, there is an ever increasing pressure on global healthcare systems to do more with less. Ironically, this will likely serve as a catalyst for change as health economic studies identify which screening and vaccination strategies are the most cost-effective and offer the highest adoption rate. Ongoing and future research should focus on answering key questions in cervical cancer program implementation such as the effect of vaccination on HPV prevalence, and the ability of extended genotyping to better stratify a patient's risk. Optimal triage strategies should also be investigated together with new studies on the long-term effects on the physical and psychological health of patients who are overtested and overtreated. As we settle into the twenty-first century of cervical cancer screening, one thing is clear, we have effective means to detect and prevent disease. The real question is: do we have the resolve to deploy these tools in an effective manner? We join others in the hope that we will learn from the past and quicken the pace of change in response to the global threat posed by cervical disease [207].

Author details

Laurence M. Vaughan*, Brian R. Faherty, Erin C. Gutierrez, James M. Harris, William A. Nussbaumer and Ryan J. Schwab

*Address all correspondence to: laurence.vaughan@bd.com

Diagnostics Systems, BD Life Sciences, Sparks, MD, USA

References

[1] Diamantis A, Magiorkinis E, Koutselini H. 50 years after the death of George Nicholas Papanicolaou (1883–1962): evaluation of his scientific work. Acta Med Hist Adriat. 2014;12(1):181–8.

[2] Classes in oncology: George Nicholas Papanicolaou's new cancer diagnosis presented at the Third Race Betterment Conference, Battle Creek, Michigan, January 2–6, 1928, and published in the Proceedings of the Conference. CA Cancer J Clin. 1973;23(3):174–9.

[3] Papanicolaou GN, Traut HF. The diagnostic value of vaginal smears in carcinoma of the uterus. 1941. Arch Pathol Lab Med. 1997;121(3):211–24.

[4] zur Hausen H. Oncogenic Herpes viruses. Biochim Biophys Acta. 1975;417(1):25–53.

[5] Gissmann L, zur Hausen H. Partial characterization of viral DNA from human genital warts (*Condylomata acuminata*). Int J Cancer. 1980;25(5):605–9.

[6] de Villiers EM, Gissmann L, zur Hausen H. Molecular cloning of viral DNA from human genital warts. J Virol. 1981;40(3):932–5.

[7] Gissmann L, deVilliers EM, zur Hausen H. Analysis of human genital warts (*Condylomata acuminata*) and other genital tumors for human papillomavirus type 6 DNA. Int J Cancer. 1982;29(2):143–6.

[8] Gissmann L, Wolnik L, Ikenberg H, Koldovsky U, Schnurch HG, zur Hausen H. Human papillomavirus types 6 and 11 DNA sequences in genital and laryngeal papillomas and in some cervical cancers. Proc Natl Acad Sci USA. 1983;80(2):560–3.

[9] Zachow KR, Ostrow RS, Bender M, Watts S, Okagaki T, Pass F, Faras AJ. Detection of human papillomavirus DNA in anogenital neoplasias. Nature. 1982;300(5894):771–3.

[10] Green M, Brackmann KH, Sanders PR, Loewenstein PM, Freel JH, Eisinger M, Switlyk SA. Isolation of a human papillomavirus from a patient with epidermodysplasia verruciformis: presence of related viral DNA genomes in human urogenital tumors. Proc Natl Acad Sci USA. 1982;79(14):4437–41.

[11] Durst M, Gissmann L, Ikenberg H, zur Hausen H. A papillomavirus DNA from a cervical carcinoma and its prevalence in cancer biopsy samples from different geographic regions. Proc Natl Acad Sci USA. 1983;80(12):3812–5.

[12] Boshart M, Gissmann L, Ikenberg H, Kleinheinz A, Scheurlen W, zur Hausen H. A new type of papillomavirus DNA, its presence in genital cancer biopsies and in cell lines derived from cervical cancer. EMBO J. 1984;3(5):1151–7.

[13] Ikenberg H, Gissmann L, Gross G, Grussendorf-Conen EI, zur Hausen H. Human papillomavirus type-16-related DNA in genital Bowen's disease and in Bowenoid papulosis. Int J Cancer. 1983;32(5):563–5.

[14] Crum CP, Ikenberg H, Richart RM, Gissman L. Human papillomavirus type 16 and early cervical neoplasia. N Engl J Med. 1984;310(14):880–3. DOI:10.1056/nejm198404053101403.

[15] Lorincz AT, Lancaster WD, Temple GF. Cloning and characterization of the DNA of a new human papillomavirus from a woman with dysplasia of the uterine cervix. J Virol. 1986;58(1):225–9.

[16] Naghashfar ZS, Rosenshein NB, Lorincz AT, Buscema J, Shah KV. Characterization of human papillomavirus type 45, a new type 18-related virus of the genital tract. J Gen Virol. 1987;68 (Pt 12):3073–9. DOI:10.1099/0022-1317-68-12-3073.

[17] Hubbard RA. Human papillomavirus testing methods. Arch Pathol Lab Med. 2003 Aug;127(8):940–5. DOI:10.1043/1543-2165(2003)127<940:hptm>2.0.co;2.

[18] Guo M, Gong Y, Deavers M, Silva EG, Jan YJ, Cogdell DE, Luthra R, Lin E, Lai HC, Zhang W, Sneige N. Evaluation of a commercialized *in situ* hybridization assay for detecting human papillomavirus DNA in tissue specimens from patients with cervical intraepithelial neoplasia and cervical carcinoma. J Clin Microbiol. 2008;46(1):274–80. DOI:10.1128/jcm.01299-07.

[19] Zhang W, Kapadia M, Sugarman M, Free H, Upchurch C, Gniewek R, White K, Miller M, Vladich F, Ferenczy A, Wright TC, Stoler MH, Pestic-Dragovich L. Adjunctive HPV in-situ hybridization (ISH) assay as an aid in the diagnosis of cervical intraepithelial neoplasia in cervical tissue specimens: an analytical and functional characterization. Int J Gynecol Pathol. 2012;31(6):588–95. DOI:10.1097/PGP.0b013e318254349a.

[20] Lorincz AT. Hybrid Capture method for detection of human papillomavirus DNA in clinical specimens: a tool for clinical management of equivocal Pap smears and for population screening. J Obstet Gynaecol Res. 1996;22(6):629–36.

[21] Cavuslu S, Mant C, Starkey WG, Bible JM, Biswas C, Kell B, Rice P, Best JM, Cason J. Analytic sensitivities of hybrid-capture, consensus and type-specific polymerase chain reactions for the detection of human papillomavirus type 16 DNA. J Med Virol. 1996;49(4):319–24. DOI:10.1002/(sici)1096-9071(199608)49:4<319::aid-jmv10>3.0.co;2-5.

[22] Reid R, Lorincz AT. Human papillomavirus tests. Baillieres Clin Obstet Gynaecol. 1995;9(1):65–103.

[23] Poljak M, Brencic A, Seme K, Vince A, Marin IJ. Comparative evaluation of first- and second-generation digene hybrid capture assays for detection of human papillomaviruses associated with high or intermediate risk for cervical cancer. J Clin Microbiol. 1999;37(3):796–7.

[24] Bruni L, Diaz M, Castellsague X, Ferrer E, Bosch FX, de Sanjose S. Cervical human papillomavirus prevalence in 5 continents: meta-analysis of 1 million women with normal cytological findings. J Infect Dis. 2010;202(12):1789–99. DOI:10.1086/657321.

[25] Patanwala IY, Bauer HM, Miyamoto J, Park IU, Huchko MJ, Smith-McCune KK. A systematic review of randomized trials assessing human papillomavirus testing in

cervical cancer screening. Am J Obstet Gynecol. 2013;208(5):343–53. DOI:10.1016/j.ajog.2012.11.013.

[26] Mullis K, Faloona F, Scharf S, Saiki R, Horn G, Erlich H. Specific enzymatic amplification of DNA *in vitro*: the polymerase chain reaction. Cold Spring Harb Symp Quant Biol. 1986;51(Pt 1):263–73.

[27] Saiki RK, Bugawan TL, Horn GT, Mullis KB, Erlich HA. Analysis of enzymatically amplified beta-globin and HLA-DQ alpha DNA with allele-specific oligonucleotide probes. Nature. 1986;324(6093):163–6. DOI:10.1038/324163a0.

[28] Mullis K, Faloona F, Scharf S, Saiki R, Horn G, Erlich H. Specific enzymatic amplification of DNA *in vitro*: the polymerase chain reaction. 1986. Biotechnology. 1992;24:17–27.

[29] Higuchi R, Fockler C, Dollinger G, Watson R. Kinetic PCR analysis: real-time monitoring of DNA amplification reactions. Biotechnology (N Y). 1993;11(9):1026–30.

[30] Heid CA, Stevens J, Livak KJ, Williams PM. Real time quantitative PCR. Genome Res. 1996;6(10):986–94.

[31] Gibson UE, Heid CA, Williams PM. A novel method for real time quantitative RT-PCR. Genome Res. 1996;6(10):995–1001.

[32] Longo MC, Berninger MS, Hartley JL. Use of uracil DNA glycosylase to control carry-over contamination in polymerase chain reactions. Gene. 1990;93(1):125–8.

[33] Kwok S, Higuchi R. Avoiding false positives with PCR. Nature. 1989;339(6221):237–8. DOI:10.1038/339237a0.

[34] Dallas PB, Flanagan JL, Nightingale BN, Morris BJ. Polymerase chain reaction for fast, nonradioactive detection of high- and low-risk papillomavirus types in routine cervical specimens and in biopsies. J Med Virol. 1989;27(2):105–11.

[35] Josefsson A, Livak K, Gyllensten U. Detection and quantitation of human papillomavirus by using the fluorescent 5' exonuclease assay. J Clin Microbiol. 1999;37(3):490–6.

[36] Cuschieri KS, Cubie HA, Whitley MW, Seagar AL, Arends MJ, Moore C, Gilkisson G, McGoogan E. Multiple high-risk HPV infections are common in cervical neoplasia and young women in a cervical screening population. J Clin Pathol. 2004;57(1):68–72.

[37] Snijders PJ, van den Brule AJ, Schrijnemakers HF, Snow G, Meijer CJ, Walboomers JM. The use of general primers in the polymerase chain reaction permits the detection of a broad spectrum of human papillomavirus genotypes. J Gen Virol. 1990;71(Pt 1):173–81. DOI:10.1099/0022-1317-71-1-173.

[38] Gravitt PE, Peyton CL, Alessi TQ, Wheeler CM, Coutlee F, Hildesheim A, Schiffman MH, Scott DR, Apple RJ. Improved amplification of genital human papillomaviruses. J Clin Microbiol. 2000;38(1):357–61.

[39] de Roda Husman AM, Walboomers JM, van den Brule AJ, Meijer CJ, Snijders PJ. The use of general primers GP5 and GP6 elongated at their 3′ ends with adjacent highly conserved sequences improves human papillomavirus detection by PCR. J Gen Virol. 1995;76(Pt 4):1057–62. DOI:10.1099/0022-1317-76-4-1057.

[40] Bulkmans NW, Rozendaal L, Snijders PJ, Voorhorst FJ, Boeke AJ, Zandwijken GR, van Kemenade FJ, Verheijen RH, v Groningen K, Boon ME, Keuning HJ, van Ballegooijen M, van den Brule AJ, Meijer CJ. POBASCAM, a population-based randomized controlled trial for implementation of high-risk HPV testing in cervical screening: design, methods and baseline data of 44,102 women. Int J Cancer. 2004;110(1):94–101. DOI: 10.1002/ijc.20076.

[41] QIAGEN. Hybrid Capture 2 High-Risk HPV DNA Test Package Insert. 2007;L00665 Rev. 2.

[42] Stoler MH, Castle PE, Solomon D, Schiffman M. The expanded use of HPV testing in gynecologic practice per ASCCP-guided management requires the use of well-validated assays. Am J Clin Pathol. 2007;127(3):335–7. DOI:10.1309/rnf3c01jkadqclkp.

[43] Kinney W, Stoler MH, Castle PE. Special commentary: patient safety and the next generation of HPV DNA tests. Am J Clin Pathol. 2010;134(2):193–9. DOI:10.1309/ajcpri8xpqueaa3k.

[44] Meijer CJ, Berkhof J, Castle PE, Hesselink AT, Franco EL, Ronco G, Arbyn M, Bosch FX, Cuzick J, Dillner J, Heideman DA, Snijders PJ. Guidelines for human papillomavirus DNA test requirements for primary cervical cancer screening in women 30 years and older. Int J Cancer. 2009;124(3):516–20. DOI:10.1002/ijc.24010.

[45] Poljak M, Kocjan BJ, Ostrbenk A, Seme K. Commercially available molecular tests for human papillomaviruses (HPV): 2015 update. J Clin Virol. 2016;76 Suppl 1:S3-S13. DOI: 10.1016/j.jcv.2015.10.023.

[46] Arbyn M, Snijders PJ, Meijer CJ, Berkhof J, Cuschieri K, Kocjan BJ, Poljak M. Which high-risk HPV assays fulfil criteria for use in primary cervical cancer screening? Clin Microbiol Infect. 2015;21(9):817–26. DOI:10.1016/j.cmi.2015.04.015.

[47] Bosch FX, Broker TR, Forman D, Moscicki AB, Gillison ML, Doorbar J, Stern PL, Stanley M, Arbyn M, Poljak M, Cuzick J, Castle PE, Schiller JT, Markowitz LE, Fisher WA, Canfell K, Denny LA, Franco EL, Steben M, Kane MA, Schiffman M, Meijer CJ, Sankaranarayanan R, Castellsague X, Kim JJ, Brotons M, Alemany L, Albero G, Diaz M, de Sanjose S. Comprehensive control of human papillomavirus infections and related diseases. Vaccine. 2013;31(Suppl 7):H1–31. DOI:10.1016/j.vaccine.2013.10.003.

[48] Munger K, Howley PM. Human papillomavirus immortalization and transformation functions. Virus Res. 2002;89(2):213–28.

[49] Doorbar J, Egawa N, Griffin H, Kranjec C, Murakami I. Human papillomavirus molecular biology and disease association. Rev Med Virol. 2015;25(Suppl 1):2–23. DOI: 10.1002/rmv.1822.

[50] Dockter J, Schroder A, Hill C, Guzenski L, Monsonego J, Giachetti C. Clinical performance of the APTIMA HPV Assay for the detection of high-risk HPV and high-grade cervical lesions. J Clin Virol. 2009;45(Suppl 1):S55–61. DOI:10.1016/s1386-6532(09)70009-5.

[51] Kacian, D.L. and T.J. Fultz. 1995. Nucleic acid sequence amplification methods. U. S. Patent 5,399,491.

[52] Arnold LJ, Jr., Hammond PW, Wiese WA, Nelson NC. Assay formats involving acridinium-ester-labeled DNA probes. Clin Chem. 1989;35(8):1588–94.

[53] GenProbe. Aptima HPV Assay. 2011;502170 Rev. A.

[54] Alaghehbandan R, Fontaine D, Bentley J, Escott N, Ghatage P, Lear A, Coutlee F, Ratnam S. Performance of ProEx C and PreTect HPV-Proofer E6/E7 mRNA tests in comparison with the hybrid capture 2 HPV DNA test for triaging ASCUS and LSIL cytology. Diagn Cytopathol. 2013;41(9):767–75. DOI:10.1002/dc.22944.

[55] Szarewski A, Mesher D, Cadman L, Austin J, Ashdown-Barr L, Ho L, Terry G, Liddle S, Young M, Stoler M, McCarthy J, Wright C, Bergeron C, Soutter WP, Lyons D, Cuzick J. Comparison of seven tests for high-grade cervical intraepithelial neoplasia in women with abnormal smears: the Predictors 2 study. J Clin Microbiol. 2012;50(6):1867–73. DOI:10.1128/JCM.00181-12.

[56] Cuzick J, Cadman L, Mesher D, Austin J, Ashdown-Barr L, Ho L, Terry G, Liddle S, Wright C, Lyons D, Szarewski A. Comparing the performance of six human papillomavirus tests in a screening population. Br J Cancer. 2013;108(4):908–13. DOI:10.1038/bjc.2013.22.

[57] Arbyn M, Roelens J, Cuschieri K, Cuzick J, Szarewski A, Ratnam S, Reuschenbach M, Belinson S, Belinson JL, Monsonego J. The APTIMA HPV assay versus the Hybrid Capture 2 test in triage of women with ASC-US or LSIL cervical cytology: a meta-analysis of the diagnostic accuracy. Int J Cancer. 2013;132(1):101–8. DOI:10.1002/ijc.27636.

[58] Reid JL, Wright TC, Jr., Stoler MH, Cuzick J, Castle PE, Dockter J, Getman D, Giachetti C. Human papillomavirus oncogenic mRNA testing for cervical cancer screening: baseline and longitudinal results from the CLEAR study. Am J Clin Pathol. 2015;144(3):473–83. DOI:10.1309/ajcphvd7mip3fyvv.

[59] Haedicke J, Iftner T. A review of the clinical performance of the Aptima HPV assay. J Clin Virol. 2016;76 Suppl 1:S40-8. DOI:10.1016/j.jcv.2015.10.027

[60] Getman D, Aiyer A, Dockter J, Giachetti C, Zhang F, Ginocchio CC. Efficiency of the APTIMA HPV Assay for detection of HPV RNA and DNA targets. J Clin Virol. 2009;45(Suppl 1):S49–54. DOI:10.1016/s1386-6532(09)70008-3.

[61] Boulet GA, Micalessi IM, Horvath CA, Benoy IH, Depuydt CE, Bogers JJ. Nucleic acid sequence-based amplification assay for human papillomavirus mRNA detection and typing: evidence for DNA amplification. J Clin Microbiol. 2010;48(7):2524–9. DOI: 10.1128/jcm.00173-10.

[62] Ong CK, Chan SY, Campo MS, Fujinaga K, Mavromara-Nazos P, Labropoulou V, Pfister H, Tay SK, ter Meulen J, Villa LL, et al. Evolution of human papillomavirus type 18: an ancient phylogenetic root in Africa and intratype diversity reflect coevolution with human ethnic groups. J Virol. 1993;67(11):6424–31.

[63] Eklund C, Zhou T, Dillner J. Global proficiency study of human papillomavirus genotyping. J Clin Microbiol. 2010;48(11):4147–55. DOI:10.1128/jcm.00918-10.

[64] Didelot MN, Boulle N, Damay A, Costes V, Segondy M. Comparison of the Papillo-Check(R) assay with the digene HC2 HPV DNA assay for the detection of 13 high-risk human papillomaviruses in cervical and anal scrapes. J Med Virol. 2011;83(8):1377–82. DOI:10.1002/jmv.22148.

[65] Stoler MH, Wright TC, Jr., Cuzick J, Dockter J, Reid JL, Getman D, Giachetti C. APTIMA HPV assay performance in women with atypical squamous cells of undetermined significance cytology results. Am J Obstet Gynecol. 2013;208(2):144 e1–8. DOI:10.1016/j.ajog.2012.12.003.

[66] Wright TC, Jr., Stoler MH, Agreda PM, Beitman GH, Gutierrez EC, Harris JM, Koch KR, Kuebler M, LaViers WD, Legendre BL, Jr., Leitch SV, Maus CE, McMillian RA, Nussbaumer WA, Palmer ML, Porter MJ, Richart GA, Schwab RJ, Vaughan LM. Clinical performance of the BD onclarity HPV assay using an adjudicated cohort of BD SurePath liquid-based cytology specimens. Am J Clin Pathol. 2014;142(1):43–50. DOI:10.1309/ajcp53kmhnrdicbl.

[67] Roche. cobas 4800 HPV Test, Instructions For Use. 2013;Reference 05641225001-10EN(Doc. Rev, 8.0).

[68] Castle PE, Hunt WC, Langsfeld E, Wheeler CM. Three-year risk of cervical precancer and cancer after the detection of low-risk human papillomavirus genotypes targeted by a commercial test. Obstet Gynecol. 2014;123(1):49–56. DOI:10.1097/aog.0000000000000013.

[69] Schiffman M, Clifford G, Buonaguro FM. Classification of weakly carcinogenic human papillomavirus types: addressing the limits of epidemiology at the borderline. Infect Agent Cancer. 2009;4:8. DOI:10.1186/1750-9378-4-8.

[70] Castle PE, Solomon D, Wheeler CM, Gravitt PE, Wacholder S, Schiffman M. Human papillomavirus genotype specificity of hybrid capture 2. J Clin Microbiol. 2008;46(8): 2595–604. DOI:10.1128/jcm.00824-08.

[71] Halec G, Alemany L, Lloveras B, Schmitt M, Alejo M, Bosch FX, Tous S, Klaustermeier JE, Guimera N, Grabe N, Lahrmann B, Gissmann L, Quint W, Bosch FX, de Sanjose S, Pawlita M. Pathogenic role of the eight probably/possibly carcinogenic HPV types 26, 53, 66, 67, 68, 70, 73 and 82 in cervical cancer. J Pathol. 2014;234(4):441–51. DOI:10.1002/path.4405.

[72] Cox JT, Castle PE, Behrens CM, Sharma A, Wright TC, Jr., Cuzick J, hena HPVSG. Comparison of cervical cancer screening strategies incorporating different combinations of cytology, HPV testing, and genotyping for HPV 16/18: results from the ATHENA HPV study. Am J Obstet Gynecol. 2013;208(3):184 e1–11. DOI:10.1016/j.ajog.2012.11.020.

[73] Lindemann ML, Dominguez MJ, de Antonio JC, Sandri MT, Tricca A, Sideri M, Khiri H, Ravet S, Boyle S, Aldrich C, Halfon P. Analytical comparison of the cobas HPV Test with Hybrid Capture 2 for the detection of high-risk HPV genotypes. J Mol Diagn. JMD. 2012;14(1):65–70. DOI:10.1016/j.jmoldx.2011.09.005.

[74] Poljak M, Kocjan BJ, Kovanda A, Lunar MM, Lepej SZ, Planinic A, Seme K, Vince A. Human papillomavirus genotype specificity of hybrid capture 2 low-risk probe cocktail. J Clin Microbiol. 2009;47(8):2611–5. DOI:10.1128/jcm.00278-09.

[75] Gillio-Tos A, De Marco L, Carozzi FM, Del Mistro A, Girlando S, Burroni E, Frayle-Salamanca H, Giorgi Rossi P, Pierotti P, Ronco G. Clinical impact of the analytical specificity of the hybrid capture 2 test: data from the New Technologies for Cervical Cancer (NTCC) study. J Clin Microbiol. 2013;51(9):2901–7. DOI:10.1128/jcm.01047-13.

[76] Bottari F, Sideri M, Gulmini C, Igidbashian S, Tricca A, Casadio C, Carinelli S, Boveri S, Ejegod D, Bonde J, Sandri MT. Comparison of the performance of the BD Onclarity HPV Assay with Hybrid Capture II in detection of CIN2+ lesions. J Clin Microbiol. 2015;53(7):2109-14. DOI:10.1128/jcm.00246-15.

[77] Cook DA, Mei W, Smith LW, van Niekerk DJ, Ceballos K, Franco EL, Coldman AJ, Ogilvie GS, Krajden M. Comparison of the Roche cobas(R) 4800 and Digene Hybrid Capture(R) 2 HPV tests for primary cervical cancer screening in the HPV FOCAL trial. BMC Cancer. 2015;15(1):968. DOI:10.1186/s12885-015-1959-5.

[78] Hologic. Cervista HPV HR, Instructions For Use. 2011;Ref. 92-011 PRD-015620 (Part number 15-3053 Revision 103).

[79] Guo M, Khanna A, Feng J, Patel S, Zhang W, Gong Y, Huo L, Staerkel G. Analytical performance of cervista HPV 16/18 in SurePath pap specimens. Diagn Cytopathol. 2015;43(4):301–6. DOI:10.1002/dc.23221.

[80] Ejegod DM, Rebolj M, Bonde J. Comparison of analytical and clinical performance of CLART HPV2 genotyping assay to Linear Array and Hybrid Capture 2: a split-sample study. BMC Cancer. 2015;15:216. DOI:10.1186/s12885-015-1223-z.

[81] Orlando G, Fasolo M, Mazza F, Ricci E, Esposito S, Frati E, Zuccotti GV, Cetin I, Gramegna M, Rizzardini G, Tanzi E. Risk of cervical HPV infection and prevalence of vaccine-type and other high-risk HPV types among sexually active teens and young women (13–26 years) enrolled in the VALHIDATE study. Hum Vaccin Immunother. 2014;10(4):986–94.

[82] Snijders PJ, Meijer CJ, Walboomers JM. Degenerate primers based on highly conserved regions of amino acid sequence in papillomaviruses can be used in a generalized polymerase chain reaction to detect productive human papillomavirus infection. J Gen Virol. 1991;72(Pt 11):2781–6. DOI:10.1099/0022-1317-72-11-2781.

[83] Ozaki S, Kato K, Abe Y, Hara H, Kubota H, Kubushiro K, Kawahara E, Inoue M. Analytical performance of newly developed multiplex human papillomavirus genotyping assay using Luminex xMAP technology (Mebgen HPV Kit). J Virol Methods. 2014;204:73–80. DOI:10.1016/j.jviromet.2014.04.010.

[84] Schalasta G, Rosenthal T, Grothe M. Roche AMPLICOR human papilloma virus (HPV) and LINEAR ARRAY HPV tests will profit from automated DNA extraction. Clin Lab. 2007;53(3–4):131–3.

[85] van Hamont D, van Ham MA, Bakkers JM, Massuger LF, Melchers WJ. Evaluation of the SPF10-INNO LiPA human papillomavirus (HPV) genotyping test and the roche linear array HPV genotyping test. J Clin Microbiol. 2006;44(9):3122–9. DOI:10.1128/JCM.00517-06.

[86] Depuydt CE, Benoy IH, Beert JF, Criel AM, Bogers JJ, Arbyn M. Clinical validation of a type-specific real-time quantitative human papillomavirus PCR against the performance of hybrid capture 2 for the purpose of cervical cancer screening. J Clin Microbiol. 2012;50(12):4073–7. DOI:10.1128/JCM.01231-12.

[87] Castle PE, Smith KM, Davis TE, Schmeler KM, Ferris DG, Savage AH, Gray JE, Stoler MH, Wright TC, Jr., Ferenczy A, Einstein MH. Reliability of the Xpert HPV assay to detect high-risk human papillomavirus DNA in a colposcopy referral population. Am J Clin Pathol. 2015;143(1):126–33. DOI:10.1309/ajcp4q0nsdhwizgu.

[88] Mesher D, Szarewski A, Cadman L, Austin J, Ashdown-Barr L, Ho L, Terry G, Young M, Stoler M, Bergeron C, McCarthy J, Wright C, Liddle S, Soutter WP, Lyons D, Cuzick J. Comparison of human papillomavirus testing strategies for triage of women referred with low-grade cytological abnormalities. Eur J Cancer. 2013;49:2179–86. DOI:10.1016/j.ejca.2013.01.018.

[89] Rebolj M, Lynge E, Ejegod D, Preisler S, Rygaard C, Bonde J. Comparison of three human papillomavirus DNA assays and one mRNA assay in women with abnormal cytology. Gynecol Oncol. 2014;135(3):474–80. DOI:10.1016/j.ygyno.2014.10.014.

[90] Heideman DA, Hesselink AT, van Kemenade FJ, Iftner T, Berkhof J, Topal F, Agard D, Meijer CJ, Snijders PJ. The Aptima HPV assay fulfills the cross-sectional clinical and reproducibility criteria of international guidelines for human papillomavirus test requirements for cervical screening. J Clin Microbiol. 2013;51(11):3653–7. DOI:10.1128/jcm.01517-13.

[91] Castle PE, Eaton B, Reid J, Getman D, Dockter J. Comparison of human papillomavirus detection by Aptima HPV and cobas HPV tests in a population of women referred for colposcopy following detection of atypical squamous cells of undetermined significance by Pap cytology. J Clin Microbiol. 2015;53(4):1277–81. DOI:10.1128/jcm.03558-14.

[92] Hesselink AT, Meijer CJ, Poljak M, Berkhof J, van Kemenade FJ, van der Salm ML, Bogaarts M, Snijders PJ, Heideman DA. Clinical validation of the Abbott RealTime High-Risk HPV assay according to the guidelines for human papillomavirus DNA test requirements for cervical screening. J Clin Microbiol. 2013;51(7):2409–10. DOI:10.1128/jcm.00633-13.

[93] Abbott. Abbott RealTime High-Risk HPV, Instructions For Use. 2010;Ref. 2N09 49-2028/R3 B2N090.

[94] Greiner-Bio-One. PapilloCheck® high-risk –Instructions For Use. Revision: BQ-065-01;2011.

[95] Castle PE, Gutierrez EC, Leitch SV, Maus CE, McMillian RA, Nussbaumer WA, Vaughan LM, Wheeler CM, Gravitt PE, Schiffman M. Evaluation of a new DNA test for detection of carcinogenic human papillomavirus. J Clin Microbiol. 2011;49(8):3029–32. DOI:10.1128/JCM.00422-11.

[96] Schiffman M, Vaughan LM, Raine-Bennett TR, Castle PE, Katki HA, Gage JC, Fetterman B, Befano B, Wentzensen N. A study of HPV typing for the management of HPV-positive ASC-US cervical cytologic results. Gynecol Oncol. 2015;138(3):573–8. DOI: 10.1016/j.ygyno.2015.06.040.

[97] Wright TC, Jr., Stoler MH, Behrens CM, Apple R, Derion T, Wright TL. The ATHENA human papillomavirus study: design, methods, and baseline results. Am J Obstet Gynecol. 2012;206(1):46 e1–11. DOI:10.1016/j.ajog.2011.07.024.

[98] Saslow D, Solomon D, Lawson HW, Killackey M, Kulasingam SL, Cain J, Garcia FA, Moriarty AT, Waxman AG, Wilbur DC, Wentzensen N, Downs LS, Jr., Spitzer M, Moscicki AB, Franco EL, Stoler MH, Schiffman M, Castle PE, Myers ER, American Cancer S, American Society for C, Cervical P, American Society for Clinical P. American Cancer Society, American Society for Colposcopy and Cervical Pathology, and American Society for Clinical Pathology screening guidelines for the prevention and early detection of cervical cancer. Am J Clin Pathol. 2012;137(4):516–42. DOI:10.1309/AJCPTGD94EVRSJCG.

[99] Carcopino X, Henry M, Mancini J, Giusiano S, Boubli L, Olive D, Tamalet C. Significance of HPV 16 and 18 viral load quantitation in women referred for colposcopy. J Med Virol. 2012;84(2):306–13. DOI:10.1002/jmv.23190.

[100] Sun Z, Zhang R, Liu Z, Liu C, Li X, Zhou W, Yang L, Ruan Q, Zhang X. Development of a fluorescence-based multiplex genotyping method for simultaneous determination of human papillomavirus infections and viral loads. BMC Cancer. 2015;15:860. DOI: 10.1186/s12885-015-1874-9.

[101] Wentzensen N, Gravitt PE, Long R, Schiffman M, Dunn ST, Carreon JD, Allen RA, Gunja M, Zuna RE, Sherman ME, Gold MA, Walker JL, Wang SS. Human papillomavirus load measured by Linear Array correlates with quantitative PCR in cervical cytology specimens. J Clin Microbiol. 2012;50(5):1564–70. DOI:10.1128/jcm.06240-11.

[102] Marongiu L, Godi A, Parry JV, Beddows S. Human Papillomavirus 16, 18, 31 and 45 viral load, integration and methylation status stratified by cervical disease stage. BMC Cancer. 2014;14:384. DOI:10.1186/1471-2407-14-384.

[103] Baron C, Henry M, Tamalet C, Villeret J, Richet H, Carcopino X. Relationship between HPV 16, 18, 31, 33, 45 DNA detection and quantitation and E6/E7 mRNA detection among a series of cervical specimens with various degrees of histological lesions. J Med Virol. 2015;87(8):1389–96. DOI:10.1002/jmv.24157.

[104] van Doorn LJ, Molijn A, Kleter B, Quint W, Colau B. Highly effective detection of human papillomavirus 16 and 18 DNA by a testing algorithm combining broad-spectrum and type-specific PCR. J Clin Microbiol. 2006;44(9):3292–8. DOI:10.1128/jcm.00539-06.

[105] van Alewijk D, Kleter B, Vent M, Delroisse JM, de Koning M, van Doorn LJ, Quint W, Colau B. A human papilloma virus testing algorithm comprising a combination of the L1 broad-spectrum SPF10 PCR assay and a novel E6 high-risk multiplex type-specific genotyping PCR assay. J Clin Microbiol. 2013;51(4):1171–8. DOI:10.1128/jcm.02831-12.

[106] Mori S, Nakao S, Kukimoto I, Kusumoto-Matsuo R, Kondo K, Kanda T. Biased amplification of human papillomavirus DNA in specimens containing multiple human papillomavirus types by PCR with consensus primers. Cancer Sci. 2011;102(6):1223–7. DOI:10.1111/j.1349-7006.2011.01922.x.

[107] Vaccarella S, Franceschi S, Snijders PJ, Herrero R, Meijer CJ, Plummer M. Concurrent infection with multiple human papillomavirus types: pooled analysis of the IARC HPV Prevalence Surveys. Cancer Epidemiol Biomarkers Prev. 2010;19(2):503–10. DOI: 10.1158/1055-9965.epi-09-0983.

[108] Struyf F, Colau B, Wheeler CM, Naud P, Garland S, Quint W, Chow SN, Salmeron J, Lehtinen M, Del Rosario-Raymundo MR, Paavonen J, Teixeira JC, Germar MJ, Peters K, Skinner SR, Limson G, Castellsague X, Poppe WA, Ramjattan B, Klein TD, Schwarz TF, Chatterjee A, Tjalma WA, Diaz-Mitoma F, Lewis DJ, Harper DM, Molijn A, van Doorn LJ, David MP, Dubin G. Post hoc analysis of the PATRICIA randomized trial of the efficacy of human papillomavirus type 16 (HPV-16)/HPV-18 AS04-adjuvanted

vaccine against incident and persistent infection with nonvaccine oncogenic HPV types using an alternative multiplex type-specific PCR assay for HPV DNA. Clin Vaccin Immunol. 2015;22(2):235–44. DOI:10.1128/cvi.00457-14.

[109] Cornall AM, Phillips S, Cummins E, Garland SM, Tabrizi SN. *In vitro* assessment of the effect of vaccine-targeted human papillomavirus (HPV) depletion on detection of non-vaccine HPV types: implications for post-vaccine surveillance studies. J Virol Methods. 2015;214:10–4. DOI:10.1016/j.jviromet.2014.12.007.

[110] Barzon L, Militello V, Lavezzo E, Franchin E, Peta E, Squarzon L, Trevisan M, Pagni S, Dal Bello F, Toppo S, Palu G. Human papillomavirus genotyping by 454 next generation sequencing technology. J Clin Virol. 2011;52(2):93–7. DOI:10.1016/j.jcv.2011.07.006.

[111] Eklund C, Wallin K-L, Forslund O, Dilllner J. Continued global improvment in HPV DNA genotyping: The 2014 HPV LabNet International Proficiency Study. International Papillomavirus Conference, Lisbon, Portugal, 17–21 September 2015.

[112] ICO. Information Centre on HPV and Cancer (Institut Català d'Oncologia). 2016; Available from: http://www.hpvcentre.net/ (accessed: 2016-01-10).

[113] Huh WK, Ault KA, Chelmow D, Davey DD, Goulart RA, Garcia FA, Kinney WK, Massad LS, Mayeaux EJ, Saslow D, Schiffman M, Wentzensen N, Lawson HW, Einstein MH. Use of primary high-risk human papillomavirus testing for cervical cancer screening: Interim clinical guidance. Gynecol Oncol. 2015;136(2):178–82. DOI:10.1016/j.ygyno.2014.12.022.

[114] Fontaine D, Narine N, Naugler C. Unsatisfactory rates vary between cervical cytology samples prepared using ThinPrep and SurePath platforms: a review and meta-analysis. BMJ Open. 2012;2(2):e000847. DOI:10.1136/bmjopen-2012-000847.

[115] Kenyon S, Sweeney BJ, Happel J, Marchilli GE, Weinstein B, Schneider D. Comparison of BD Surepath and ThinPrep Pap systems in the processing of mucus-rich specimens. Cancer Cytopathol. 2010;118(5):244–9. DOI:10.1002/cncy.20096.

[116] Chen G, Kobayashi L, Nazarenko I. Effect of sample aliquot size on the limit of detection and reproducibility of clinical assays. Clin Chem. 2007;53(11):1962–5. DOI:10.1373/clinchem.2007.089854.

[117] Becton-Dickinson. BD Onclarity™ HPV Assay, CE Mark Instructions for use, Ref. 442946, 8089899(02). 2014.

[118] Power Y, Bowes C. Reprocessing bloodstained ThinPrep Papanicolaou cervical cytology samples using glacial acetic acid increases the satisfactory rate in previously unsatisfactory smears. Br J Biomed Sci. 2013;70(3):130.

[119] Depuydt CE, Jonckheere J, Berth M, Salembier GM, Vereecken AJ, Bogers JJ. Serial type-specific human papillomavirus (HPV) load measurement allows differentiation between regressing cervical lesions and serial virion productive transient infections. Cancer Med. 2015;4(8):1294–302. DOI:10.1002/cam4.473.

[120] Stoler MH, Ronnett BM, Joste NE, Hunt WC, Cuzick J, Wheeler CM. The interpretive variability of cervical biopsies and its relationship to HPV status. Am J Surg Pathol. 2015;39(6):729–36. DOI:10.1097/pas.0000000000000381.

[121] Clinton LK, Miyazaki K, Ayabe A, Davis J, Tauchi-Nishi P, Shimizu D. The LAST guidelines in clinical practice: implementing recommendations for p16 use. Am J Clin Pathol. 2015;144(6):844–9. DOI:10.1309/ajcpuxlp7xd8oqyy.

[122] Badaracco G, Venuti A, Sedati A, Marcante ML. HPV16 and HPV18 in genital tumors: significantly different levels of viral integration and correlation to tumor invasiveness. J Med Virol. 2002;67(4):574–82. DOI:10.1002/jmv.10141.

[123] Cullen AP, Reid R, Campion M, Lorincz AT. Analysis of the physical state of different human papillomavirus DNAs in intraepithelial and invasive cervical neoplasm. J Virol. 1991;65(2):606–12.

[124] Hu Z, Zhu D, Wang W, Li W, Jia W, Zeng X, Ding W, Yu L, Wang X, Wang L, Shen H, Zhang C, Liu H, Liu X, Zhao Y, Fang X, Li S, Chen W, Tang T, Fu A, Wang Z, Chen G, Gao Q, Li S, Xi L, Wang C, Liao S, Ma X, Wu P, Li K, Wang S, Zhou J, Wang J, Xu X, Wang H, Ma D. Genome-wide profiling of HPV integration in cervical cancer identifies clustered genomic hot spots and a potential microhomology-mediated integration mechanism. Nat Genet. 2015;47(2):158–63. DOI:10.1038/ng.3178.

[125] Liu Y, Lu Z, Xu R, Ke Y. Comprehensive mapping of the human papillomavirus (HPV) DNA integration sites in cervical carcinomas by HPV capture technology. Oncotarget. 2016;2;7(5):5852-64. DOI:10.18632/oncotarget.6809.

[126] Cullen M, Boland JF, Schiffman M, Zhang X, Wentzensen N, Yang Q, Chen Z, Yu K, Mitchell J, Roberson D, Bass S, Burdette L, Machado M, Ravichandran S, Luke B, Machiela MJ, Andersen M, Osentoski M, Laptewicz M, Wacholder S, Feldman A, Raine-Bennett T, Lorey T, Castle PE, Yeager M, Burk RD, Mirabello L. Deep sequencing of HPV16 genomes: A new high-throughput tool for exploring the carcinogenicity and natural history of HPV16 infection. Papillomavirus Res. 2015;1:3–11. DOI:10.1016/j.pvr.2015.05.004.

[127] Chandrani P, Kulkarni V, Iyer P, Upadhyay P, Chaubal R, Das P, Mulherkar R, Singh R, Dutt A. NGS-based approach to determine the presence of HPV and their sites of integration in human cancer genome. Br J Cancer. 2015;112(12):1958–65. DOI:10.1038/bjc.2015.121.

[128] Tjalma WA, Depuydt CE. Cervical cancer screening: which HPV test should be used-L1 or E6/E7? Eur J Obstet Gynecol Reprod Biol. 2013;170(1):45–6. DOI:10.1016/j.ejogrb.2013.06.027.

[129] Tjalma WA, Depuydt CE. Cervical atypical glandular cells and false negative HPV testing: a dramatic reality of the wrong test at the right place. Eur J Gynaecol Oncol. 2014;35(2):117–20.

[130] Morris BJ. Cervical human papillomavirus screening by PCR: advantages of targeting the E6/E7 region. Clin Chem Lab Med. 2005;43(11):1171–7. DOI:10.1515/CCLM.2005.203.

[131] Einstein MH, Cruz Y, El-Awady MK, Popescu NC, DiPaolo JA, van Ranst M, Kadish AS, Romney S, Runowicz CD, Burk RD. Utilization of the human genome sequence localizes human papillomavirus type 16 DNA integrated into the TNFAIP2 gene in a fatal cervical cancer from a 39-year-old woman. Clin Cancer Res. 2002;8(2):549–54.

[132] Karlsen F, Kalantari M, Jenkins A, Pettersen E, Kristensen G, Holm R, Johansson B, Hagmar B. Use of multiple PCR primer sets for optimal detection of human papillomavirus. J Clin Microbiol. 1996;34(9):2095–100.

[133] Hagmar B, Johansson B, Kalantari M, Petersson Z, Skyldberg B, Walaas L. The incidence of HPV in a Swedish series of invasive cervical carcinoma. Med Oncol Tumor Pharmacother. 1992;9(3):113–7.

[134] Walboomers JM, Jacobs MV, Manos MM, Bosch FX, Kummer JA, Shah KV, Snijders PJ, Peto J, Meijer CJ, Munoz N. Human papillomavirus is a necessary cause of invasive cervical cancer worldwide. J Pathol. 1999;189(1):12–9. DOI:10.1002/(SICI)1096-9896(199909)189:1<12::AID-PATH431>3.0.CO;2-F.

[135] Hopenhayn C, Christian A, Christian WJ, Watson M, Unger ER, Lynch CF, Peters ES, Wilkinson EJ, Huang Y, Copeland G, Cozen W, Saber MS, Goodman MT, Hernandez BY, Steinau M, Lyu C, Tucker TT, Saraiya M. Prevalence of human papillomavirus types in invasive cervical cancers from 7 US cancer registries before vaccine introduction. J Low Genit Tract Dis. 2014;18(2):182–9. DOI:10.1097/LGT.0b013e3182a577c7.

[136] Molijn A, Jenkins D, Chen W, Zhang X, Pirog E, Enqi W, Liu B, Schmidt J, Cui J, Qiao Y, Quint W. The complex relationship between human papillomavirus and cervical adenocarcinoma. Int J Cancer. 2015;15;138(2):409-16. DOI:10.1002/ijc.29722.

[137] Holl K, Nowakowski AM, Powell N, McCluggage WG, Pirog EC, Collas De Souza S, Tjalma WA, Rosenlund M, Fiander A, Castro Sanchez M, Damaskou V, Joura EA, Kirschner B, Koiss R, O'Leary J, Quint W, Reich O, Torne A, Wells M, Rob L, Kolomiets L, Molijn A, Savicheva A, Shipitsyna E, Rosillon D, Jenkins D. Human papillomavirus prevalence and type-distribution in cervical glandular neoplasias: results from a European multinational epidemiological study. Int J Cancer. 2015;137(12):2858–68. DOI:10.1002/ijc.29651.

[138] Adegoke O, Kulasingam S, Virnig B. Cervical cancer trends in the United States: a 35-year population-based analysis. J.Women's Health (2002). 2012;21(10):1031–7. DOI: 10.1089/jwh.2011.3385.

[139] Mbatani N, Adams T, Wijk LV, Behrens C, Tam T, Wright T, Jr., Stoler M, Denny L. Performance of an Human Papillomavirus Test in Samples From Women With Histolopathologically Confirmed Invasive Cervical Cancer. J Low Genit Tract Dis. 2016;20(2):151-3. DOI:10.1097/lgt.0000000000000183.

[140] Cuzick J, Clavel C, Petry KU, Meijer CJ, Hoyer H, Ratnam S, Szarewski A, Birembaut P, Kulasingam S, Sasieni P, Iftner T. Overview of the European and North American studies on HPV testing in primary cervical cancer screening. Int J Cancer. 2006;119(5): 1095-101. DOI:10.1002/ijc.21955.

[141] Pileggi C, Flotta D, Bianco A, Nobile CG, Pavia M. Is HPV DNA testing specificity comparable to that of cytological testing in primary cervical cancer screening? Results of a meta-analysis of randomized controlled trials. Int J Cancer. 2014;135(1):166–77. DOI:10.1002/ijc.28640.

[142] Ronco G, Segnan N, Giorgi-Rossi P, Zappa M, Casadei GP, Carozzi F, Dalla Palma P, Del Mistro A, Folicaldi S, Gillio-Tos A, Nardo G, Naldoni C, Schincaglia P, Zorzi M, Confortini M, Cuzick J. Human papillomavirus testing and liquid-based cytology: results at recruitment from the new technologies for cervical cancer randomized controlled trial. J Natl Cancer Inst. 2006;98(11):765–74. DOI:10.1093/jnci/djj209.

[143] Ronco G, Giorgi-Rossi P, Carozzi F, Confortini M, Dalla Palma P, Del Mistro A, Ghiringhello B, Girlando S, Gillio-Tos A, De Marco L, Naldoni C, Pierotti P, Rizzolo R, Schincaglia P, Zorzi M, Zappa M, Segnan N, Cuzick J. Efficacy of human papillomavirus testing for the detection of invasive cervical cancers and cervical intraepithelial neoplasia: a randomised controlled trial. Lancet Oncol. 2010;11(3):249–57. DOI:10.1016/s1470-2045(09)70360-2.

[144] Kitchener HC, Almonte M, Gilham C, Dowie R, Stoykova B, Sargent A, Roberts C, Desai M, Peto J. ARTISTIC: a randomised trial of human papillomavirus (HPV) testing in primary cervical screening. Health Technol Assess. 2009;13(51):1–150, iii–iv. DOI: 10.3310/hta13510.

[145] Leinonen M, Nieminen P, Kotaniemi-Talonen L, Malila N, Tarkkanen J, Laurila P, Anttila A. Age-specific evaluation of primary human papillomavirus screening vs conventional cytology in a randomized setting. J Natl Cancer Inst. 2009;101(23):1612–23. DOI:10.1093/jnci/djp367.

[146] Sankaranarayanan R, Nene BM, Shastri SS, Jayant K, Muwonge R, Budukh AM, Hingmire S, Malvi SG, Thorat R, Kothari A, Chinoy R, Kelkar R, Kane S, Desai S, Keskar VR, Rajeshwarkar R, Panse N, Dinshaw KA. HPV screening for cervical cancer in rural India. N Engl J Med. 2009;360(14):1385–94. DOI:10.1056/NEJMoa0808516.

[147] Mayrand MH, Franco EL. Integrating novel primary- and secondary-prevention strategies: the next challenge for cervical cancer control. Future Oncol. 2010;6(11):1725–33. DOI:10.2217/fon.10.141.

[148] Rijkaart DC, Berkhof J, Rozendaal L, van Kemenade FJ, Bulkmans NW, Heideman DA, Kenter GG, Cuzick J, Snijders PJ, Meijer CJ. Human papillomavirus testing for the detection of high-grade cervical intraepithelial neoplasia and cancer: final results of the POBASCAM randomised controlled trial. Lancet Oncol. 2012;13(1):78–88. DOI:10.1016/s1470-2045(11)70296-0.

[149] Blatt AJ, Kennedy R, Luff RD, Austin RM, Rabin DS. Comparison of cervical cancer screening results among 256,648 women in multiple clinical practices. Cancer Cytopathol. 2015;123(5):282–8. DOI:10.1002/cncy.21544.

[150] Castle PE. Comparison of cervical cancer screening results among 256,648 women in multiple clinical practices. Cancer Cytopathol. 2015;123(9):566. DOI:10.1002/cncy.21572.

[151] Carozzi FM, Del Mistro A, Cuschieri K, Frayle H, Sani C, Burroni E. HPV testing for primary cervical screening: Laboratory issues and evolving requirements for robust quality assurance. J Clin Virol. 2016;76 Suppl 1:S228. DOI:10.1016/j.jcv.2015.10.025.

[152] El-Zein M, Richardson L, Franco EL. Cervical cancer screening of HPV vaccinated populations: cytology, molecular testing, both or none. J Clin Virol. 2016;76 Suppl 1:S62-8. DOI:10.1016/j.jcv.2015.11.020.

[153] Wright TC, Stoler MH, Behrens CM, Sharma A, Zhang G, Wright TL. Primary cervical cancer screening with human papillomavirus: end of study results from the ATHENA study using HPV as the first-line screening test. Gynecol Oncol. 2015;136(2):189–97. DOI:10.1016/j.ygyno.2014.11.076.

[154] Stoler MH, Austin RM, Zhao C. Point-counterpoint: cervical cancer screening should be done by primary human papillomavirus testing with genotyping and reflex cytology for women over the age of 25 years. J Clin Microbiol. 2015;53(9):2798–804. DOI:10.1128/jcm.01087-15.

[155] Uijterwaal MH, Polman NJ, Van Kemenade FJ, Van Den Haselkamp S, Witte BI, Rijkaart D, Berkhof J, Snijders PJ, Meijer CJ. Five-year cervical (pre)cancer risk of women screened by HPV and cytology testing. Cancer Prev Res (Phila). 2015;8(6):502–8. DOI: 10.1158/1940-6207.capr-14-0409.

[156] Gage JC, Schiffman M, Katki HA, Castle PE, Fetterman B, Wentzensen N, Poitras NE, Lorey T, Cheung LC, Kinney WK. Reassurance against future risk of precancer andcancer conferred by a negative human papillomavirus test. J Natl Cancer Inst. 2014;106(8)1-4. DOI:10.1093/jnci/dju153.

[157] Wright TC, Jr., Stoler MH, Behrens CM, Sharma A, Sharma K, Apple R. Interlaboratory variation in the performance of liquid-based cytology: insights from the ATHENA trial. Int J Cancer. 2014;134(8):1835–43. DOI:10.1002/ijc.28514.

[158] Rijkaart DC, Berkhof J, van Kemenade FJ, Coupe VM, Hesselink AT, Rozendaal L, Heideman DA, Verheijen RH, Bulk S, Verweij WM, Snijders PJ, Meijer CJ. Evaluation of 14 triage strategies for HPV DNA-positive women in population-based cervical screening. Int J Cancer. 2012;130(3):602–10. DOI:10.1002/ijc.26056.

[159] van Ballegooijen M, van den Akker-van Marle E, Patnick J, Lynge E, Arbyn M, Anttila A, Ronco G, Dik J, Habbema F. Overview of important cervical cancer screening process

values in European Union (EU) countries, and tentative predictions of the corresponding effectiveness and cost-effectiveness. Eur J Cancer. 2000;36(17):2177–88.

[160] Peto J, Gilham C, Fletcher O, Matthews FE. The cervical cancer epidemic that screening has prevented in the UK. Lancet. 2004;364(9430):249–56. DOI:10.1016/s0140-6736(04)16674-9.

[161] Kinney W, Sung HY, Kearney KA, Miller M, Sawaya G, Hiatt RA. Missed opportunities for cervical cancer screening of HMO members developing invasive cervical cancer (ICC). Gynecol Oncol. 1998;71(3):428–30. DOI:10.1006/gyno.1998.5135.

[162] Dugue PA, Lynge E, Rebolj M. Mortality of non-participants in cervical screening: register-based cohort study. Int J Cancer. 2014;134(11):2674–82. DOI:10.1002/ijc.28586.

[163] Virtanen A, Nieminen P, Malila N, Luostarinen T, Anttila A. Self-sampling and reminder letters increase participation in the Finnish cervical cancer screening programme. Duodecim. 2013;129(16):1709–17.

[164] Broberg G, Jonasson JM, Ellis J, Gyrd-Hansen D, Anjemark B, Glantz A, Soderberg L, Ryd ML, Holtenman M, Milsom I, Strander B. Increasing participation in cervical cancer screening: telephone contact with long-term non-attendees in Sweden. Results from RACOMIP, a randomized controlled trial. Int J Cancer. 2013;133(1):164–71. DOI:10.1002/ijc.27985.

[165] Racey CS, Gesink DC, Burchell AN, Trivers S, Wong T, Rebbapragada A. Randomized intervention of self-collected sampling for human papillomavirus testing in underscreened rural women: uptake of screening and acceptability. Journal of Women's Health. November 2015, ahead of print. doi:10.1089/jwh.2015.5348.

[166] Rychla L. New self-sampling device for cervical cancer screening tested in Denmark. Copenhagen Post(2015) December 8. Available from CPH POST ONLINE: http://cphpost.dk/news/new-self-sampling-device-for-cervical-cancer-screening-tested-in-denmark.html

[167] ICO. HPV Information Center (Institut Català d'Oncologia): Human Papillomavirus and Related Diseases Report –Denmark. Available from: http://wwwhpvcentrenet/statistics/reports/DNKpdf (accessed: 2015-12-30. 2015).

[168] Verdoodt F, Jentschke M, Hillemanns P, Racey CS, Snijders PJ, Arbyn M. Reaching women who do not participate in the regular cervical cancer screening programme by offering self-sampling kits: a systematic review and meta-analysis of randomised trials. Eur J Cancer. 2015;51(16):2375–85. DOI:10.1016/j.ejca.2015.07.006.

[169] Othman NH, Mohamad Zaki FH. Self-collection tools for routine cervical cancer screening: a review. Asian Pac J Cancer Prev. 2014;15(20):8563–9.

[170] Snijders PJ, Verhoef VM, Arbyn M, Ogilvie G, Minozzi S, Banzi R, van Kemenade FJ, Heideman DA, Meijer CJ. High-risk HPV testing on self-sampled versus clinician-collected specimens: a review on the clinical accuracy and impact on population

attendance in cervical cancer screening. Int J Cancer. 2013;132(10):2223–36. DOI: 10.1002/ijc.27790.

[171] Petignat P, Faltin DL, Bruchim I, Tramer MR, Franco EL, Coutlee F. Are self-collected samples comparable to physician-collected cervical specimens for human papillomavirus DNA testing? A systematic review and meta-analysis. Gynecol Oncol. 2007;105(2):530–5. DOI:10.1016/j.ygyno.2007.01.023.

[172] Arbyn M, Verdoodt F, Snijders PJ, Verhoef VM, Suonio E, Dillner L, Minozzi S, Bellisario C, Banzi R, Zhao FH, Hillemanns P, Anttila A. Accuracy of human papillomavirus testing on self-collected versus clinician-collected samples: a meta-analysis. Lancet Oncol. 2014;15(2):172–83. DOI:10.1016/s1470-2045(13)70570-9.

[173] Chernesky M, Jang D, Gilchrist J, Elit L, Lytwyn A, Smieja M, Dockter J, Getman D, Reid J, Hill C. Evaluation of a new APTIMA specimen collection and transportation kit for high-risk human papillomavirus E6/E7 messenger RNA in cervical and vaginal samples. Sex Transm Dis. 2014;41(6):365–8. DOI:10.1097/olq.0000000000000125.

[174] Eperon I, Vassilakos P, Navarria I, Menoud PA, Gauthier A, Pache JC, Boulvain M, Untiet S, Petignat P. Randomized comparison of vaginal self-sampling by standard vs. dry swabs for human papillomavirus testing. BMC Cancer. 2013;13:353. DOI: 10.1186/1471-2407-13-353.

[175] Lorenzi AT, Fregnani JH, Possati-Resende JC, Neto CS, Villa LL, Longatto-Filho A. Self-collection for high-risk HPV detection in Brazilian women using the careHPV test. Gynecol Oncol. 2013;131(1):131–4. DOI:10.1016/j.ygyno.2013.07.092.

[176] Forslund O, Hansson BG, Rymark P, Bjerre B. Human papillomavirus DNA in urine samples compared with that in simultaneously collected urethra and cervix samples. J Clin Microbiol. 1993;31(8):1975–9.

[177] Geddy PM, Wells M, Lacey CJ. Lack of detection of human papillomavirus DNA in male urine samples. Genitourin Med. 1993;69(4):276–9.

[178] Bianchi S, Frati ER, Panatto D, Martinelli M, Amicizia D, Zotti CM, Martinese M, Bonanni P, Boccalini S, Coppola RC, Masia G, Meloni A, Castiglia P, Piana A, Gasparini R, Tanzi E. Detection and genotyping of human papillomavirus in urine samples from unvaccinated male and female adolescents in Italy. PLoS One. 2013;8(11):e79719. DOI: 10.1371/journal.pone.0079719.

[179] Enerly E, Olofsson C, Nygard M. Monitoring human papillomavirus prevalence in urine samples: a review. Clin Epidemiol. 2013;5:67–79. DOI:10.2147/clep.s39799.

[180] Vorsters A, Van Keer S, Van Damme P. The use of urine in the follow-up of HPV vaccine trials. Hum Vaccin Immunother. 2015;11(2):350–2. DOI:10.4161/21645515.2014.995058.

[181] Vorsters A, Van Damme P, Clifford G. Urine testing for HPV: rationale for using first void. BMJ. 2014;349:g6252. DOI:10.1136/bmj.g6252.

[182] Pathak N, Dodds J, Zamora J, Khan K. Accuracy of urinary human papillomavirus testing for presence of cervical HPV: systematic review and meta-analysis. BMJ. 2014;349:g5264. DOI:10.1136/bmj.g5264.

[183] Vorsters A, Van den Bergh J, Micalessi I, Biesmans S, Bogers J, Hens A, De Coster I, Ieven M, Van Damme P. Optimization of HPV DNA detection in urine by improving collection, storage, and extraction. Eur J Clin Microbiol Infect Dis. 2014;33(11):2005–14. DOI:10.1007/s10096-014-2147-2.

[184] Vorsters A, Micalessi I, Bilcke J, Ieven M, Bogers J, Van Damme P. Detection of human papillomavirus DNA in urine. A review of the literature. Eur J Clin Microbiol Infect Dis. 2012;31(5):627–40. DOI:10.1007/s10096-011-1358-z.

[185] Senkomago V, Des Marais AC, Rahangdale L, Vibat CR, Erlander MG, Smith JS. Comparison of urine specimen collection times and testing fractions for the detection of high-risk human papillomavirus and high-grade cervical precancer. J Clin Virol. 2016;74:26–31. DOI:10.1016/j.jcv.2015.11.005.

[186] Santiago-Rodriguez TM, Ly M, Bonilla N, Pride DT. The human urine virome in association with urinary tract infections. FrontMicrobiol. 2015;6:14. DOI:10.3389/fmicb. 2015.00014.

[187] Bryzgunova OE, Laktionov PP. Extracellular nucleic acids in urine: sources, structure, diagnostic potential. Acta Naturae. 2015;7(3):48–54.

[188] Vorsters A, Vankerckhoven V, Beyers K, Van Damme P, Long D, Schwab R, Gutierrez G, Nussbaumer W, Harris J, Vaughan L. Performance of an automated HPV genotyping assay using first void urine specimens. International Papillomavirus Conference, Lisbon, Portugal, 17–21 September 2015.

[189] Zhang SH, Zhao SM, Zhao ZM, Li CT. Genotyping of urinary samples stored with EDTA for forensic applications. Genetics Mol Research. 2012;11(3):3007–12. DOI: 10.4238/2012.May.10.5.

[190] Musante L, Tataruch D, Gu D, Liu X, Forsblom C, Groop PH, Holthofer H. Proteases and protease inhibitors of urinary extracellular vesicles in diabetic nephropathy. J Diabetes Res. 2015;2015:289734. DOI:10.1155/2015/289734.

[191] Milde A, Haas-Rochholz H, Kaatsch HJ. Improved DNA typing of human urine by adding EDTA. Int J Legal Med. 1999;112(3):209–10.

[192] Ducancelle A, Reiser J, Pivert A, Le Guillou-Guillemette H, Le Duc-Banaszuk AS, Lunel-Fabiani F. Home-based urinary HPV DNA testing in women who do not attend cervical cancer screening clinics. J Infect. 2015;71(3):377–84. DOI:10.1016/j.jinf. 2015.05.001.

[193] Thomsen LT, Frederiksen K, Munk C, Junge J, Iftner T, Kjaer SK. Long-term risk of cervical intraepithelial neoplasia grade 3 or worse according to high-risk human

papillomavirus genotype and semi-quantitative viral load among 33,288 women with normal cervical cytology. Int J Cancer. 2015;137(1):193–203. DOI:10.1002/ijc.29374.

[194] Schiffman M, Wentzensen N, Wacholder S, Kinney W, Gage JC, Castle PE. Human papillomavirus testing in the prevention of cervical cancer. J Natl Cancer Inst. 2011;103(5):368–83. DOI:10.1093/jnci/djq562.

[195] Cuzick J, Ho L, Terry G, Kleeman M, Giddings M, Austin J, Cadman L, Ashdown-Barr L, Costa MJ, Szarewski A. Individual detection of 14 high risk human papilloma virus genotypes by the PapType test for the prediction of high grade cervical lesions. J Clin Virol. 2014;60(1):44–9. DOI:10.1016/j.jcv.2014.02.002.

[196] Joste NE, Ronnett BM, Hunt WC, Pearse A, Langsfeld E, Leete T, Jaramillo M, Stoler MH, Castle PE, Wheeler CM. Human papillomavirus genotype-specific prevalence across the continuum of cervical neoplasia and cancer. Cancer Epidemiol Biomarkers Prev. 2015;24(1):230–40. DOI:10.1158/1055-9965.epi-14-0775.

[197] Monsonego J, Cox JT, Behrens C, Sandri M, Franco EL, Yap PS, Huh W. Prevalence of high-risk human papilloma virus genotypes and associated risk of cervical precancerous lesions in a large U.S. screening population: data from the ATHENA trial. Gynecol Oncol. 2015;137(1):47–54. DOI:10.1016/j.ygyno.2015.01.551.

[198] de Sanjose S, Quint WG, Alemany L, Geraets DT, Klaustermeier JE, Lloveras B, Tous S, Felix A, Bravo LE, Shin HR, Vallejos CS, de Ruiz PA, Lima MA, Guimera N, Clavero O, Alejo M, Llombart-Bosch A, Cheng-Yang C, Tatti SA, Kasamatsu E, Iljazovic E, Odida M, Prado R, Seoud M, Grce M, Usubutun A, Jain A, Suarez GA, Lombardi LE, Banjo A, Menendez C, Domingo EJ, Velasco J, Nessa A, Chichareon SC, Qiao YL, Lerma E, Garland SM, Sasagawa T, Ferrera A, Hammouda D, Mariani L, Pelayo A, Steiner I, Oliva E, Meijer CJ, Al-Jassar WF, Cruz E, Wright TC, Puras A, Llave CL, Tzardi M, Agorastos T, Garcia-Barriola V, Clavel C, Ordi J, Andujar M, Castellsague X, Sanchez GI, Nowakowski AM, Bornstein J, Munoz N, Bosch FX. Human papillomavirus genotype attribution in invasive cervical cancer: a retrospective cross-sectional worldwide study. Lancet Oncol. 2010;11(11):1048–56. DOI:10.1016/s1470-2045(10)70230-8.

[199] Joura EA, Ault KA, Bosch FX, Brown D, Cuzick J, Ferris D, Garland SM, Giuliano AR, Hernandez-Avila M, Huh W, Iversen OE, Kjaer SK, Luna J, Miller D, Monsonego J, Munoz N, Myers E, Paavonen J, Pitisuttithum P, Steben M, Wheeler CM, Perez G, Saah A, Luxembourg A, Sings HL, Velicer C. Attribution of 12 high-risk human papillomavirus genotypes to infection and cervical disease. Cancer Epidemiol Biomarkers Prev. 2014;23(10):1997–2008. DOI:10.1158/1055-9965.epi-14-0410.

[200] Katki HA, Schiffman M, Castle PE, Fetterman B, Poitras NE, Lorey T, Cheung LC, Raine-Bennett T, Gage JC, Kinney WK. Benchmarking CIN3+ risk as the basis for incorporating HPV and Pap cotesting into cervical screening and management guidelines. J Low Genit Tract Dis. 2013;17(5 Suppl 1):S28–35. DOI:10.1097/LGT.0b013e318285423c.

[201] Joura EA, Giuliano AR, Iversen OE, Bouchard C, Mao C, Mehlsen J, Moreira ED, Jr., Ngan Y, Petersen LK, Lazcano-Ponce E, Pitisuttithum P, Restrepo JA, Stuart G, Woelber L, Yang YC, Cuzick J, Garland SM, Huh W, Kjaer SK, Bautista OM, Chan IS, Chen J, Gesser R, Moeller E, Ritter M, Vuocolo S, Luxembourg A. A 9-valent HPV vaccine against infection and intraepithelial neoplasia in women. N Engl J Med. 2015;372(8): 711–23. DOI:10.1056/NEJMoa1405044.

[202] Khan MJ, Castle PE, Lorincz AT, Wacholder S, Sherman M, Scott DR, Rush BB, Glass AG, Schiffman M. The elevated 10-year risk of cervical precancer and cancer in women with human papillomavirus (HPV) type 16 or 18 and the possible utility of type-specific HPV testing in clinical practice. J Natl Cancer Inst. 2005;97(14):1072–9. DOI:10.1093/jnci/dji187.

[203] Larson H. The world must accept that the HPV vaccine is safe. Nature. 2015;528(7580): 9. DOI:10.1038/528009a.

[204] Schiffman M, Wentzensen N. A Suggested Approach to Simplify and Improve Cervical Screening in the United States. J Low Genit Tract Dis. 2016;20(1):1–7. DOI:10.1097/lgt.0000000000000170.

[205] Wentzensen N, Schiffman M, Palmer T, Arbyn M. Triage of HPV positive women in cervical cancer screening. JClin Virol. 2015. DOI:10.1016/j.jcv.2015.11.015.

[206] Wentzensen N, Schiffman M, Palmer T, Arbyn M. Triage of HPV positive women in cervical cancer screening. J Clin Virol. 2016;76 Suppl 1:S49-55. DOI:10.1016/j.jcv.2015.11.015.

7

Preventive Strategies against Human Papillomaviruses

Naveed Shahzad, Muhammad Umer, Memoona Ramzan and Bilal Aslam

Abstract

Human papillomavirus (HPV) infection is among the most common viral infections of the reproductive tract. Out of more than 100 different types of HPV identified so far, only a few (termed as "high-risk" subtypes) are associated with cervical cancer. On the other hand, "low-risk" subtypes are associated with genital warts and other benign changes in cervical and oral mucosa. Majority of the HPV infections usually clear up without any intervention within a few months. However, a fraction of HPV infections, such as those with types 16 and 18, can become persistent which may lead to the development of anogenital or cervical cancers. HPV subtypes 16 and 18 together are responsible for approximately 70% of all cervical cancer cases, the fourth major cause of cancer-related deaths in women. In the absence of any specific treatment options, preventive measures are considered as cornerstone of strategies aimed at curbing the burden of this disease. This chapter presents a comprehensive review of strategies that can be employed to prevent and eradicate HPV infection. Minimizing the exposure to HPV risk factors such as unprotected sex, multiple sex partners, early age sex, and not being circumcised, can reduce the chances of getting HPV infection to a significant level. Mass screening programs have also been effective in HPV eradication. Nevertheless, immunization against HPV has proven to be the most promising strategy in fight against HPV. Virus-like particles based on bivalent, quadrivalent, and nonavalent anti-HPV vaccines have been licensed and are available in market under the trade names of Cervarix®, Gardasil®, and Gardasil9®, respectively. Various clinical trials and population-based studies have demonstrated high levels of efficacy for all the three vaccines in preventing type-specific malignancies.

Keywords: human papillomavirus (HPV), prevention of HPV, immunization, HPV vaccines, cervical cancer

1. Introduction

Although genital warts, papillomatous, and verrucous lesions of skin have been known to human beings since ancient times [1, 2], it was not until the dawn of twentieth century that infectious nature of these warts could be demonstrated [3]. Toward the end of twentieth century, data started to emerge that hinted toward a link between papillomavirus infection and cervical cancer [4]. It is now well established that this heterogeneous family of epitheliotropic viruses is responsible for a spectrum of diseases that range from mild self-limiting anogenital warts and rare recurrent respiratory papillomatosis (RRP) to the penile, vaginal, vulvar, cervical, anal as well as pharyngeal carcinomas [5, 6].

Disease	Commonly associated HPV subtypes
Cutaneous lesions	
Verrucae vulgares, verrucae palmares et plantares	1, 2, 4
Bowen's disease	16
Butcher's warts	7
Verrucae planae	3, 10
EV-squamous cell carcinomas	5, 8
Epidermodysplasia verruciformis (EV)	3, 5, 8
Mucosal lesions	
Condylomataacuminata	6, 11
Laryngeal papillomatosis	6, 11
Buschke–Löwenstein tumor	6, 11
Bowenoidpapulosis, erythroplasia of Queyrat	16
Squamous intraepithelial neoplasias and invasive carcinomas of the anogenital tract	16
Heck's disease	13, 32

Table 1. Diseases caused by HPV Infection and associated subtypes.

More than a 100 types of Human papillomaviruses (HPV) have so far been identified and are classified into five genera; alpha beta, gamma, mu, and nu [7]. HPV genus alpha, also known as genital or mucosal HPV, comprises of about 40 different subtypes and is the most important genus from medical point of view. These genital or mucosal HPV types are further categorized as low-risk (non-oncogenic) and high-risk (oncogenic) types [8] and infect epithelial cells of skin as well as mucosa of anogenital and upper aerodigestive tracts. There are about 15 high-risk subtypes associated with various cancers of anogenital tract as well as head and neck cancer [7]. Notable high-risk HPV genotypes include subtypes 16 and 18 which together account for more than 90% of cervical cancer cases worldwide [9]. Low-risk subtypes, such as subtypes 6 and 11, on the other hand, are responsible for benign changes in cervical tissue as well as genital warts [10]. The beta genus of HPV includes various cutaneous subtypes some of which might act as a cofactor in the development of non-melanoma skin cancer [11]. The genera gamma, mu, and nu also have cutaneous tropism and are rare [12]. **Table 1** summarizes the diseases caused by HPV infection and associated subtypes.

HPV is the most commonly occurring sexually transmitted infection [5] and around 300 million women worldwide are HPV carriers [13]. In USA, around 14 million people acquire HPV infection every year [14]. Young women are the most commonly affected with highest prevalence in <25 years age group [15, 16]. The incidence of HPV infection is directly correlated with the start of sexual activity as well as the number of sex partners. However, even the persons who remain monogamous for their whole lives are still at the risk of contracting this infection. The major route of HPV transmission is oro-genital and genital–genital contact, and it does not necessarily involve sexual intercourse [5]. More than 90% of HPV infections are cleared within 2 years without any major consequences on the health of patients [17]. A petite fraction of infections with certain types of HPV can persist and progress to cancer, however, this progression usually takes many years. Only persistent viral infection turns into tumors or cancer in the body [18].

Cervical cancer is the fourth major cause of cancer-related deaths in women, and more than 90% of cases are associated with high-risk HPV infection [19]. Infection with any of the 15 high-risk HPV types, particularly subtypes 16 and 18, is considered as necessary but not a sufficient cause of cervical cancer [20]. More than 500,000 new cases of cervical cancer are diagnosed every year out of which about 80% live in developing countries [10] and about 250,000 women die of this malignancy every year [15]. More than 90% of cervical cancer cases are curable with surgical and radiochemotherapeutic interventions if diagnosed at early stages.

Recent years have seen phenomenal success in fight against HPV infection and related cancers. However, the major focus of these efforts remained to be cancerous subtypes or at the best only a couple of warts causing subtypes like 6 and 11. Therefore, there is an urgent need to broaden the scope of preventive strategies to other clinically relevant subtypes as well. This chapter covers an expert commentary on various preventive as well as eradication strategies against HPV and methods being practiced routinely in developed and underdeveloped countries. Guidelines and bottlenecks established by WHO and other-related bodies in prevention and control of HPV will also be a part of this commentary in order to highlight strengths and shortcomings of prevention strategies currently in practice in various regions of the world. Since immunization has been proved the most promising method for HPV prevention, this chapter will focus mainly on the components of the immune system, passive and active immunity, mechanisms of vaccines for immune stimulation, and types of HPV vaccines available.

2. Preventive strategies for HPV

As no specific treatments are available against HPV yet, therefore, more emphasis is put on the prevention rather than treating the infection. Many developed countries including USA,

Australia, Canada, Brazil, Sweden, and United Kingdom have established national guidelines to defeat the HPV and associated cancers [21]. Notably, the established guidelines in mentioned countries altogether focus mainly on the HPV-related cervical cancer in women only. There is no recommendation to screen men particularly and women under the age of 30 years. Similarly, only a small portion of management guidelines refer to other HPV-associated infections/cancers in both genders.

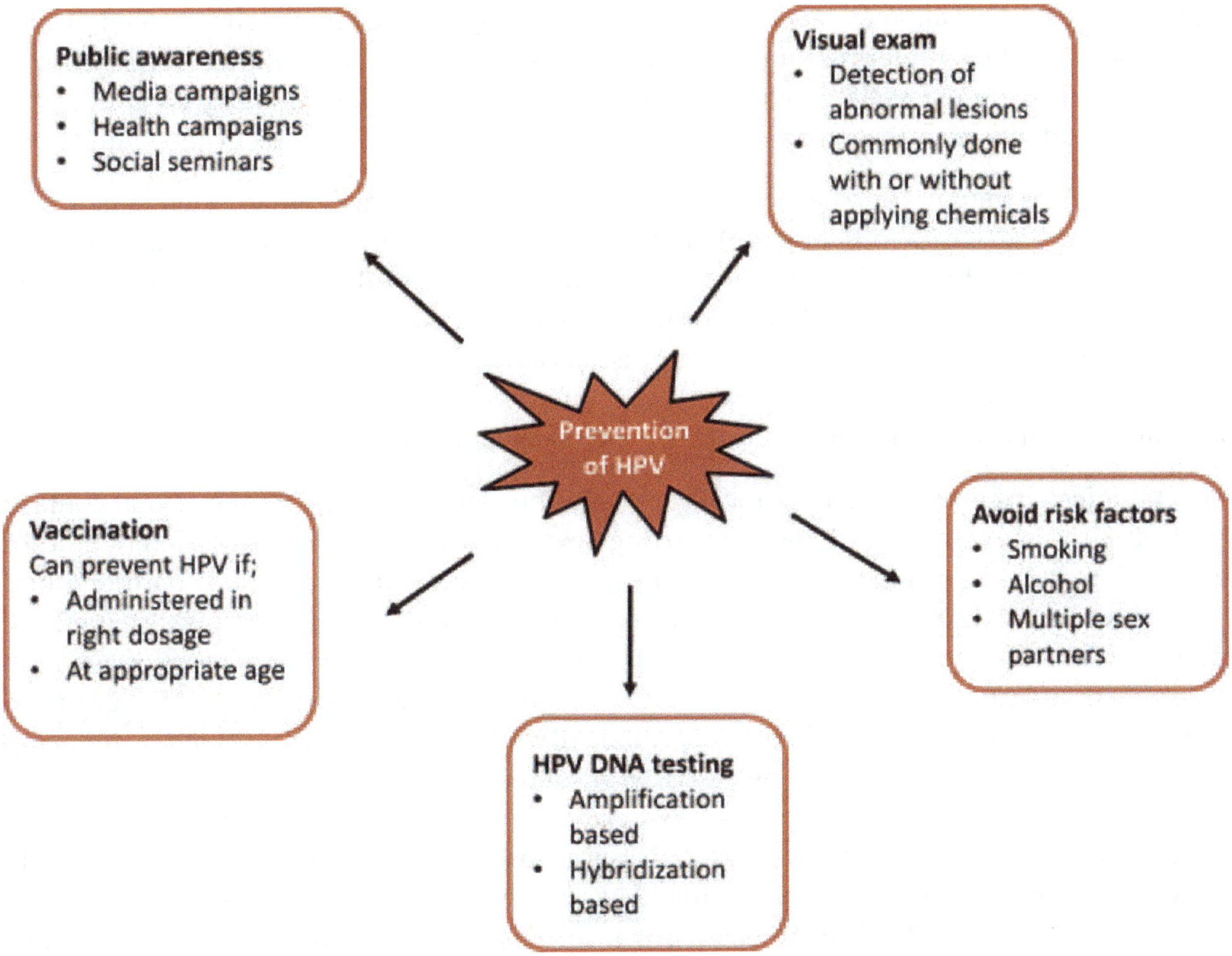

Figure 1. The possible ways for prevention and eradication of the HPV infections.

Despite millions of new HPV infections cases every year, only a few women infected even with hrHPV types manifest precancerous lesions and even fewer develop invasive cervical cancer. This difference in the ratio between HPV infections and HPV-related cancers clearly indicates the role of other risk factors that might be involved in the development of cervical cancer [22]. Current guidelines suggest that HPV infections can be avoided by minimizing the exposure to risk factors such as unprotected sex, multiple sex partners, early age sex, and not being circumcised. In addition to that, practice of mass screening in women aged 21–65 years has been declared a promising strategy to combat the burden of HPV [23].

Above all, vaccination against HPV in both men and women has proven to be the most critical way in preventing the HPV infection. The possible way forward in handling the HPV infections are depicted in **Figure 1**.

2.1. Reduction of exposure to the risk factors

Almost all HPV infections are transmitted from skin to skin and sexual contact [5]. To the best of our knowledge, HPV transmission through body fluids and secretions has never been reported. However, HPV can be transferred vertically from infected mother to child during birth such as in papillomatosis [18, 22]. Risk factors associated with HPV infection and development of its long-term sequelae, particularly cancers, can be broadly categorized into two categories: those associated with HPV infection of mucosal layers lining the oral cavity and lungs and the second category that is associated with warts and cancers of anogenital tract.

Factors, such as smoking, alcoholism, drugs, and direct skin contact with infected person, can play a supportive role for initiating HPV infection, and thus cancer, in the mucosal layers lining the oral cavity and lungs. These types of cancers already constitute a smaller fraction among HPV-associated cancers. Nonetheless, oropharynx cancer has exhibited increasing trend in USA and other parts of the world since the last decade. The cancer of mucosal layers can be prevented by avoiding direct skin contact with infected person. Further, decrease of tobacco and alcohol can also be helpful in reducing head, neck, and oropharyngeal cancer [22].

Genital infections and ultimately cancers are commonly transmitted through sexual contact. Indeed, HPV is the most commonly occurring sexually transmitted virus. Different studies revealed that the sexual behavior including early age sex, multiple sexual partners, oral contraceptives, and co-infection with other sexually transmitted diseases predispose the HPV infection [5]. Data show that risk of HPV infection among women of 18–25 years of age with three life time sexual partners is more than double as compared to women of same age group with one life time partner [24]. Therefore, genital HPV infections can be prevented by reducing the number of sexual partners. Likewise, HPV burden is also linked with certain risk factor in male; for instance, circumcised males are associated with a lower risk of penile HPV infection [25]. Various cohort studies carried out for cervical cancer prevention has demonstrated that the use of alcohol and smoking along with poor and unhealthy sexual practices lead to cervical cancer in early ages [24, 26]. Vulvar, vaginal anal, and penile cancers are also attributed to same risk factors. Altogether, safe and ethical practices can reduce the spread of disease among population.

2.2. Screening methodologies

Up till now, no precise guidelines have been put forward by medical organizations for the surveillance of all HPV types except for those associated with cancer. The available guidelines vary with the severity of pathogenesis and the level of gender involved. There is no requirement of HPV screening for anogenital warts or papillomatosis. However, cervical cancer and precancerous lesions are strongly recommended to be screened at regular intervals for suspicion of cancer. In this regard, the mass screening is helpful in order to detect the virus at early stages before becoming drastic and uncontrollable. It is also helpful to diagnose the silent HPV infection where virus does not produce any disease symptoms. Common methods available for HPV screening are visual examination, cytology-based tests, and a few molecular assays. Although these methods are equally beneficial for detection of HPV in any part of the body, they are commonly practiced for the screening of cervical cancer only [27]. Researchers have also endorsed the implementation of these methods for the screening of HPV in anogenital warts and cancer, oropharyngeal cancer/infection, lung cancer, vaginal, and vulvar or penile cancer.

2.2.1. *Cytology-based screening*

Since the most commonly performed HPV screening involves the cervical cancer, therefore, most of the tests and data are available in this regard. The Papanicolaou test usually known as Pap test is the most common method of cervical screening. This test is applied to detect abnormal cervical cells, precancerous lesions, or early stage cancerous lesions among women between ages of 30 and 65 years. Moreover, it is practiced equally for both non-HPV and HPV-infected cervix. Due to accuracy and ease of performance, this test has become the cornerstone of cervical HPV screening strategies [28]. Unfortunately, no Pap-like test is available for the screening of HPV among men [29]. Similarly, histopathological examination is the only method carried out for anogenital, vulvar, vaginal, or oropharyngeal cancers to detect the involvement of HPV in these cases.

2.2.2. *Visual examination*

Regularly repeated Pap smears followed by appropriate treatment has saved the lives of millions of women in developed countries [27]. But HPV infections and associated cancers still pose a burden in less developed countries where poor socioeconomic conditions prevail. Therefore, in such low resource set ups such as Africa, Asia, South and Central America visual examination is recommended in screening programs [14]. This paradigm shift in screening programs has occurred due to the moderate sensitivity of cytology-based tests. Moreover, quality assurance and high possibility of false positives has led to the evaluation of alternative methods such as visual examination and HPV DNA testing. Visual inspection with 3–5% acetic acid or Lugol's iodine is performed to observe abnormal lesions in HPV associated cervical and penile cancers. However, the application of acetic acid has been most widely evaluated as compared to visual inspection with iodine as most of the cohort and field studies in the areas of Africa, India, Bangladesh, Thailand, China, and Philippines, report the utilization of acetic acid before visual examination. Altogether, these studies have suggested visual screening as an effective, acceptable, safe, accurate, and cost-effective method for the screening of cervical cancer [14].

However, visual inspection is not feasible for the detection of HPV in oropharyngeal or anogenital cancers. But genital warts or other HPV warts can be identified by their peculiar characteristics on visual examination [30]. In addition to all the merits of visual exam, one needs to be sure for the HPV genotype involved in the infection. For this purpose, some tests with high accuracy and efficiency are required such as nucleic acid testing.

2.2.3. Molecular testing of HPV

Molecular tests offer more rapid and robust screening of HPV and its particular genotype involved in the infection. Based on the nucleic acid detection of virus in clinical specimen, these tests are helpful to detect the virus before the appearance of any cellular abnormalities [27]. Numerous molecular screening modalities have been developed for the detection of hrHPV and lrHPV types among the subjects showing abnormal Pap test. These tests include Hybrid Capture 2 assay, Cervista High Risk HPV assay, Cobas 4800 HPV test, Abbot real Time High Risk HPV test, Papillocheck HPV screening, APTIMA HPV assay, E6/E7 quantitative PCR, GP5+/6+ PCR, and Matrix-assisted laser desorption/ionization time-of-light (MALDI-TOF). Despite the availability of a large number of commercial assays, only Hybrid Capture 2 assay, GP5+/6+ PCR, Cobas 4800 HPV test and APTIMA HPV assay are commonly applied [9, 31]. These four tests were validated in various cohort studies and large randomized trials carried out for 8 years or more in different parts of the world. Moreover, FDA and WHO have recommended these tests to be used in first-line primary screening. They can be used both in adjunct to cytology assays or alone for screening purpose [32]. Other mentioned tests are in the process of validation on large and small cohorts but they still need approval from FDA and other relevant governing bodies.

Usually, HPV testing with above-mentioned assays is not practiced in mass screening of men where simple PCR is performed for the detection of HPV in penile and anal cancer. Most of the testing data constitutes the cross-sectional studies on patients with sexually transmitted diseases (STDs), men having HPV infected partner, military recruits, and few small-scale studies [5]. Similarly, no research or analytical data have been found in support of practicing nucleic acid based assays for the detection of HPV in other associated cancers. But there lies a great potential in these methods for the detection of HPV due to high sensitivity and specificity as compared to visual or cytological examination.

2.3. Immunization

2.3.1. Immunity and principles of vaccine development

A fair comprehension on the basic function of the immune system is absolutely necessary in order to understand the mechanism of vaccines preparation and the prescribed ways to use them. However, the detailed discussion is beyond the scope of this chapter. The immune system is a multifaceted system comprising of interacting cells, tissues, and organs whose prime purpose is to identify and protect the body from pathogens and other potentially damaging foreign objects known as antigens. It is generally divided into two categories: "Innate" and "Adaptive" Immune systems that interact with each other to provide an effective immune response. The Innate immune system is first line of defense against invading pathogens and is equipped with physical and chemical barriers and some non-specific immune cells such as phagocytic leukocytes, dendritic cells, and natural killer cells which come into action immediately (within hours) after the manifestation of the antigens in the body [33]. Though non-specific but innate immunity plays a significant role in controlling infections until the initial adaptive response takes place [34], the adaptive immune response is composed of two arms: the humoral and cell-mediated response. The humoral response involves the production of antibodies by B-lymphocytes; whereas, cell-mediated response includes the specific cells known as T-lymphocytes which facilitate the elimination of foreign substances. The adaptive immune system provides a more versatile means of security as it manifests wonderful specificity for its target antigens and confers increased protection against subsequent re-infection with the same pathogen [30].

The active and passive ways are two basic mechanisms for acquiring the immunity. Active immunity emerges from the person's own immune response either as a result of exposure to a live pathogen or induced by the vaccine. It involves the production of antigen specific antibody or cellular response of T-lymphocytes. This kind of immunity is very long lasting, usually continues for life time in the form of immunologic memory mediated by memory B cells which survive in the blood after infection, and generate antibodies very quickly in case of re-exposure to the same antigen providing the rapid protection [35]. Some vaccines create the immune response analogous to natural infection without causing a disease signs and symptoms. Likewise, vaccine-mediated immune response also involve production of immunologic memory similar to the natural infection [36]. Unlike active immunity, passive immunity is a short-term immunization in which antibodies from another organism are transferred to the recipient. that is, antibodies are not generated by the immune cells of recipient. This type of immunity protects the host temporarily as the injected antibodies will be degraded over the short time span (weeks to months) leaving the host no more protected. Numerous host factors such as age, genetics, co infection of other disease, immune status, and nutritional factors may influence the response of passive immunization [37, 38].

2.3.2. *Classification of vaccines*

As a matter of fact, the immune response extremely diverges with antigenic variation. Therefore, a fundamental information of antigen properties; for instance, how it infect cells and what is the response of immune system to that antigen, must be considered for designing vaccines. The most efficient immune response is produced against live antigens. However, purified products from the microbes may also be used to formulate vaccines, though the immune response will not be much effective [39]. Likewise, recent developments in molecular biology enabled scientists to devise the alternative methods of vaccine production. Followings are different possibilities:

- Whole organism vaccines (Live attenuated and inactivated vaccines)
- Subunit vaccines (Subvirion, toxoid, and capsule polysaccharides vaccines)
- DNA vaccines
- Recombinant vaccines

Greater part of the vaccines being used today is based on the use of whole virus, whether, live attenuated or killed. Live attenuated vaccines contain the laboratory prepared version of the viruses which are usually attenuated by passaging in cultures. The attenuated virus retains the replication ability inside the host and induces immunity but lacks pathogenecity. In fact, the live-attenuated vaccines generate nearly identical immune response to that of natural infection [35]. Conversely, inactivated vaccines consist of pathogens that are usually inactivated by the effect of heat or chemicals. Inactivated strains lack replication ability within the host and cannot produce disease even in the immunocompromised individuals. Unlike, live-attenuated vaccines, inactive vaccines produce only humoral but not the cellular response. The protection in case of inactive vaccine is for limited time period because the antibody titer declines after some time [37].

Subunit vaccines include purified macromolecules (antigens) rather than the entire organism. More precisely, major antigenic sites of viral antigens that are recognized efficiently by antibodies or T cells are identified and subjected to purification. These purified molecules are often coupled to an immunogenic carrier protein or adjuvant, for instance, an aluminum salt in order to enhance their immunogenic potential. Immunologists obtain subunit vaccines either by breaking the microbes with chemicals in the laboratory or using recombinant DNA technology [40].

The development of DNA vaccines has ushered the immunization technology into a new exciting era. Precisely, DNA vaccines employ only the genes encoding the immunogenic antigen. Genes of interest are injected either alone (naked) or mixed with molecules that facilitate their entry into the cell, by taking up some cells which prepare the antigen under the instructions of foreign DNA. This way the host cells become vaccines making factories producing the antigens required to evoke the immune response [31]. The immune response to DNA vaccines is very strong and involves cellular and antibodies reaction. Some serious concerns are also linked with DNA vaccine, for instance, the integration of foreign DNA in host chromosome where it can manipulate the expression of onco- or tumor suppressor genes [41].

Only a handful of viral infections can be prevented using conventional live attenuated or killed vaccines. However, advances in recombinant DNA technology have opened up novel avenues for the development of vaccines against organisms for which development of conventional vaccines has so far proved unsuccessful. Virus-like particles (VLPs) are an efficient recombinant DNA technology-based tool which have been used as carriers of other organisms' genes. Immunogenic protein/s of a particular microorganism is introduced into harmless and weakened viruses which act as a vehicle to carry these proteins of interest to the desired site/organ inside the body. Similarly, attenuated bacteria are used as a vector where they display the antigens of other microbes on their surface and induce a strong immune response [42]. Recombinant vaccines mimic the natural infection in producing the immune response and stimulate both humoral and cellular immunity [15]. Five genetically engineered vaccines including Human papillomavirus (HPV) vaccine are being used in USA these days. The pros and cons of all above discussed vaccine types are summarized in the **Table 2**.

Type of vaccines	Features						
	Dose	Booster shots	Requirement of adjuvant	Virulence	Duration of efficacy	Potential advantages	Limitations
Live attenuated vaccines	Low	Single	No	Possible	More than 10 years	Produce immunity like natural infection	Instable, heat labile
Killed vaccines	High	Multiple	Yes	No	Temporary	Can be administered to immune-compromised patients	Can only activate humoral immune response
Subunit vaccines	High	Multiple	Yes	No	Short	Safe as compared to live attenuated vaccines	Sometimes may produce toxins, initiate hypersensitivity response
DNA vaccines	Low	Single	No	No	Long lasting	Safe, cost-effective, no side effects	May trigger the expression of onco-genes
Recombinant vaccines	Low	Single	No	Possible	Long lasting	Cost-effective, easy production	May cause contagious spread of virus

Table 2. General features of various vaccines used for immunization against HPV.

2.3.3. *HPV vaccines*

The HPV vaccines in use are based on recombinant DNA technology where the major capsid proteins L1 of HPV strains are synthesized and expressed in *in vitro* system. This protein is capable of self-assembling into HPV virus-like particles (VLPs) which display the morphological and antigenic properties similar to HPV virion but lack the viral DNA, therefore not capable of producing cancer. These HPV VLPs are used to synthesize HPV subunit vaccines [43]. All HPV vaccines being used today contain an adjuvant but not a preservative. The VLPs-based vaccines are highly immunogenic and generate even stronger response than the natural HPV infection [44]. All HPV vaccines available today and some other viral vaccines for instance Hepatitis B vaccine are VLP based.

2.3.4. *Currently available HPV vaccines*

An explosion of interest has been observed in vaccine production against HPV in recent years. Unfortunately, after many scientific endeavors, vaccines are not available against all strains of HPV; however, scientists are manufacturing newer vaccines including more strains of HPV.

Till now, three HPV vaccines have been licensed by Food and Drug Administration (FDA) and equally recommended by Advisory Committee on Immunization Practices (ACIP).

2.3.4.1. CervarixTM

The CervarixTM is a bivalent HPV vaccine marketed by GlaxoSmithKline Biologicals, Belgium, which protects the host from two most lethal types of HPV, 16 and 18, that are responsible for 70% cases of cervical cancer. These HPV types are also responsible for genital warts as well as head and neck cancer [21]. The CervarixTM contains L1 capsid proteins from HPV 16 and 18 in the form of VLPs and an adjuvant AS04 containing: 3-O-desacyl-4'-monophosphoryl lipid A. In fact, the L1 protein from HPV 16 and 18 strains are cloned in a baculovirus vector and expressed in Hi-5 Rix4446 cells that are derived from insect Trichoplusia. The VLPs for these strains are generated separately and then combined together. In addition to protection against HPV16 and 18, this vaccine has manifested cross reactivity with HPV 45 and 31. However, it does not provide protection in case the women have previously been exposed to one of the HPV strains. Clinical data in 2009 have shown that Cervarix TM was still affective after 7 years of vaccine administration showing that protection provided by this vaccine is long lasting [45].

2.3.4.2. Gardasil®

The quadrivalent HPV vaccine Gardasil® is being marketed by Merck & Co. Inc, against 4 HPV types: 16, 18, 6, and 11. The HPV strains 6 and 11 altogether are responsible for 90% of genital warts burden [46]. The VLPs from L1 capsid protein of each strain are produced using a recombinant Saccharomyces Pombe vector and mixed with alum adjuvant for better delivery. In addition to contributing protection against mentioned HPV types, this vaccine manifested a fractional protection against some other HPV types which are responsible for anal, vulvar, and vaginal cancer as well as genital warts [47].

2.3.4.3. Gardasil 9®

Very recently, in 2014, another HPV vaccine namely Gardsil9® was approved by US Food and Drug Administration. It is 9-valent recombinant vaccine which provides protection against wide range of HPV strains. It was recommend for the prevention of cervical, vulvar, anal, and vaginal cancers caused by HPV 16, 18, 31, 33, 45, 52, and 58, genital warts caused by HPV 6 and 11 and dysplastic lesions caused by HPV types: 16, 18, 31, 33, 45, 52, and 58 [12, 48]. Both Gardasil and Gardasil9 HPV vaccines are recommended for males also. In addition, both Gardasil and Gardasil 9 are recommended by FDA for males against the HPV-caused precancerous and cancerous lesions, and genital warts.

All three available HPV vaccines are administered into the body by a series of three intramuscular shots during a period of 6 months. The first shot is followed by second and third shots after 2 and 6 months, respectively.

3. Effective implementation of HPV vaccines

3.1. Age for HPV vaccination

The Centers for Disease Control and Prevention (CDC) recommends the routine administration of HPV vaccines in preteen boys and girls at the age of 11 or 12 before their first potential exposure to HPV [38]. Likewise, a more vigorous immune response is produced against vaccines at this age. However, if they are not fully vaccinated at this age, it is also recommended that women can get vaccinated at age 26 and boys and men at age 21. Recently, FDA has approved the Gardasil® and Gardsil®9 use in both male and female ages 9 through 26 [49]. Young homosexual men with weakened immune response may also get vaccine until they are 27. No vaccine is licensed yet in both male and female over the age of 27 years. However, the HPV vaccines can be given at the same age, similar to other age-specific vaccines for instance, tetanus toxoid, acellular pertussis vaccine, influenza vaccine, and hepatitis B vaccine. The HPV vaccine-targeted population is further enlisted in **Table 3**.

Persons who can receive HPV vaccine	Persons who cannot receive HPV vaccine
Patients with HPV positive test	Patients with history of hypersensitivity
Females with abnormal Pap test	Patients with acute illness
Lactating mothers	Pregnant woman
Patients suffering from any mild disease/immunocompromised	Persons who may develop allergies to yeast, latex or any vaccine component

Table 3. List of possible candidates who may or may not be safely administered with HPV vaccines.

3.2. HPV vaccine efficacy

The available HPV vaccines target the HPV types that most commonly cause cervical cancer and genital warts. Several studies have been conducted for bivalent and quadrivalent HPV vaccines to check their efficacy in young women of age between 15 and 25 years. These studies demonstrated that antibody response against the included types of HPV is generated approximately 1 month after the 3 shots of HPV vaccines in 99% of studied female population [38]. Clinical trials have demonstrated that the bivalent vaccine is 93% efficient in preventing cervical cancers caused by HPV 16 and 18 in women who had not been previously exposed to those strains [50]. The quadrivalent HPV vaccines have demonstrated more promising results as they were found 100% efficient in women for preventing cervical, vulvar, vaginal cancers along with genital warts due to HPV types 16, 18, 6, and 11 [48, 51]. The quadrivalent vaccine was equally effective in controlling genital warts and anal precancerous lesions of male. Besides that HPV vaccines have no therapeutic effects on HPV caused diseases and do not confer protection to the host already infected with those HPV types [52].

3.3. HPV vaccines safety

Large-scale clinical trials have confirmed the safety of vaccine [53]. However, common minor side effects such as pain, redness, fever, dizziness, and nausea could be observed. The medical procedure of injecting HPV vaccines may cause syncope (to faint) in teens or preteens such as other medical procedures. Being safe to use, 46 million doses of HPV vaccine have been distributed in United States as of June 2012 [54].

3.4. Impact of HPV vaccination

In general, vaccines are considered the most victorious medical intervention because they have provided protections against various diseases axf nd saved the death of millions of people [55]. In fact, HPV vaccines have been proved to be an important strategy for a notable decrease in the global burden of cervical cancer and genital warts. According to an estimate, the common use of vaccine during last decade has reduced cervical cancer deaths by 50% [56]. In addition, some additional long-term benefits are also associated with HPV vaccination such as it shows marked reduction in the prevalence of high-grade lesions CIN grade 2 and 3 [57]. The reduction in percentage of cervical associated deaths are further anticipated to rise up to 70% by next few decades when more vaccines would be available against a wide range of HPV strains.

4. Public awareness

Biomedical scientists have succeeded to develop reasonable approaches to cope with the obnoxious HPV infection. However, the success of these methods relies largely in creating awareness among general public about HPV infection and cervical cancer particularly in countries where inadequate attention is paid to the health problems. At first, the knowledge about HPV infection and its relation to anogenital as well as cervical cancer must be tailored in a very comprehensive and easily understandable way for general public in the form of booklets and brochures. The cultural and religious aspects should also be considered while devising an HPV prevention strategy. The dissemination of information should be ensured as much as possible through medical practitioners, teachers, and other sectors of the society. Likewise, the parents should be convinced and encouraged to get their child vaccinated at preteen ages. Both paper and electronic media should play a constructive role in spreading the information about HPV.

5. Conclusions

HPV is the main sexually transmitted viral infection which is associated with the cancers of oral cavity and reproductive tract of both male and female. In the absence of particular treatment for obnoxious HPV infection, the prevention strategies have been centered upon. The prevention paradigm against HPV infection must be multipronged. Briefly, to fend off HPV infection systematically the armamentarium should include avoiding risk factors which support the establishment of HPV infection such as multiple sex partners, early age sex, and unprotected sex, regular screening for cervical cancer, and administration of HPV vaccines.

Indeed, during last few years, it has been revealed that early and specific diagnosis in combination with effective therapeutic intervention could be the pragmatic and preeminent choice to overcome HPV-related diseases. In addition to that, several molecular therapeutic strategies can prove to be the indispensable allies in this quest against HPV infection. However, vaccination at the age of 10–12 in both genders is even a better choice since it provides immunity even before the first exposure to HPV lethal strains. The bivalent, quadrivalent, and nanovalent HPV vaccines have been successfully used in developed countries during last decade and proved to be highly efficient and safe to use. Theses vaccines not only provided a significant protection against highly virulent HPV strains against which they were designed, but also showed considerable seroconversion rate and lowered the occurring of other HPV-related abnormalities such as CIN and genital warts.

6. Future perspectives

Currently, no specific therapies are available for HPV infected patients. Therefore, there is an urgent need to invest our efforts in developing novel drugs against HPV. Moreover, the costs associated with HPV prevention and therapy is so far among the major hurdles in eradication of this problem. Considering the fact that more than 80% of HPV positive cases reside in low- and middle-income countries, accessibility and cost-effectiveness of any new drugs should also be kept in consideration. Any future HPV strategies must also take into account the cultural and religious stigma attached to vaccination in general and HPV in particular. Necessary measures should be devised and implemented in order to do away with these stigmas. There is also a need to devise and implement global anti-HPV vaccination campaigns for women of developing countries.

Development of new, sensitive, and cost-effective diagnostic tests is also one of the areas which demands high attention. To overcome this issue in developing countries, a sufficient advancement in diagnostics is mandatory. Although, screening and vaccination are being applied successfully in different parts of the world, HPV is still causing a significant number of deaths per year [58]. Likewise, quality control and assurance is another great hurdle towards the success of currently proposed modalities for elimination of HPV [20]. Keeping in view the given scenario, updated screening, and management guidelines are needed.

Author details

Naveed Shahzad[1*], Muhammad Umer[2], Memoona Ramzan[1] and Bilal Aslam[3]

*Address all correspondence to: hnaveed.shahzad@gmail.com

1 School of Biological Sciences, University of the Punjab, Lahore, Pakistan

2 National Institute for Biotechnology and Genetic Engineering, Faisalabad, Pakistan

3 Department of Microbiology, Government College University Faisalabad, Pakistan

References

[1] Bafverstedt B. Condylomata acuminata past and present. Acta Dermato-Venereologica. 1967; 47: 376–381.

[2] Zur Hausen H. Papillomaviruses in the causation of human cancers—a brief historical account. Virology. 2009; 384: 260–265.

[3] Giuffo, G. Positive engagement with filtered verruca vulgaris. Ital Mal Newspaper Venereol Skin. 1907; 48: 12–17.

[4] Zur Hausen H. Human papillomaviruses and their possible role in squamous cell carcinomas. Current Topics in Microbiology and Immunology. 1977; 78: 1–30.

[5] Dunne EF, Nielson CM, Stone KM, Markowitz LE, Giuliano AR. Prevalence of HPV infection among men: a systematic review of the literature. Journal of Infectious Diseases. 2006; 194(8): 1044–1057.

[6] Muñoz N, Castellsagué X, de González AB, Gissmann L. Chapter 1: HPV in the etiology of human cancer. Vaccine. 2006; 24: 1–10.

[7] Handisurya A, Schellenbacher C, Kirnbauer R. Diseases caused by human papillomaviruses (HPV). Journal der Deutschen Dermatologischen Gesellschaft. 2009; 7: 453–467.

[8] Ramzan M, Ain Nu, Ilyas S, Umer M, Bano S, Sarwar S, Shahzad N, Shakoori AR. A cornucopia of screening and diagnostic techniques for human papillomavirus associated cervical carcinomas. Journal of Virological Methods. 2015; 222: 192–201.

[9] Burger EA, Kornor H, Klemp M, Lauvrak V, Kristiansen IS. HPV mRNA tests for the detection of cervical intraepithelial neoplasia: a systematic review. Gynecologic Oncology. 2011; 120: 430–438.

[10] Cutts F, Franceschi S, Goldie S, Castellsague X, De Sanjose S, Garnett G, Edmunds W, Claeys P, Goldenthal K, Harper D. Human papillomavirus and HPV vaccines: a review. Bulletin of the World Health Organization. 2007; 85: 719–726.

[11] Pfister H. Chapter 8: human papillomavirus and skin cancer. Journal of the National Cancer Institute of Mongoraphs. 2003; 31: 52–56.

[12] Galloway DA, Laimins LA. Human papillomaviruses: shared and distinct pathways for pathogenesis. Current Opinion in Virology. 2015; 14: 87–92.

[13] Soohoo M, Blas M, Byraiah G, Carcamo C, Brown B. Cervical HPV infection in female sex workers: a global perspective. Open AIDS Journal. 2013; 7: 58–66.

[14] Satterwhite CL, Torrone E, Meites E, Dunne EF, Mahajan R, Ocfemia MCB, Su J, Xu F, Weinstock H. Sexually transmitted infections among US women and men: prevalence and incidence estimates. Sexually Transmitted Diseases. 2013; 40: 187–193.

[15] Castle PE, Schiffman M, Herrero R, Hildesheim A, Rodriguez AC, Bratti MC, Sherman ME, Wacholder S, Tarone R, Burk R. A prospective study of age trends in cervical

human papillomavirus acquisition and persistence in Guanacaste, Costa Rica. The Journal of Infectious Diseases. 2005; 191: 1808–1816.

[16] Franceschi S, Herrero R, Clifford GM, Snijders PJF, Arslan A, Anh PTH, Bosch FX, Ferreccio C, Hieu NT, Lazcano-Ponce E, Matos E, Molano M, Qiao YL, Rajkumar R, Ronco G, de Sanjosé S, Shin HR, Sukvirach S, Thomas JO, Meijer CJLM, Muñoz N. Variations in the age-specific curves of human papillomavirus prevalence in women worldwide. International Journal of Cancer. 2006; 119: 2677–2684.

[17] Moscicki AB, Schiffman M, Kjaer S, Villa LL. Chapter 5: updating the natural history of HPV and anogenital cancer. Vaccine. 2006; 24: 42–51.

[18] Giuliano AR Nyitray AG, Kreimer AR, Pierce Campbell CM, Goodman MT, Sudenga SL, Monsonego J, Franceschi S. EUROGIN 2014 roadmap: differences in human papillomavirus infection natural history, transmission and human papillomavirus-related cancer incidence by gender and anatomic site of infection. International Journal of Cancer. 2015; 136: 2752–2760.

[19] Ferlay J, Soerjomataram I, Ervik M, Dikshit R, Eser S, Mathers C, Rebelo M, Parkin D, Forman D, Bray F. Cancer Incidence and Mortality Worldwide: IARC Cancer Base No. 11. International Agency for Research on Cancer. 2013.

[20] Woodman CBJ, Collins SI, Young LS. The natural history of cervical HPV infection: unresolved issues. Nature Reviews Cancer. 2007; 7(1): 11–22.

[21] Östensson E, Fröberg M, Leval A, Hellström A-C, Bäcklund M, Zethraeus N, Andersson S. Cost of preventing, managing, and treating human papillomavirus (HPV)-related diseases in Sweden before the introduction of quadrivalent HPV vaccination. Plos One. 2015; 10: 9, e0139062.

[22] Bosch FX, de Sanjose S. Chapter 1: human papillomavirus and cervical cancer burden and assessment of causality. Journal of the National Cancer Institute of Monographs. 2003: 3–13.

[23] Vuyst HD, Dillner J, Dillner L, Franceschi S, Patnick J, Ronco G, Segnan N, Tornberg S, Antilla A. European guidelines for quality assurance in cervical cancer screening. Summary of the supplements on HPV screening and vaccination. Papillomavirus Research. 2015; 1: 22–31.

[24] Winer RL, Feng Q, Hughes JP, O'Reilly S, Kiviat NB, Koutsky LA. Risk of female human papillomavirus acquisition associated with first male sex partner. Journal of Infectious Diseases. 2008; 197: 279–282.

[25] Lowndes CM. Vaccines for cervical cancer. Epidemiology and Infection. 2006; 134(1): 1–12.

[26] Wiley DJ, Douglas J, Beutner K, Cox T, Fife K, Moscicki AB, Fukumoto L. External genital warts: diagnosis, treatment, and prevention. Clinical Infectious Diseases. 2002; 35: 210–224.

[27] Arbyn M, Snijders PJ, Meijer CJ, Berkhof J, Cuschieri K, Kocjan B, Poljak J. Which high-risk HPV assays fulfil criteria for use in primary cervical cancer screening? Clinical Microbiology and Infection. 2015; 21(9): 817–826.

[28] Coldman AJ, Phillips N, van Niekerk D, Smith L, Krajden M, Cook D, Peacock S. Projected impact of HPV and LBC primary testing on rates of referral for colposcopy in a Canadian cervical cancer screening program. Journal of Obstetrics and Gynaecology Canada. 2015; 37(5): 412–420.

[29] Giuliano AR, Nielson CM, Flores R, Dunne EF, Abrahamsen M, Papenfuss MR, Harris RB. The optimal anatomic sites for sampling heterosexual men for human papillomavirus (HPV) detection: the HPV detection in men study. Journal of Infectious Diseases. 2007; 196(7): 1146–1152.

[30] The Merck Manuals Online Medical Library. Components of the Immune System. 2008. Available from: http://www.merck.com/mmpe/sec13/ch163/ch163b.html.

[31] Bins AD, Van Den Berg JH, Oosterhuis K, Haanen JB. Recent advances towards the clinical application of DNA vaccines. Netherlands Journal of Medicine. 2013; 71: 109–117.

[32] Flores YN, Bishai DM, Lőrincz A, Shah KV, Lazcano-Ponce E, Hernández M, Salmerón J. HPV testing for cervical cancer screening appears more cost-effective than Papanicolau cytology in Mexico. Cancer Causes & Control. 2011; 22(2): 261–272.

[33] Pashine A, Valiante NM, Ulmer JB. Targeting the innate immune response with improved vaccine adjuvants. Nature Medicine. 2005; 11: 63–68.

[34] Margolick JB, Markham RB, Scott AL. Infectious disease epidemiology: theory and practice. Chapter 10. In: Nelson KE, Masters CF, editors. The immune system and host defense against infections. Boston, MA: Jones and Bartlett, 2006: 317–343.

[35] Clem AS. Fundamentals of vaccine immunology. Journal of Global Infectious Diseases. 2011; 3: 73–78.

[36] Plotkin S. Correlates of vaccine-induced immunity. Clinical Infectious Disease. 2008; 47: 401–409.

[37] Bovier PA. Recent advances with virosomal hepatitis A vaccine. Expert Opinion on Biological Therapy. 2008; 8: 1177–1185.

[38] Centers for Disease Control and Prevention. Immunity Types. [Last cited on 2009 Dec 20]. 2009. Available from: http://www.cdc.gov/vaccines/vacgen/ immunitytypes.html.

[39] Huang DB, Wu JJ, Tyring SK. A review of licensed viral vaccines, some of their safety concerns, and the advances in the development of investigational viral vaccines. Journal of Infectious Diseases. 2004; 49: 179–209.

[40] Dudek NL, Perlmutter P, Aguilar MI, Croft NP, Purcell AW. Epitope discovery and their use in peptide based vaccines. Current Pharmaceutical Design. 2010; 16: 3149–3157.

[41] Senovilla L, Vacchelli E, Garcia P, Eggermont A, Fridman WH, Galon J, Zitvogel L, Kroemer G, Galluzzi L. Trial watch: DNA vaccines for cancer therapy. Oncoimmunology. 2013; 2(4): e23803.

[42] Bachmann MF, Jennings GT. Vaccine delivery: a matter of size, geometry, kinetics and molecular patterns. Nature Reviews Immunology. 2010; 11: 787–796.

[43] Stanley M, Lowy DR, Frazer I. Prophylactic HPV vaccines: underlying mechanisms. Vaccine. 2006; 24: 106–113.

[44] Roldão A, Mellado MC, Castilho LR, Carrondo MJ, Alves PM. Virus-like particles in vaccine development. Expert Review of Vaccines. 2010; 10: 1149–1176.

[45] Schwarz TF. Clinical update of the AS04-adjuvanted human papillomavirus-16/18 cervical cancer vaccine, cervarix®. Advances in Therapy. 2009; 11: 983–998.

[46] Insinga RP, Dasbach EJ, Elbasha EH, Liaw KL, Barr E. Incidence and duration of cervical human papillomavirus 6, 11, 16, and 18 infections in young women: an evaluation from multiple analytic perspectives. Cancer Epidemiology Biomarkers Prevention. 2007; 16(4): 709–715.

[47] Garland SM, Hernandez-Avila M, Wheeler CM, Perez G, Harper DM, Leodolter S. Quadrivalent vaccine against human papillomavirus to prevent anogenital diseases. The New England Journal of Medicine. 2007; 19: 1928–1943.

[48] Group FIIS, Dillner J, Kjaer SK, Wheeler CM, Sigurdsson K, Iversen OE, Hernandez-Avila M, Perez G, Brown DR, Koutsky LA, Tay EH, García P, Ault KA, Garland SM, Leodolter S, Olsson SE, Tang GWK, Ferris DG, Paavonen J, Lehtinen M, Steben M, Bosch FX, Joura EA, Majewski S, Muñoz N, Myers ER, Villa LL, Taddeo FJ, Roberts C, Tadesse A, Bryan JT, Maansson RLS, Vuocolo S, Hesley TM, Barr E, Haupt R. Four year efficacy of prophylactic human papillomavirus quadrivalent vaccine against low grade cervical, vulvar, and vaginal intraepithelial neoplasia and anogenital warts: randomised controlled trial. Biomedical Journal. 2010; 341: 3493.

[49] Petrosky E, Bocchini JA, Hariri S, Chesson H, Curtis CR, Saraiya M, Unger ER, Markowitz LE. Use of 9-valent human papillomavirus (HPV) vaccine: updated HPV vaccination recommendations of the advisory committee on immunization practices. MMWR Morbidity and Mortality Weekly Report. 2015; 64(11): 300.

[50] Deleré Y, Wichmann O, Klug SJ, van der Sande M, Terhardt M, Zepp F, Harder T. The efficacy and duration of vaccine protection against human papillomavirus: a systematic review and meta-analysis. Deutsches Ärzteblatt International. 2014; 111(35–36): 584–591.

[51] Paavonen J, Naud P, Salmerón J, Wheeler CM, Chow SN, Apter D, Kitchener H, Castellsague X, Teixeira JC, Skinner SR, Hedrick J, Jaisamrarn U, Limson G, Garland S,

Szarewski A, Romanowski B, Aoki FY, Schwarz TF, Poppe WAJ, Bosch FX, Jenkins D, Hardt K, Zahaf T, Descamps D, Struyf F, Lehtinen M, Dubin G, Group HPS. Efficacy of human papillomavirus (HPV)-16/18 AS04-adjuvanted vaccine against cervical infection and precancer caused by oncogenic HPV types: final analysis of a double-blind, randomised study in young women. The Lancet. 2009; 374: 301–314.

[52] Noronha AS, Markowitz LE, Dunne EF. Systematic review of human papillomavirus vaccine coadministration. Vaccine. 2014; 32: 2670–2674.

[53] Harper, DM, Franco EL, Wheeler CM, Moscicki AB, Romanowski B, Roteli-Martins CM, Jenkins D, Schuind A, Costa Clemens SA, Dubin G. Sustained efficacy up to 4.5 years of a bivalent L1 virus-like particle vaccine against human papillomavirus types 16 and 18: follow-up from a randomised control trial. Lancet. 2006; 367: 1247–1255.

[54] Megan C, Diana Z, Brandel FB, Janet A, Phoenix MD. A closer look at HPV and the HPV vaccine. Cancer Prevention and Treatment. 2010; 28: 3149–3157.

[55] Bloom DE, Canning D, Weston M. The value of vaccination. World Economics. 2005; 6: 15.

[56] Dempsey AF, Koutsky LA, Golden M. Potential impact of human papillomavirus vaccines on public STD clinic workloads and on opportunities to diagnose and treat other sexually transmitted diseases. Sexually Transmitted Diseases. 2007; 34(3): 1–5.

[57] Kohli M, Ferko N, Martin A, Franco EL, Jenkins D, Gallivan S. Estimating the long-term impact of a prophylactic human papillomavirus 16/18 vaccine on the burden of cervical cancer in the UK. British Journal of Cancer. 2007; 96(1): 143–150.

[58] Brouwer AF, Eisenberg MC, Carey TE, Meza R. Trends in HPV cervical and seroprevalence and associations between oral and genital infection and serum antibodies in NHANES 2003–2012. BMC Infectious Diseases. 2015; 15: 575.

8

Genital Human Papillomavirus (HPV) Infections in Men as a Factor for the Development of Cervical Cancer

Slawomir A. Dutkiewicz, Anna Rezner,
Witold Rezner and Jack Chalasinski

Abstract

The prevalence of human papillomavirus (HPV) infection in males is comparable to females, although in men it is largely unknown. HPV infections may be connected with the development of carcinomas and other dermoepithelial changes such as intraepithelial neoplasia. Multidirectional studies have shown that chronic HPV infection is a necessary, though insufficient factor for the development of cervical cancer. Although men are regarded as the dominant vector of HPV transmission to their female sexual partners, they do not develop clinically significant HPV-related lesions and are usually asymptomatic during relatively short infections.

Analysis of data from a multicenter, clinical preventive trial was to estimate the incidence of type-specific genital infection among men and HPV transmission dynamics. The routine clinical examination included a peniscopy and detection of HPV DNA in smears using hybrid capture and in biopsy material using PCR.

It is necessary to establish prevention strategies for HPV infection in men whose female sexual partners have cervical cancer. Cervical cancer prevention strategies are likewise needed and should include the use of prophylactic HPV vaccines.

Keywords: human papillomavirus, genital infection, sexually transmitted disease, cervical cancer, HPV free

1. Introduction

Numerous infectious, inflammatory, and neoplastic diseases arise in male sexual organs. Infection of the genitalia with human papillomavirus (HPV) is worldwide and is currently the most frequent sexually transmitted infection [1]. For unknown reasons, clinical changes are absent in most infected individuals as the virus remains in a latent phase until spontaneous elimination occurs by unknown mechanisms. On the other hand, immuno-suppressed individuals frequently present with the clinical changes caused by HPV. Their clinical course is more severe, and their therapy is impeded since the immune system is compromised. Furthermore, genital HPV infections in women and subclinical changes of various degrees of cervical intraepithelial neoplasia (CIN 1–3) that can pave the way for the development of cervical cancer are relatively well understood. However, little is known about the subclinical infections in men that cause penile intraepithelial neoplasia (PIN). The significance of PIN is clear, since men who are carriers of HPV can be frequently undiscovered sources of infection for their female sexual partners [2, 3].

2. The risk of HPV infections

HPV is known for its characteristic heterogeneity, and the viral infection can run its course asymptomatically, subclinically, or symptomatically. Thanks to the polymerase chain reaction (PCR), over 200 types of HPV have been identified and subsequently classified according to changes induced, that is high risk (e.g., types 16, 18, 31, and 33) and low risk (e.g., 6 and 11) [2, 4]. Infection with HPV types 16 and 18 carries a large risk of precancerous and cancerous changes, while the appearance of genital warts caused by HPV types 6 and 11 is accompanied by a small risk of cancer development. Evaluation of risk and detection of HPV infection when clinical symptoms are absent is possible with a number of investigations, which include peniscopy, hybrid capture II (HC2), and PCR. The results of tested specimens, however, are variable and largely depend on anatomic sampling site and method of investigation [5, 6]. For instance, HPV DNA was found around the glans penis and external prepuce in 24% of individuals studied, while in 44% it was found on the inner (mucosal) prepuce where low-risk HPV types predominated. When material was collected using a brush, 70–92% of obtained samples were positive and 33% of which were high-risk types [6]. Furthermore, the results of a peniscopy only suggest the probability of HPV infection, since the presence of HPV DNA was not confirmed in 57% of positive peniscopy results [5, 7]. Nonetheless, peniscopy is necessary for gross identification of lesions, and the biopsy allows for histopathologic assessment of character to differentiate inflammatory changes (e.g., lichen sclerosus) from neoplastic changes of low- and high-grade PIN. PCR and HC2 examinations together with peniscopy allow for evaluation of the infection and defining its risk group. Also, positive findings upon acetowhitening, PCR, and HC2 are sufficient to establish diagnosis [7].

3. The risk of HPV infection transmission to partners depending on type of changes

3.1. Genital warts

HPV DNA is detected in approximately 5–11% of sexually active and healthy men aged 16–35 years [8]. The HPV types responsible for the development of genital warts (mainly types 6 and 11) are the predominant cause of infection. Other viral types are strongly associated with cancer of the cervix and are therefore termed "high-risk" types, and they include 16, 18, 31, 33, 39, 42, and 51–54 [9]. HPV viruses 16 and 18 are diagnosed most often in infections running subclinical courses in genital cancer patients. The risk of infecting sexual partners is estimated at 60%. However, although the peak of infection detection is in the age of 18–25 years, peak incidence of cervical cancer occurs around the fifth decade of life. Thus, the process of tumor progression is slow, and additional factors, so-called cocarcinogens, are necessary for the development of the cancer [10, 11].

Warts are most often multifocal. The following are three main types affecting the genital region:

1. genital warts (condyloma acuminata) are the most infectious lesions; they are pedunculated with a cauliflower-like appearance; depending on location and degree of irritation, they can be flesh-colored or various shades of red; and in uncircumcised men, they are localized on the inner (mucosal) prepuce, but can also be found on the glans penis, coronal sulcus, frenulum, external prepuce, shaft of penis, and scrotum [12].
2. papular, flesh-colored warts, and
3. flat warts—flattened papules of various colors such as red, pink on red, and brown [8, 13].

Warts may also occur at the urethral meatus or navicular fossa, where they are diagnosed in approximately 28% of patients [8]. In men who use condoms, warts are often localized in the suprapubic area. Interestingly, apart from prevention, condoms may accelerate the regression of flat warts on the penis [14]. In addition, they prevent reinfection and formation of new growths on the penis, but only when the same type of HPV occurs in partners. When different HPV types are present in the female partner, condoms do not protect against infection [15]. Condoms minimize the risk of so-called neoplasm transmission because they block the transmission of oncogenic HPV [16]. By minimizing the risk of penile cancer formation, the risk of cervical cancer is significantly limited. Moreover, with circumcision, the risk of penile cancer is decreased from 19.6 to 5.5% and subsequently the risk of cervical cancer formation in female sexual partners is also decreased [17, 18].

In a study of a large number of patients and a group of healthy controls, HPV DNA was found in 25% of men whose female partners had been diagnosed with CIN. HPV DNA was found in 6% of healthy women, but there was often discord with the results in their partners. Consequently, it has been proposed that no investigations are required in the absence of clinical changes in the partner of a woman with diagnosed CIN. It is also emphasized that HPV DNA results be assessed diligently because HPV DNA was not found in 25% of positive acetowhitening and 57% of those diagnosed with peniscopy [19]. In addition, up to 30% of warts have been found to regress spontaneously over the course of 3 months owing to immune system functions dominated by a cell-mediated response [10].

The treatment of warts includes the use of podofilox in 0.5% gel or solution, dichloroacetic acid or trichloroacetic acid, 5% imiquimod cream, cryotherapy with liquid nitrogen, destruction of tissue with electrofulguration, and laser ablation [20].

3.2. Buschke-Lowenstein tumor

Large warts resembling tumors were first described in 1925 by Buschke and Lowenstein—the Buschke and Lowenstein tumor [21]. This rare wart variant is associated with HPV infection types 6 and 11 and is characterized by deep rooting into the stroma that results in damage to deep-lying tissues. Its aggressive growth produces tumors of large dimensions. Histopathologically, typically mild warts are found alternating in coexistence with foci of atypical epithelial cells or cells of highly differentiated squamous cell carcinoma. Patient history is positive for inflammation or ulceration and phimosis of the glans penis. The warts may ulcerate or cause fistulation. Diagnosis of this tumor may require multiple biopsies or imaging studies that include computed tomography (CT) and magnetic resonance imaging (MRI) [22].

3.3. Changes in female partners of men having intraepithelial neoplasia

Intraepithelial neoplasia may involve both male and female genitalia—penile intraepithelial neoplasia (PIN), cervical intraepithelial neoplasia (CIN), vulvar intraepithelial neoplasia (VIN), and vaginal intraepithelial neoplasia (VaIN), respectively. Additionally, the anus may be involved in either gender—anal intraepithelial neoplasia (AIN). The changes can have a character of bowenoid papulosis or Bowen's disease. Moreover, female sexual partners of men with diagnosed PIN can have changes corresponding to CIN, VIN, or VaIN in various degrees of advancement. They require long-term observation over several months because these changes often resolve spontaneously. Fortunately, neoplastic transformation of PIN is very rare [23]. Although the infection status of female partners of men with subclinical infection of the penis is not determined, it has been accepted that subclinical changes and latent infections do not require treatment, which would be ineffective in such cases.

3.4. Risk of bowenoid papulosis (BP) development in sexual partners

Bowenoid papulosis (BP), also described as Bowen's atypia, is an advanced phase of intraepithelial changes with features of PIN. These warts are generally numerous and tend to form clusters on the penile shaft and scrotum [22]. In young men, BP resolves spontaneously, but in the elderly it can maintain itself for years with a tendency to progression. Progression to squamous cell carcinoma is marked. BP characterizes itself with the occurrence of flat warts (papulae) of skin color, but they may also be pink or sometimes brown. In men, it mainly occurs on the glans, while in women on the labia, groin, and around the anus. It is evoked by HPV 16, but other types (e.g., 18 and 31) may be culprits. The threat to infected women is the development of cervical cancer; for men, it is that they can infect their female partners and in doing so predispose them to cervical cancer [24]. Since the presence of BP is entwined with great risk of cancer development, treatment is considered crucial; excision of the change is most effective. Cryoablation with liquid nitrogen or laser ablation is also used. Recurrence should be taken into consideration since it has been estimated as high as 33% [20].

3.5. Erythroplasia of Queyrat

Erythroplasia of the glans penis is a form of carcinoma *in situ* occurring in uncircumcised men. Macroscopically, the change is erythematous, well demarcated, and slightly raised above the level of the skin on the glans penis or on the internal (mucosal) prepuce.

Histologically, it resembles Bowen's disease; it occurs on mucosal surfaces. The changes are singular or multiple and painless. Their surface tends to be smooth, scaly, or verrucous. The most frequent patient complaints are itching and bleeding with difficulties in retracting the prepuce. Diagnosis is made on the basis of biopsy specimen evaluation. Transformation of erythroplasia into penile squamous cell carcinoma occurs in 10–33% of patients [25]. Treatment of choice is surgical excision of the lesions.

3.6. Bowen's disease

Bowen's disease is most often observed as a solitary focus that is demarcated, flat, and reddish in color. Histopathological assessment reveals a squamous cell carcinoma in situ (corresponding to changes of PIN 3 and VIN 3). The disease is mainly caused by HPV 16 and 18, but sometimes also by HPV 31, 33, 45, and other oncogenic types. It occurs less often in women, growing slowly over years though it does not resolve spontaneously. The possibility of progression to invasive cancer should be considered when induration of the base, ulceration, or bleeding occurs, or the lesions increase in size. Changes on the vulva classified as intraepithelial neoplasia VIN 1–3 occur particularly in young women. The possible risk of progression of VIN3 to invasive cancer should be considered during therapy [22, 26]. In men who are partners of women with CIN 1–3 or VIN 1–3, changes consistent with PIN 1–3 are relatively frequent (up to 40%) in comparison with partners of women with genital warts (approximately 5%) [22]. Advanced changes corresponding to PIN 3 are diagnosed more often in older men in comparison with PIN 1–2. Clinical observations show that BP occurs more often than Bowen's disease in younger men [22].

3.7. Penile cancer

Penile cancer is not analogous to cervical cancer. While the detection of HPV DNA approaches 100% in cervical cancer cases, it is found in approximately 40% of penile cancer cases. Differences in frequency of finding HPV DNA (50–70%) exist and it depends on the type of cancer. HPV DNA is diagnosed most often in early premalignant changes corresponding to PIN 3, and in warts undergoing malignant transformation. For female sexual partners, infectivity is greater in cases with PIN 2 and 3 than in those with invasive cancers. The risk of infecting male partners of women with invasive cancer is not greater than when compared to women with CIN 2 [27].

Penile cancer is a rarely diagnosed neoplasm (<1% of neoplasms in men) occurring mainly in older individuals. In recent years, however, this cancer is being diagnosed in younger men. It predominantly arises on preexisting PIN 3, but, in addition to infection with high-risk oncogenic HPV types, other factors play a significant role: tobacco smoking, poor hygiene, phimosis, and changes consistent with lichen sclerosus [28, 29]. When PIN lesions are sustained, circumcision should be performed for its protective effect.

Chronic infection with oncogenic HPV types, specifically 16 and 18, is the most significant factor favoring penile cancer. Depending on the method used, HPV DNA is found in up to 90% of penile cancer in such cases. The risk of developing cervical cancer is increased in female partners of men having penile cancer [30]. As in women, an association between lichen sclerosus and cancer of genital organs has also been described in men [29, 31]. In one study, it was shown that neoplastic changes of the penis occur in approximately 8% of men with lichen sclerosus localized there for 10–23 years [32]. In subsequent studies, it was concluded that lesions consistent with lichen sclerosus coexisted or preceded penile squamous cell carcinoma in eight of 20 cases [33]. The etiopathogenesis of lichen sclerosus is unknown, but genetic, immunologic, infectious (bacteria such as Borrelia), or environmental factors may be possible. The disease is chronic in character. An association between lichen sclerosus and squamous cell carcinoma, which is diagnosed in 6% of patients with lesions on the labia, exists in women. Lichen sclerosus is an inflammatory disease in which involved tissues are affected by atrophic changes and indurations. Secondary phimosis or induration of the urethral meatus may be observed in men [31, 33]. In a study of 86 uncircumcised men affected by lichen sclerosus (the disease most often concerns the uncircumcision of middle age), malignant changes occurred in five (6%) [32]. The presence of HPV 16 was found in PCR studies while another study found histologic features of lichen sclerosus in 10 of 20 patients with diagnosed penile squamous cell carcinoma [33]. A significant role is attributed to genital HPV types. Men affected by lichen sclerosus report to physicians due to itching and burning sensations, they have painful erections and difficulties retracting the prepuce, and also they complain of voiding symptoms. If lichenification involves the glans penis, there is often bleeding, ulceration, and fistulas, and hemorrhagic bullae may also occur. Progression of changes often expands to involve the glans penis and prepuce, as well as the frenulum. An indurated white ring around the rim of the prepuce is a significant finding. It can present with strangulation of the prepuce (paraphimosis) or phimosis [34, 35]. Genital HPV types are regarded as dominating in the development of cancer on preexisting lichen sclerosus [36]. It is possible that the long-term inflammation favors proliferation of epidermal cells and causes activation of the HPV life cycle. Another favoring factor is local immunosuppression caused by use of preparations containing potent corticosteroids [36]. Due to the risk of phimosis, especially in young men, circumcision is most often performed following diagnosis of lichen sclerosis.

Since HPV is a proliferating virus, it should be remembered that it multiplies only in proliferating cells. Therefore, an underlying inflammatory state or irritation in the genital region increases the proliferation of epidermis, which in this way supports infection and multiplication of the virus. Significantly more often, infections with genital HPV types occur in immunosuppressed patients, such as those undergoing treatment with cytostatic agents, those after organ transplant, and also women during pregnancy [37–39]. The clinical course of HPV infection in patients infected with HIV is very aggressive [40]. The changes caused by HPV are more extensive in such cases. The risk of progression of preneoplastic lesions into invasive cancer increases, and the changes occur rapidly. The risk of neoplasm development increases fivefold in patients after organ transplant [41, 42]. This is linked to HPV infection and impairment of T lymphocyte and natural killer (NK) cell function by the immunosuppressive preparations. T lymphocytes and NK cells are responsible for elimination of neoplastic cells in early oncogenesis [43].

4. Discussion

Most men infected with HPV are naive, either because they have no signs and symptoms or because the signs and symptoms are so mild that they persist unrecognized or ignored. Men with HPV infection are a frequent source of infection for their female sexual partners who are at great risk of death resulting from the development of cervical cancer. Identification of infected men may reduce transmission and subsequent preneoplastic and neoplastic changes; however, numerous factors reduce the plausibility of testing men. Unlike the consistent sampling site in women (the cervix), the sampling site in men varies from anus and perianal area to the scrotum up to the urethral meatus and into the navicular fossa. Incomplete anogenital sampling is a major factor contributing to the variability in HPV prevalence estimates [44]. This variability together with spontaneous elimination of the virus will pose difficulties for recommendations regarding duration of abstinence and frequency of follow-up. It has been suggested that for optimal detection, scrotal, perianal, or anal samples should be included together with the minimum protocol of penile shaft, glans penis, and coronal sulcus [44].

Surely, we may infer that the knowledge of the presence of HPV infection in the man may reduce the incidence of cervical cancer in woman by reducing transmission resulting from proper condom use or sexual abstinence until the virus is eradicated. However, how can the man be inspired to do comply with such recommendations and what findings can be used to determine when the man is HPV free and allowed to resume unrestricted coitus? For what duration and frequency should the man be tested to determine the continued presence of HPV after the initial positive result? When and for how long should he be tested after changing partners? This can be considered a serious issue since HPV can be deadly for the woman who contracts HPV from the unsuspecting man and develops cervical cancer as a result. Yearly PAP testing for women is already a standard of care in many countries, but what can be done in developing and underdeveloped countries? How can illiterate populations be educated about the risks of HPV infection and consequences, and also how they can avoid it? What solutions can we implement in poor communities, whose women may not visit their gynecologists yearly, or ever? HPV is currently the leading sexually transmitted infection. In countries where resources are limited or women must travel hours or days by foot to visit their physician, the implications of late diagnosis may be deadly.

5. Conclusion

In summary, it must be stated that chronic immunosuppression favors HPV infection, allows for its self-preservation, and also favors activation of the viral life cycle, which is a primary factor triggering proliferative changes on genital organs. The therapeutic options for HPV-related changes are numerous (superficial preparations, cryotherapy, laser therapy, surgical excision) but are unfortunately burdened with recurrence and complications to a large degree. The changes caused by genital HPV types in the region of the sexual organs demand elimination of coexisting inflammatory states and treatment of sexual partners when indicated. It also appears that using a polyvalent HPV vaccine may prove effective in preventing benign and malignant changes, especially in groups of patients at increased risk [45]. Vaccination strategies, however, may be met with difficulties given geographic (e.g., access to facilities), cultural (e.g., core beliefs), and socio-demographic limitations (e.g., access to information) [46].

Author details

Slawomir A. Dutkiewicz[1], Anna Rezner[1], Witold Rezner[2] and Jack Chalasinski[3*]

*Address all correspondence to: drjackmd@live.com

1 Department of Prevention and Epidemiology of Neoplasms, Medical School and Faculty of Health Sciences, Institute of Public Health, Jan Kochanowski University, Kielce, Poland

2 Neoplasm Pathology Department, The Holycross Cancer Centre in Kielce, Kielce, Poland

3 Atlantic University School of Medicine, Gros Islet Highway, Rodney Bay, Saint Lucia, West Indies

References

[1] Centers for Disease Control (CDC) Fact Sheet: HPV and Men; February 4, 2015, accessed at www.cdc.gov, on February 21, 2016.

[2] Schiffman M, Kjaer SK. Natural history of anogenital human papillomavirus infection and neoplasia. Chapter 2. J Nat Cancer Inst Monogr 2003; 31: 14–19.

[3] Bleeker MCG, Hogewoning CJA, van den Brule AJC, et al. Penile lesions and human papillomavirus in male sexual partners of women with cervical intraepithelial neoplasia, J Am Acad Dermatol 2002; 47: 351–357.

[4] Dupin N. Genitals warts. Clin Dermatol 2004; 22: 481–486.

[5] Rosenblatt C, Lucon AM, Pereyra EAG, et al. HPV prevalence among partners of women with cervical intraepithelial neoplasia. Int J Gynecol Obst 2004; 84: 156–161.

[6] Nicolau SM, Camargo CGC, Stavale JN, et al. Human papillomavirus DNA detection in male sexual partners of women with genital human papillomavirus infection. Urology 2005; 65: 251–255.

[7] Markos AR. The management of penile intraepithelial neoplasia in genitourinary medicine. Int J STD AIDS 2003; 14: 314–319.

[8] Von Krogh G, Horenblas S. Diagnosis and clinical presentation of premalignant lesions of the penis. Scand J Urol Nephrol Suppl 2000; 205: 201–214.

[9] Severson J, Evans T, Lee P, et al. Human papillomavirus infections. Epidemiology, pathogenesis and therapy. J Cutan Med Surg 2001; 5: 43–60.

[10] Brown T, Yen-Moore A, Tyring S. An overview of sexually transmitted diseases. Part II. J Am Acad Dermatol 1999; 41: 661–677.

[11] Brady R, Bernstein DI. Treatment of herpes simplex virus infections. Antiv Res 2004; 61: 73–81.

[12] Moscicki A. Genital human papillomavirus infections in children and adolescents. Curr Probl Dermatol 2000; 28: 134–140.

[13] Bleeker MC, Hogewoning CJ, Voorhorst FJ, et al. Condom use promotes regression of human papillomavirus-associated penile lesions in male sexual partners of women with cervical intraepithelial neoplasia. Int J Cancer 2003; 107: 804–810.

[14] Bleeker MCG, Berkhof J, Hogewonin CJA, et al. HPV type concordance in sexual couples determines the effect of condoms on regression of flat penile lesions. Br J Cancer 2005; 92: 1388–1392.

[15] Baldwin SB, Wallace DR, Papenfuss MR, et al. Condom use and other factors affecting penile human papillomavirus detection in men attending a sexually transmitted disease clinic. Sex Trans Dis 2004; 31:601–607.

[16] Castellsague X, Bosch FX, Munoz N, et al. Male circumcision in female partners. N Engl J Med 2002; 346: 1105–1113.

[17] Witeska A, Dutkiewicz S, Walczak L, et al. HPV prevalence among partners of women with cervical intraepithelial neoplasia. Int J Gynecol Obst 2004; 84: 156–161.

[18] Rosenblatt C, Lucon AM, Pereyra EAG, et al. HPV prevalence among partners of women with cervical intraepithelial neoplasia. Int J Gynecol Obst 2004; 84: 156–161.

[19] Von Krogh G, Horenblas S. The management and prevention of premalignant penile lesions. Scand J Urol Nephrol Suppl 2000; 205: 220–229.

[20] Buschke A, Loewenstein L. Uber carcinomahnliche condylomata accuminata des penis. Klin Wochenschr 1925; 41: 726–728.

[21] Partidge JM, Koutsky LA. Genital human papillomavirus infection in men. Lancet Infect Dis 2006; 6: 21–31.

[22] Park KC, Kim KH, Youn SW, et al. Heterogeneity of human papillomavirus DNA in a patient with bowenoid papulosis that progressed to squamous cell carcinoma. Br J Dermatol 1998; 139: 1087–1091

[23] Obalek S, Jablonska S, Orth G, et al. Bowenoid papulosis of the male and female genitalia: risk of cervical neoplasia. J Am Acad Dermatol 1986; 14: 433–444.

[24] Micali G, Innocenzi D, Nasca M, et al. Squamous cell carcinoma of the penis. J Am Acad Dermatol 1996; 35: 432–451.

[25] McNally OM, Mulvany NJ, Pagano R, et al. VIN 3: a clinicopathologic review. Int J Gynecol Cancer 2002; 12: 490–495.

[26] Rubin MA, Kleter B, Zhou M, et al. Detection and typing of human papillomavirus DNA in penile carcinoma. Am J Pathol 2001; 159: 1211–1218.

[27] Micali G, Nasaca MR, Innocenzi D, Schwarrz RA. Penile cancer. J Am Acad Dermatol 2006; 54: 369–391.

[28] Nasca MR, Panetta C, Micali G, Innocensi D. Microinvasive squamous cell carcinoma arising on lichen sclerosus of the penis. JEADV 2003; 17: 337–339.

[29] Maiche AG, Pyrhonen S. Risk of cervical cancer among wives of men with carcinoma of the penis. Acta Oncol 1990; 29: 569–571.

[30] Micali G, Nasca MR, Innocenzi D. Lichen sclerosus of the glans is significantly associated with penile carcinoma. Sex Transm Infect 2001; 77: 226.

[31] Nasca MR, Innocenzi D, Micali G. Penile cancer among patients with genital lichen sclerosus. J Am Acad Dermatol 1999; 41: 911–914.

[32] Powell J, Robson A, Cranston D, et al. High incidence of lichen sclerosis in patients with squamous cell carcinoma of the penis. Br J Dermatol 2001; 145: 85–89.

[33] Barbagli G, Lazzeri M, Palminteri E, Turini D. Lichen sclerosus of male genitalia involving anterior urethra. Lancet 1999; 354: 429.

[34] Powell J, Wojnarowska F. Lichen sclerosus. Lancet 1999; 353: 1777–1783.

[35] Lau PW, Cook N, Andrews H, et al. Detection of human papillomavirus types in balanitis xerotica obliterans and other penile conditions. Genitourin Med 1995; 71: 228–230.

[36] Meffert JJ, Davis BM, Grimwood RE. Lichen sclerosus. J Am Acad Dermatol 1995; 32: 393–416.

[37] Bosch FX, de Sanjose S, Castellsague X, et al. Epidemiology of human papillomavirus infection and association with cervical cancer: new opportunities for prevention. Papillomavirus Res 2006; 19–39.

[38] Scheurer ME, Tortolero-Luna G, Adler-Storthz K. Human papillomavirus infection: biology, epidemiology, and prevention. Int J Gynecol Cancer 2005; 15: 727–746.

[39] Zur Hausen H. Papillomavirus and cancer: from basic to clinical application. Nat Rev Cancer 2002; 2: 342–350.

[40] Chin-Hong PV, Palefsky JM, Human papillomavirus anogenital disease in HIV-infected individuals. Dermatol Ther 2005; 18: 67–76.

[41] Adami J, Gabel H, Lidelof B, et al. Cancer risk following organ transplantation: a nationwide cohort study in Sweden. Br J Cancer 2003; 89: 1221–1227.

[42] Somers GR, Chow CW. Infections and tumors associated with iatrogenic immunosuppression. Curr Diag Pathol 2003; 9: 114–123.

[43] Stanley M. Immune responses to human papillomavirus. Vaccine 2006; 24 (Suppl 1): S1–S22.

[44] Giuliano AR, Nielson CM, Flores R, et al. The Optimal anatomic sites for sampling heterosexual men for HPV detection: the HPV detection in men study. JID 2007; 196: 1146–52.

[45] Lacey CJN. Therapy for genital human papillomavirus-related disease. J Clin Virol 2005; 32 (Suppl 1): S82-–S90

[46] Smith MA, Canfell K. Incremental benefits of male HPV vaccination: accounting for inequality in population uptake. Plos One 2014; 9(8): e101048

9

Diagnosis and Prevalence of High-Risk Human Papillomavirus Infection in Heterosexual Men

Elena López-Díez, Sonia Pérez and Amparo Iñarrea

Abstract

A better understanding of human papillomavirus (HPV) infection in men is an essential component of prevention programs aimed to reduce cervical cancer and other HPV-related diseases. A screening test capable of detecting asymptomatic/subclinical genital HPV infection in men at a reasonable price and causing minimal discomfort to the patient would be very valuable. The following chapter focuses on acetowhite test usefulness in the detection of asymptomatic/subclinical genital high-risk (HR) HPV infection in high-risk men populations, HR-HPV prevalence in sexually active healthy male partners of women diagnosed of high-grade cervical intraepithelial neoplasia and genotype-specific concordance between partners, addressing the preventive strategies that would reduce HPV infection in men. We present data from 125 men, sexual partners of women with preneoplastic cervical lesions. Prevalence of HR-HPV infection in male was high (50, 24% HPV16) and genotype concordance within the 60 infected couples was remarkable (62% shared at least one genotype). Acetowhite (AW) test was positive in 27% patients, showing low sensitivity for the identification of HR-HPV infection but allowed the diagnosis of subclinical HPV-related lesions in more than 10%. Current smoking and genital warts were associated with an increased risk of HR-HPV infection in men (OR: 2.4 and 5.6, respectively).

Keywords: human papillomavirus DNA test, prevention, prevalence, cervical intraepithelial neoplasia, male, mass screening, genital warts, diagnosis

1. Introduction

Human papillomavirus (HPV) infections are one of the most common sexually transmitted infections worldwide [1], representing a significant health problem due to their high prevalence and transmissibility. HPVs are a very large family of double-stranded DNA viruses (dsDNA), very resistant that can survive in the environment without a host and is able to infect humans. These viruses are not classified as serotypes, but as genotypes on the basis of DNA sequence. Currently, over 120 genotypes have been identified and about 40 genotypes (the alpha genus) can be transmitted through sexual contact and infect the anogenital region. HPV genotypes have been classified into low-risk genotypes, associated with anogenital warts, low-grade cervical lesions and recurrent respiratory papillomatosis, and high-risk genotypes (HR-HPV) [1] (**Table 1**), which eventually can lead to malignant transformation. HR-HPV are strongly associated with cancer and high-grade neoplasia of the anogenital tract, including the anus (AIN), penis (PeIN), uterine cervix (CIN), and vulva (VIN), and also a proportion of oropharyngeal cancer [2]. Although these infections are typically transient and asymptomatic, some of them will result in anogenital warts, and dysplastic and/or neoplastic lesions, which cause a substantial disease burden in both sexes and generate a considerable economic distress within society [3].

IARC classification	HPV genotypes
HR-HPV	16, 18, 31, 33, 35, 39, 45, 51, 52, 56, 58, 59
pHR-HPV	26, 34, 53, 66, 67, 68, 69, 70, 73, 82

Classification of oncogenic HPV genotypes detected in this work.
IARC, International Agency for Research on Cancer; HR-HPV, high-risk HPV genotypes; pHR, probable/possible high-risk genotypes.

Table 1. Oncogenic HPV genotypes.

The virus may remain inactive for a long time and produce asymptomatic infection of the skin. It can be transmitted from one individual to another directly (by sexual contact) or indirectly. The dynamics of heterosexual transmission of HPV are still being investigated [4].

About one-third to one-quarter of invasive penile cancers (Alemany et al.) and nearly 99.7% of cervical cancer worldwide and in 96.8% of cervical preneoplastic and neoplastic lesions in our community (Perez et al.) may be related to HPV according to the retrospective studies. Although rare, penile cancer is associated with a high morbidity and mortality. The carcinogenesis of penile cancer is thought to involve two pathways: one related to inflammation and other dermatological conditions of the penis, and other related to HPV infection (López-Romero et al.). HPV DNA prevalence in invasive penile cancer varied geographically, with the highest prevalence in Oceania (55.6%), North America (48.7), Africa (36.8%), South America (39.7%), and Europe (45.9%), being the most common HR-HPV types: HPV16 (30.8%) and HPV18 (6.6%) [5]. So that, it is important to be cautious and not to consider overall prevalence as universal because the role of HPV in penile cancer etiology could be strongly influenced by histologic distribution and geographic region as it is also true for other HPV malignancies such as vulvar and head and neck cancers [6].

Genital warts (GWs) represent a significant public health problem associated with clinical symptoms (burning, bleeding, and pain) and psychosocial problems (embarrassment, anxiety, and decreased self-esteem). Several studies have suggested that the occurrence of genital warts has been increasing over time [7]. Approximately 65% of people who have sex with an infected partner will develop warts themselves [8].

There has been immense progress in understanding the natural history of HPV infection in women disease. HPV is the primary cause of cervical cancers. Recently, there has been an interest in understanding the relationship between HPV infection and disease in men [9]. The male sexual partner`s role and in his partner's genital warts or high-grade cervical intraepithelial neoplasia (CIN II, CIN III-Ca in situ) lesions is also undefined. The diagnosis of most cutaneous and external genital wart (GW) can be made on clinical examination or with AW test and biopsy. In case of genital intraepithelial neoplasia, determining the extent of diseases is essential.

2. HR-HPV transmission among sexual partners

Epidemiological studies show that the HR-HPV infection is necessarily the sexual transmitted cause of invasive cervical cancer in women and its precursor lesion, cervical intraepithelial neoplasia (CIN) [10].

Direct genital mucosa contact during sexual intercourse is the principal route of HPV transmission [11]. About 80% of newly sexual couples will develop HPV-related lesions within 3 years after commencing sexual activity, most of whom will spontaneously regress within 1–2 years or until the age of 30–35 years [12]. The biology and dynamics of HPV transmission among sexual partners is still a cause for debate and has not already been completely established. Models have shown that HPV transmissibility is substantially higher than that of other viral sexually transmitted pathogens [13], but data on the natural history of HPV transmission between heterosexual partners are limited. Many studies [14–17] analyzed the prevalence and genotypes of high-risk infections of the foreskin before first sexual intercourse found asymptomatic infection in 12–83.3% [14, 16], speculating that non-sexual routes play significant roles in HPV transmission. In this regard, HPV transmission may occur upon contact with infected towels or other objects. In contrast to these findings, Pilatz et al. [15] did not find HPV in the foreskin of boys.

Despite the recommendation of the guidelines on sexually transmitted diseases, investigation of the presence of HPV in men who are sexual partners of infected woman has not been agreed. Previous studies suggested that the cancer of the penis and cervix may share the same etiological factor(s), because significant numbers of invasive cervical cancer were detected in partners of patients with penile cancer [18, 19]. It was assessed the contribution of the males' genital HPV DNA status to the risk of development of cervical neoplasia in their sexual partners, confirming that men could be vectors of HPV types typically observed in cervical cancer [20]. However, another studies did not confirm the findings of these investigators [21]. As the process of HPV infection can take more than 15 years, the current partner could not be necessarily the source of infection.

3. HR-HPV prevalence in heterosexual men populations

HPV infection causes substantial morbidity and its incidence is similar in both genders. The ongoing HPV in men study (HIM) provides the most current data on HPV infection and lesion development in men [9, 22–24]. Assessing HPV prevalence in men and investigating the sources of variation are essential for understanding the epidemiology of HPV infection.

The pooled HPV in the general population is significantly higher (20.4–36.3%) [25, 26] in studies published after 2000 (8.8%) [27]. The lower pooled prevalence in earlier publications might therefore be due to the detection method used and potentially not to a change in HPV prevalence over time. Age-specific prevalence curves among men are flatter [19, 28, 29] in contrast to the pattern observed in women [30]. The prevalence of genital infection in men does not differ significantly among age groups as it does in females [30]. In general population, HPV infection has a consistently higher prevalence within the penile epithelium of asymptomatic men than within the cervix of women with normal cytological testing [29].

Several factors have been suggested to influence HPV prevalence, varying substantially between sampling sites, techniques [31, 32], and different populations [33]. HPV prevalence is higher when samples are collected from a greater number of anatomic sites [29]. Hebnes et al. [27] in meta-analysis of studies examining HPV prevalence among men found a wide heterogeneity between general and high-risk populations. HIV-positive men, men with sexually transmitted infection and male sexual partners of women with HPV, CIN, CIS, or invasive cervical cancer are considered a high-risk population [34, 35]. Number of types tested for varies between articles. In studies reporting prevalence estimates for more than one HPV type, the commonest detected types were HPV16 [20, 24, 26, 27, 36, 37] and HPV18 [27].

From a socio-epidemiological standpoint, it is important to note that HPV-infected men play a key role in the transmission of the HPV virus to their female sexual partners. The range reported in other studies for sexual partners of women with CIN was 30–68% [19, 24, 26, 36, 38]. Geographical region, anatomical sampling site, or HPV detection methods have not explained the wide heterogeneity of results [27]. In contrast, Franceschi et al. [39] showed the strongest variation by countries, with a higher prevalence of HPV infection among Brazilian sexual partners of woman with CIN compared with those detected in other countries (Colombia, Mexico, Spain).

The natural course of disease in men by establishing rates of acquisition and time to clearance of HPV infection has not been investigated properly. Although fewer data of infection duration have been reported in men, findings suggest that HPV infection clear more quickly for men than for women and that men have similar duration of infection for oncogenic and non-oncogenic types [7, 28]. Mean clearance time, defined as time to elimination of 50% of all infections, was estimated to be 5.9 months (patridge JM). HPV infections in women tend to have a longer duration and are estimated to clear at average of 12.2 months [40].

4. Concordance between sexual partners

Positive concordance is defined as both partners having the HPV outcome of interest. HPV concordance in heterosexual couples has important clinical and public health implications. In terms of HR-HPV detection, the percentage of couples harboring HR-HPV was 32–65% [28, 36, 37, 41]. In couples where both members were HPV positive, more than 60% were infected with one or more of the same HPV types. This level of concordance was observed independently of HPV prevalence and is consistent with the high transmissibility of HPV [25, 28, 36, 38, 41]. Studies over the past 20 years evaluating HPV infection concordance among heterosexual partners have shown many inconsistencies, reporting concordances of type-specific infection between 2 and 87% [20, 42–44]. Such heterogeneous findings may be due to diverse laboratory DNA detection techniques, methods for study population selection and different anatomical sites sampling, among other factors [25].

Positive concordance was usually higher for female partners of men with HPV infection than for male partners of women with HPV infection. Men with HPV-positive female partners had one or more of the same HPV types more often in studies that recruited men with HPV-related diseases compared with studies without this inclusion criterion for men (65.8 vs. 27.2%) [28]. These findings suggest that the epithelial cells of the penile skin are more resistant to HPV infection than the cervical epithelium and the duration of HPV infection is shorter in men than in women [28, 38].

5. Acetowhite test versus molecular detection of HR-HPV infection

Infection with one or more of the 40 HPV detected at the genitals is common among men aged 18–70 years. Only 5% of these HPV infections progressed to an external genital lesions during follow-up. There were observed substantially higher rates of progression for certain HPV types [45].

Most genital infections in men are asymptomatic, detectable only by viral DNA testing and become undetectable over time. Subclinical lesions, including those related with HR-HPV types, are more than 10 times common than clinical (apparent) infection and are identified on examination after application of acetic acid solution, a procedure known as acetowhite test (AW test, peniscopy). Since the American Society for Colposcopy and Cervical Pathology recommended the use of HPV DNA testing for the triage and management of women with atypical squamous cells of undetermined significance result of Pap test, an increasing number of female patients are requesting HPV DNA testing for their partners. Although the current gold standard for HPV genotyping is a genetic sequencing targeting the product of gene amplification (Heidegger), a screening test capable of detecting asymptomatic and subclinical genital HPV infection in men at a reasonable price and causing minimal discomfort to the patient would be very valuable.

To date, economic data have primarily focused on the more common HPV-related cervical cancer and its precursor lesions, as well as the benign, very common condition of genital warts.

Nevertheless, available data indicate that HPV-related disease is associated with a significant economic burden in males. Specifically, in men, the total direct cost of HPV infection acquired through the age of 24 years was estimated at 62 million dollars per year, the comparable figure for women being 2.8 billion [46].

Studies of the psychosocial effects of HPV-related disease in males are lacking. However, there is a significant psychosocial burden reported in women being screened for, or diagnosed, with HPV-related disease [47].

The currently available methods for evaluating HPV infection in male are HPV DNA test and AW test [12]. This is full description of our study procedures: The entire penis and scrotum of the patient were examined under magnification, and the presence of genital warts was recorded. After this examination, we sprayed them with 5% acetic acid solution. After 5 min, we enhanced the visualization of the skin by a colposcope under fourfold and sevenfold magnification, respectively. AW lesions were classified as typical for the presence of well-demarcated lesions with a slightly elevated border and the occurrence centrally of punctuated capillaries with or without an associated epithelial depression (Groove) and non-typical for the presence of lesions exhibiting a ragged border and lacking punctuated capillaries. Regardless of AW test result, the specimen for HPV DNA detection was obtained. Samples were taken with three cytobrushes from the preputial cavity (the inner part of the foreskin, the glans and the sulcus coronarius, scrotum, and urethral meatus) rotated 360 grades and suspended together into one single vial containing TE buffer pH 8.0 Molecular Biology grade (AppliChem GmbH, Darmstadt, Germany). Samples were maintained at 2–8°C and processed within 24–72 h after collection. The brushings were collected without spraying the genital region with saline solution. DNA was isolated using QIAamp MinElute Media Kit (Qiagen, Hilden, Germany). Extracted nucleic acids were stored at −20°C. An aliquot of the original sample was also stored at −20°C. Amplification and detection were carried out using the Linear Array HPV Genotyping Test (Linear Array. Roche Diagnostics, Mannheim, Germany) according to the manufacturer's instructions. We described the distribution of 22 HPV genotypes classified as HR (HR-HPV, IARC Group 1 carcinogens) or probable/possible HR (pHR-HPV, IARC Group 2A/B carcinogens) by the International Agency for Research on Cancer Monograph Working Group (**Table 1**). This test also detects human beta-globin in order to test the adequate sample cellularity and absence of inhibitors. Linear Array does not have individual probe for HPV52 but uses a probe that simultaneously detects HPV52, HPV33, HPV35 and HPV58. Additional specific PCR was performed in case of HPV33, HPV35 and/or HPV58 infection in order to properly detect confections of these three genotypes with HPV52 [48].

In our study, around 30% of positive AW results were not related with HR-HPV infection [49–51]. False-positive results may be due to low-risk HPV infection or inflammatory conditions, common in patients with sexually transmitted diseases [52]. Nevertheless, the need for detecting subclinical genital HPV infection, associated with detectable AW lesions [53], has been emphasized and these population would need follow-up or biopsy. Afonso et al. [37] found that 50% of sexual partners of women with CIN harbored HPV in lesions and these were predominantly subclinical. The diagnosis and treatment of acetowhite lesions in men do not seem to alter or improve the progress of the squamous intraepithelial lesions in their female partners [54]. Nevertheless, these acetowhite lesions on male genitalia are in fact squamous intraepithelial alterations and should not be left due to the risk of their further development [37] as Sudenga et al. [45]. have presented the first estimates of genital HPV infection progression to PeIN. They are the first authors that follow these HPV infections and their progress to lesion in men. We encourage the importance of the clinical follow-up of this men and perhaps of taking a biopsy afterwards, in case of HPV infection persistence.

Problems associated with screening techniques in men include inadequate collection of cells for the detection of HPV DNA by use of swabs and brushes, poor specificity, and patient discomfort during peniscopy. When lesions are not visible, sampling at multiple penile sites could increase the sensitivity of the HPV [41, 55]. In addition, the use of acetic acid and a colposcope requires specific training, clinical experience, and significant costs associated with the procedure and training. Polymerase chain reaction (PCR) has emerged as the most sensitive available method for the detection of latent HPV infection. The infectious diseases literature supports the lack of the US Food and Drug Administration (FDA) approval of HPV tests for HPV detection in men and the absence of adequate therapy for established HPV infection in this population.

6. Our results of HPV prevalence in a high-risk population of heterosexual men and concordance between heterosexual partners

A cross-sectional study was conducted by the Urology Department of the University Hospital of Vigo, Spain, from January 2013 to June 2015 (López Díez et al., Enf Infecc Microbiol Clin, 2016 *in press*). We recruited 125 asymptomatic men, aged 18 years, whose SP (sexual partner, regular sexual intercourse for more than 1 year) had presented high-grade squamous cervical lesions (CIN grade 2 or CIN grade 3-carcinoma in situ) in the previous 6 months. Prevalence of HR-HPV infection in men was 50.4% (63/125). Multiple HR-HPV infections were detected in 30.4% (38/125) of this population. Data of HPV genotype were available in 120 women. HPV16 was the most frequent genotype, detected in 47.6% (30/63) of infected men and 67.5% (81/120) women (**Table 2**). HR-HPV infection was detected in both partners in 50% (60/120). Among these infected couples, 62% (37/60) harbored at least one genotype in common. The HPV16-specific concordance was as follows: 41.7% (25/60) couples were concordantly HPV16 positive and 18.3% (11/60) were concordantly HPV16 negative (Kappa value: 0.21).

The proportion of women with the same genotype as their male partner was 58.7% (37/63). The proportion of men sharing the same genotype as their female partner was 30.8% (37/120), $p < 0.0001$.

AW procedure was positive in 34/125 (27.2%) patients. AW procedure showed 25.4% (95% CI 13.8–36.9) sensitivity, 71.0% (95% CI 58.9–83.1) specificity, 47.1% (95% CI 28.8–65.3) positive predictive value and 48.3% (95% CI 37.5–59.2) negative predictive value for the identification of HR-HPV infection (**Table 3**). AW lesions and HR-HPV were detected at the same time in 16/125 (12.8%) males.

IARC classification	Genotype	Infected men (n)	Global prevalence (N = 125) %	Prevalence in HPV-positive men (N = 63) %
HR-HPV	HPV16	30	24.0	47.6
	HPV18	4	3.2	6.3
	HPV31	9	7.2	14.3
	HPV33	2	1.6	3.2
	HPV39	6	4.8	9.5
	HPV45	5	4.0	7.9
	HPV51	11	8.8	17.5
	HPV52	12	9.6	19.0
	HPV56	8	6.4	12.7
	HPV58	3	2.4	4.8
	HPV59	6	4.8	9.5
pHR-HPV	HPV53	13	10.4	20.6
	HPV66	10	8.0	15.9
	HPV67	1	0.8	1.6
	HPV68	2	1.6	3.2
	HPV69	1	0.8	1.6
	HPV70	4	3.2	6.3
	HPV73	3	2.4	4.8

HR-HPV, high-risk HPV genotypes; pHR, probable/possible high-risk genotypes; IARC, International Agency for Research on Cancer.
Crude HPV prevalence calculated in 63 HPV-positive patients: 25 single and 38 multiple infections (López Díez et al., Enf Infecc Microbiol Clin, 2016 *in press*).

Table 2. Type-specific HPV prevalence in men.

		HR-HPV DNA detection			
		Yes	No		
		n (%)	n (%)	p	OR (95% CI)
AW lesion	Yes	16 (25.4)	18 (29.0)	0.648	0.83 (0.38–1.83)
	No	47 (74.6)	44 (71.0)	–	–

Genital lesions detected by peniscopy in asymptomatic sexual partners of women with high-grade cervical lesions, according to the presence of HR-HPV.
HR-HPV DNA, high-risk HPV; AW, acetowhite test; OR, odd ratio; 95% CI, confidence interval.
Statistically significant, $p < 0.05$ (chi-square test).

Table 3. Acetowhite lesions according to HR-HPV DNA detection.

Genital warts were present in 17/125 (13.6%) patients. AW procedure showed sensitivity 82.3 (95% CI 55.8–95.3), specificity 81.4% (95% CI 72.6–88.6), positive predictive value 41.1% (95% CI 25.1–59.1) and negative predictive value 96.7% (95% CI 89.9–99.1) for genital warts' detection (**Table 4**).

		Genital warts			
		Yes	**No**		
		n (%)	**n (%)**	p	**OR (95% CI)**
AW lesion	Yes	14 (82.3)	20 (18.5)	<0.0001	20.53 (5.39–78.27)
	No	3 (17.6)	88 (81.5)	–	–

AW: Acetowhite test, OR: odd ratio, 95% CI: confidence interval.
Statistically significant, $^*p < 0.05$ (chi-square test).

Table 4. Acetowhite lesions according to genital warts' detection.

HR-HPV prevalence was 6/15 (40.0%) in circumcised men and 57/110 (51.8%) in not circumcised men ($p > 0.05$).

7. Risk factors for HR-HPV prevalence in men

Coexistence of non-oncogenic and oncogenic HPV-types is frequent [56, 57], which may itself predispose to cancer. A Danish study of 50,000 people with GW found an elevated risk of HPV-associated cancers in people with GW compared with the general population [56]. Although test for the presence of HPV are not recommended for the diagnosis of GW [58] in our study, the AW test was sensitive and specific for genital warts' detection, showing a high negative predictive value. This procedure could avoid missing small clinical lesions. They are generally regarded as a benign condition not associated with mortality, but they can be difficult to treat and recurrence is often observed. Visible warts represent only the tip of the iceberg, and low- and high-risk HPV infections contribute to the genital lesion burden in men [24]. Healthcare providers should have a higher suspicion for HPV-associated cancers in immunocompromised patients with GW. AW test can be helpful in the diagnosis of GW. In particular, soaking acetic acid into suspicious lesions can enhance the degree of suspicion in lesions without classic features. Taking a biopsy might also be indicated if diagnosis is uncertain, the lesions do not respond to standard therapy or the disease worsens during therapy [58].

Limited data exist on the association between HPV infection and smoking in men. In this study, current smoking could increase 2.3-fold the risk of HPV-prevalent infection in males, as found in the HIM study. At present, it is unclear how smoking may influence HPV infection in men, but many possible mechanisms exist. Smoking could potentially increase viral load by weakening the cellular immune response [59].

Sexual behavior has been strongly associated with HPV infection and seropositivity in men [60]. Features previously associated with HR-HPV were as follows: young age at first sexual intercourse (FSI), a higher number of lifetime sexual partners (LSP) and a higher number of recent SP. Contradictory results about the influence of lifetime number of SP were reported [26, 41, 55, 61, 62]. This data could be attributable not only to the range of birth year of men but also to geographical characteristics [27, 33]. In Western population, the numbers of lifetime sexual partners in men and women are both relatively high, and little gender difference could be observed. Burchell et al. reported that the proportion of ≥5 lifetime sexual partners was 64.4% for men, in line with our results (55.2% in men).

The risk of having one or more SP in the preceding year was has been poorly evaluated. The risk of HPV re-infection between a monogamous couple is still a matter of debate [63]. In contrast, Rombaldi et al. [64] and Parada [25] found a high association between both variables.

In the National Questionnaire of Sexual Health, published by Spanish Government in 2009, it was found that the mean age of FSI was 17–18 years (29.3%) for Spanish men. In our study, younger age at FSI was not a risk factor for HPV infection as other authors have previously reported [27, 64]. There are contradictory data that could be attributable not only to the range of birth year of men but also to geographical characteristics [55, 60].

Similar to other studies [55, 65], we did not find the expected protective effect of circumcision on HPV acquisition. Circumcision seems to be associated with reduced persistence in men [66] even though the mechanism of protection is unclear. Removal of the foreskin could minimize the chance of acquisition of new infections or could result in an increased clearance of preexisting infections [28, 67]. Our different results could be due to the fact that circumcision is not very common in our geographical area and that analysis could not assess specific associations in the glans penis, the area expected to be most likely protected by removal of the foreskin [68].

8. HR-HPV risk factors found in our study

Epidemiological characteristics of the studied high-risk population are shown in **Table 5.** Current smoking status was associated with an increased risk of HR-HPV infection in men: 38.2% (21/55) versus 60% (42/70), OR 2.3 (95% CI 1.1–4.7), $p = 0.016$.

Variable	HPV detection (n = 125)		*p*-value	
	Positive	**Negative**	**Bivariate analysis**	**Multivariate analysis**
Age at FSI	16.9 ± 2.7	17.4 ± 2.4	0.382	
Lifetime SP				
1–5 SP	10 (34.5%)	19 (65.5%)	0.050	
>5 SP	53 (55.2%)	43 (44.8%)		

Variable	HPV detection (n = 125)		*p*-value	
	Positive	**Negative**	**Bivariate analysis**	**Multivariate analysis**
Recent SP				
1 SP	51 (49.0%)	53 (51.0%)	0.498	
>1 SP	12 (57.1%)	9 (42.9%)		
Current smoking				
Yes	42 (60.0%)	28 (40.0%)	0.015*	0.016* (OR 2.3, 95% CI 1.1–4.7)
No	21 (38.2%)	34 (61.8%)		
CIN grade in partner				
CIN 2	30 (54.5%)	25 (45.5%)	0.411	
CIN 3-CIS	33 (47.1%)	37 (52.9%)		

FSI, first sexual intercourse;, SP, sexual partners; CIN, cervical intraepithelial neoplasia; CIS: carcinoma *in situ*.
Age was expressed as mean ± standard deviation.
* $p < 0.05$, statistically significant.

Table 5. HPV detection in men according to epidemiological characteristics.

Prevalence of HR-HPV infection was 14/17 (82.4%) in patients with genital warts versus 49/108 (45.4%) in patients without genital warts (OR 5.6, 95% CI 1.5–20.7, $p = 0.008$) (**Figure 1**).

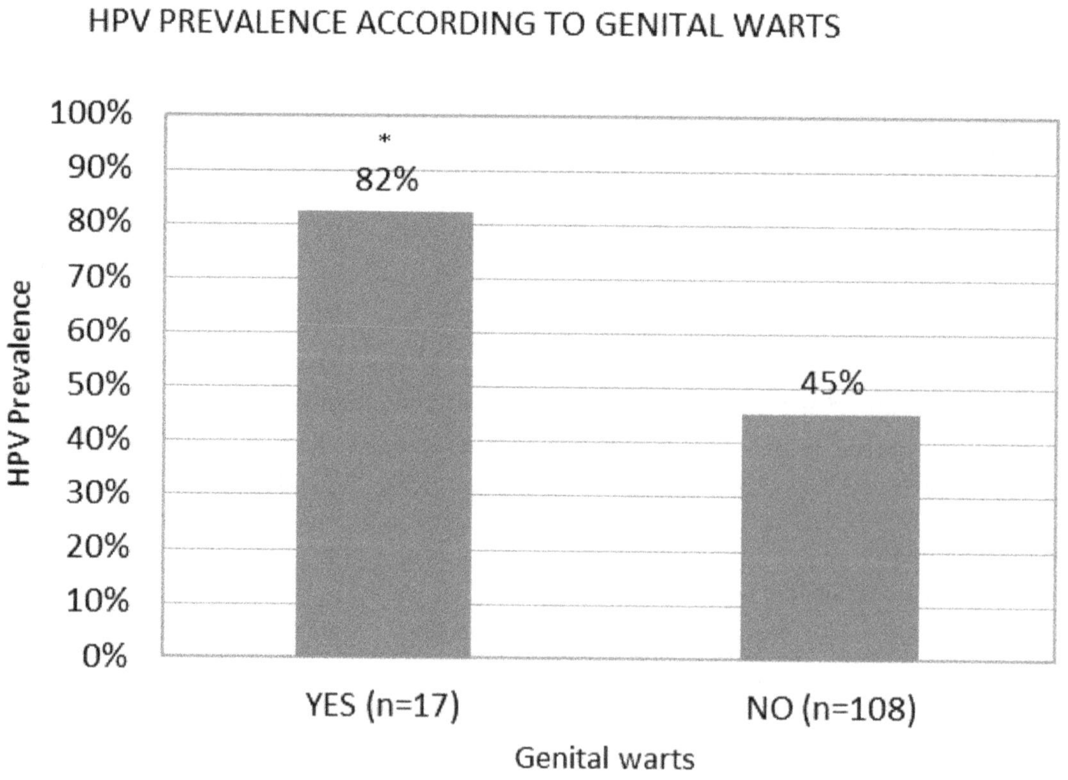

Figure 1. Statistically significant, *$p < 0.05$ (chi-square test).

9. Prevention of HPV infection in men

Until recently, no highly effective primary prevention strategy to reduce the risk of HPV acquisition existed. However, research has demonstrated that nonavalent, quadrivalent and bivalent HPV vaccines stimulate immunogenicity in males and females [69]. On October 16, 2009, the FDA approved the use of quadrivalent vaccine in males aged 9–26 years for the prevention of genital warts. Subsequently, the Advisory Committee on immunization Practices (ACID) declined to recommend the quadrivalent vaccine for routine immunization in men [70], providing a permissive recommendation in this age range for HPV vaccination. Most European countries offer HPV vaccination for girls, but vaccine recommendations for boys are warranted. HPV vaccination of girls will in theory also benefit the male population through herd immunity.

Uninfected sexual partners may be an important target population for HPV vaccination [71]. Potential interventions such as a therapeutic HPV vaccine may avert new HPV infections. Moreover, vaccinating boys would reduce HPV-related diseases in both sexes to a greater extent than herd immunity, which depends on high vaccination rates among females.

The benefits of vaccination to individuals seronegative to HPV types included in the vaccine are clear, and emerging studies suggest that HPV vaccine may also help people who previously had and cleared an infection [72] although additional researches in this population are needed. While prophylactic HPV vaccine does not have substantial impact on established infection, it may have cross-protection against non-vaccine genotypes [73]. However, if these vaccines could also be successful in lowering the HPV load, they may also assist in lowering transmission [13].

There is no direct evidence for protection by HPV vaccines against penile cancer because penile cancer is so rare that there could never be a clinical trial large enough to measure the effect [74]. HPV vaccines have not been around long enough to measure the population impact on penile cancer. However, the observed HPV type distribution reinforces the potential benefit of current and new vaccines in reduction in HPV-related penile neoplasia lesions [6].

Future trials of HPV vaccines in men should take into account not only the presence of penile HPV infection but also the presence of penile subclinical lesions as an outcome measure for the efficacy of a vaccine. More complex study designs would also allow researchers to better understand first transmission, reinfection and back and forth passage within couples, concordance in couples in which one partner has received HPV vaccine and concordance after treatment for HPV-related lesions is an essential component of prevention programs aimed to reduce cervical cancer and other HPV-related diseases in men and women.

10. Final considerations

HPV causes cancer in both men and women. The HPV-related cancer burden remains higher in women than men, even in countries that have effective cervical cancer screening programs.

It is clear that males have poor knowledge of HPV infection, morbidity, transmission, and prevention. Moreover, several issues are controversial and should be addressed by adopting a multidisciplinary and multiprofessional approach. Regardless of vaccination strategies adopted, efforts should be made to educate males about HPV and its health implications.

Currently, there is no licensed test for HPV detection in men and there are no recommendations for male screening. Although routine HPV testing is not necessary for men in general population, findings from emerging research in high-risk population suggest that HPV infection is pervasive and persistent in these groups, warranting the adoption of additional screening and prevention policies. Our findings suggest the need for greater attention to sexual partners of HPV-infected individuals. Male sexual partners of female with high-grade lesions should be referred for evaluation and combined peniscopy, and HPV DNA test will ensure accurate detection of HPV status among males. Female partners of men with HPV-related diseases should be encouraged to get screened for HPV-related disease given that they have a high likelihood of concomitant infection and that most infection in couples are of the same viral type. Screening may also benefit male partners of HPV-infected women. Interventions that study the true prevalence of HPV infection in asymptomatic men and try to reduce HPV-associated penile lesions could be important to both men and women.

Further prospective and controlled studies in different populations are needed to provide adequate counseling to men that demand to know whether they are infected by HR-HPV. Long-term follow-up will contribute to the knowledge about the influence of persistent HPV infection in male and the potential recurrence of his sexual partner after treatment. We assume that the faster way to achieve greatest protection for cervical cancer and its precursors is to vaccinate males as well as female because both genders contribute to the transmission of HPV infection.

The prevention, diagnosis, and treatment of HPV-associated diseases in men will reduce the disease burden not only in males, but also in females, and help destigmatize the focus of the HPV-related disease on women.

Acknowledgements

We thank nursery team, especially Carmen Garcia from the Urology Department of the University Hospital of Vigo, for their excellent help in this research, collecting patients. We thank M. Consuelo Reboredo from the Gynecology Department and the laboratory technicians of the Microbiology Department of the University Hospital of Vigo, for their support of the study. We are also grateful to Angel de la Orden for the revision of the manuscript.

Author details

Elena López-Díez[1], Sonia Pérez[2*] and Amparo Iñarrea[3]

*Address all correspondence to: elena.lopez.diez@sergas.es

1 Department of Urology, University Hospital of Vigo, Vigo, Spain

2 Department of Microbiology, University Hospital of Vigo, Vigo, Spain

3 Department of Obstetrics and Gynecology, University Hospital of Vigo, Vigo, Spain

References

[1] Bouvard V, Baan R, Straif K, Grosse Y, Secretan B, El Ghissassi F, et al. A review of human carcinogens—part B: biological agents. Lancet Oncol. 2009;10(4):321–2.

[2] de Sanjose S, Quint WG, Alemany L, Geraets DT, Klaustermeier JE, Lloveras B, et al. Human papillomavirus genotype attribution in invasive cervical cancer: a retrospective cross-sectional worldwide study. Lancet Oncol. 2010;11(11):1048–56.

[3] Chesson HW, Ekwueme DU, Saraiya M, Dunne EF, Markowitz LE. The cost-effectiveness of male HPV vaccination in the United States. Vaccine. 2011;29(46):8443–50.

[4] Gavillon N, Vervaet H, Derniaux E, Terrosi P, Graesslin O, Quereux C. [How did I contract human Papillomavirus (HPV)?]. Gynecol Obstet Fertil. 2010;38(3):199–204.

[5] Backes DM, Snijders PJ, Hudgens MG, Bailey RC, Bogaarts M, Agot K, et al. Sexual behaviour and less frequent bathing are associated with higher human papillomavirus incidence in a cohort study of uncircumcised Kenyan men. Sex Transm Infect. 2013;89(2):148–55.

[6] Alemany L, Cubilla A, Halec G, Kasamatsu E, Quirós B, Masferrer E, et al. Role of human papillomavirus in penile carcinomas worldwide. Eur Urol. 2016 Jan 4. pii: S0302-2838(15)01215-4. doi: 10.1016/j.eururo.2015.12.007.

[7] Giuliano AR, Lu B, Nielson CM, Flores R, Papenfuss MR, Lee JH, et al. Age-specific prevalence, incidence, and duration of human papillomavirus infections in a cohort of 290 US men. J Infect Dis. 2008;198(6):827–35.

[8] Giuliano AR, Anic G, Nyitray AG. Epidemiology and pathology of HPV disease in males. Gynecol Oncol. 2010;117(2 Suppl):S15–9.

[9] Giuliano AR, Lee JH, Fulp W, Villa LL, Lazcano E, Papenfuss MR, et al. Incidence and clearance of genital human papillomavirus infection in men (HIM): a cohort study. Lancet. 2011;377(9769):932–40.

[10] Bosch FX, Lorincz A, Muñoz N, Meijer CJ, Shah KV. The causal relation between human papillomavirus and cervical cancer. J Clin Pathol. 2002;55(4):244–65.

[11] Liu M, He Z, Zhang C, Liu F, Liu Y, Li J, et al. Transmission of genital human papillomavirus infection in couples: a population-based cohort study in rural China. Sci Rep. 2015;5:10986.

[12] Bar-Am A, Niv J. The role of HPV DNA in the evaluation and follow-up of asymptomatic male sexual partners of females with CIN3. Eur J Gynaecol Oncol. 2007;28(3):207–10.

[13] Grabowski MK, Kong X, Gray RH, Serwadda D, Kigozi G, Gravitt PE, et al. Partner human papillomavirus viral load and incident human papillomavirus detection in heterosexual couples. J Infect Dis. 2016 Mar 15;213(6):948–56.

[14] de Martino M, Haitel A, Wrba F, Schatzl G, Klatte T, Waldert M. High-risk human papilloma virus infection of the foreskin in asymptomatic boys. Urology. 2013;81(4): 869–72.

[15] Pilatz A, Altinkilic B, Rusz A, Izykowski N, Traenkenschuh W, Rische J, et al. Role of human papillomaviruses in persistent and glucocorticoid-resistant juvenile phimosis. J Eur Acad Dermatol Venereol. 2013;27(6):716–21.

[16] Verit A, Verit FF. Re: de Martino et al. High-risk human papilloma virus infection of the foreskin in asymptomatic boys (Urology 2013;81:869–872). Urology. 2013;82(3):750–1.

[17] Klinglmair G, Pichler R, Zelger B, Dogan HS, Becker T, Esterbauer J, et al. Prevalence of the human papillomavirus (HPV) expression of the inner prepuce in asymptomatic boys and men. World J Urol. 2013;31(6):1389–94.

[18] Graham S, Priore R, Graham M, Browne R, Burnett W, West D. Genital cancer in wives of penile cancer patients. Cancer. 1979;44(5):1870–4.

[19] Smith JS, Gilbert PA, Melendy A, Rana RK, Pimenta JM. Age-specific prevalence of human papillomavirus infection in males: a global review. J Adolesc Health. 2011;48(6): 540–52.

[20] Bosch FX, Castellsagué X, Muñoz N, de Sanjosé S, Ghaffari AM, González LC, et al. Male sexual behavior and human papillomavirus DNA: key risk factors for cervical cancer in Spain. J Natl Cancer Inst. 1996;88(15):1060–7.

[21] de Bruijn RE, Heideman DA, Kenter GG, van Beurden M, van Tinteren H, Horenblas S. Patients with penile cancer and the risk of (pre)malignant cervical lesions in female partners: a retrospective cohort analysis. BJU Int. 2013;112(7):905–8.

[22] Schabath MB, Villa LL, Lazcano-Ponce E, Salmerón J, Quiterio M, Giuliano AR, et al. Smoking and human papillomavirus (HPV) infection in the HPV in Men (HIM) study. Cancer Epidemiol Biomarkers Prev. 2012;21(1):102–10.

[23] Giuliano AR, Lazcano-Ponce E, Villa LL, Flores R, Salmeron J, Lee JH, et al. The human papillomavirus infection in men study: human papillomavirus prevalence and type

distribution among men residing in Brazil, Mexico, and the United States. Cancer Epidemiol Biomarkers Prev. 2008;17(8):2036–43.

[24] Ingles DJ, Pierce Campbell CM, Messina JA, Stoler MH, Lin HY, Fulp WJ, et al. Human papillomavirus virus (HPV) genotype- and age-specific analyses of external genital lesions among men in the HPV Infection in Men (HIM) Study. J Infect Dis. 2015;211(7): 1060–7.

[25] Parada R, Morales R, Giuliano AR, Cruz A, Castellsagué X, Lazcano-Ponce E. Prevalence, concordance and determinants of human papillomavirus infection among heterosexual partners in a rural region in central Mexico. BMC Infect Dis. 2010;10:223.

[26] Álvarez-Argüelles ME, Melón S, Junquera ML, Boga JA, Villa L, Pérez-Castro S, et al. Human papillomavirus infection in a male population attending a sexually transmitted infection service. PLoS One. 2013;8(1):e54375.

[27] Hebnes JB, Olesen TB, Duun-Henriksen AK, Munk C, Norrild B, Kjaer SK. Prevalence of genital human papillomavirus among men in Europe: systematic review and meta-analysis. J Sex Med. 2014;11(11):2630–44.

[28] Reiter PL, Pendergraft WF, Brewer NT. Meta-analysis of human papillomavirus infection concordance. Cancer Epidemiol Biomarkers Prev. 2010;19(11):2916–31.

[29] Flaherty A, Kim T, Giuliano A, Magliocco A, Hakky TS, Pagliaro LC, et al. Implications for human papillomavirus in penile cancer. Urol Oncol. 2014;32(1):53:e1–8.

[30] Pérez-Castro S, Lorenzo-Mahía Y, Iñarrea Fernández A, Lamas-González MJ, Sarán-Díez MT, Rubio-Alarcón J, et al. Cervical intraepithelial neoplasia grade 2 or worse in Galicia, Spain: HPV 16 prevalence and vaccination impact. Enferm Infecc Microbiol Clin. 2014 Oct;32(8):479–85.

[31] Weaver BA, Feng Q, Holmes KK, Kiviat N, Lee SK, Meyer C, et al. Evaluation of genital sites and sampling techniques for detection of human papillomavirus DNA in men. J Infect Dis. 2004;189(4):677–85.

[32] Giuliano AR, Nielson CM, Flores R, Dunne EF, Abrahamsen M, Papenfuss MR, et al. The optimal anatomic sites for sampling heterosexual men for human papillomavirus (HPV) detection: the HPV detection in men study. J Infect Dis. 2007;196(8):1146–52.

[33] Dunne EF, Gift TL, Stamm WE. What about the men? Sex Transm Dis. 2008;35(11 Suppl):S1–2.

[34] Castellsagué X, Bosch FX, Muñoz N. The male role in cervical cancer. Salud Publica Mex. 2003;45(Suppl 3):S345–53.

[35] Barzon L, Militello V, Pagni S, Franchin E, Dal Bello F, Mengoli C, et al. Distribution of human papillomavirus types in the anogenital tract of females and males. J Med Virol. 2010;82(8):1424–30.

[36] Lorenzon L, Terrenato I, Donà MG, Ronchetti L, Rollo F, Marandino F, et al. Prevalence of HPV infection among clinically healthy Italian males and genotype concordance between stable sexual partners. J Clin Virol. 2014;60(3):264–9.

[37] Afonso LA, Rocha WM, Carestiato FN, Dobao EA, Pesca LF, Passos MR, et al. Human papillomavirus infection among sexual partners attending a Sexually Transmitted Disease Clinic in Rio de Janeiro, Brazil. Braz J Med Biol Res. 2013;46(6):533–8.

[38] Giuliano AR, Nyitray AG, Kreimer AR, Pierce Campbell CM, Goodman MT, Sudenga SL, et al. EUROGIN 2014 roadmap: differences in human papillomavirus infection natural history, transmission and human papillomavirus-related cancer incidence by gender and anatomic site of infection. Int J Cancer. 2015;136(12):2752–60.

[39] Franceschi S, Castellsagué X, Dal Maso L, Smith JS, Plummer M, Ngelangel C, et al. Prevalence and determinants of human papillomavirus genital infection in men. Br J Cancer. 2002;86(5):705–11.

[40] Anic GM, Giuliano AR. Genital HPV infection and related lesions in men. Prev Med. 2011;53(Suppl 1):S36–41.

[41] Nyitray AG, Iannacone MR. The epidemiology of human papillomaviruses. Curr Probl Dermatol. 2014;45:75–91.

[42] Bleeker MC, Hogewoning CJ, Voorhorst FJ, van den Brule AJ, Snijders PJ, Starink TM, et al. Condom use promotes regression of human papillomavirus-associated penile lesions in male sexual partners of women with cervical intraepithelial neoplasia. Int J Cancer. 2003;107(5):804–10.

[43] Benevolo M, Mottolese M, Marandino F, Carosi M, Diodoro MG, Sentinelli S, et al. HPV prevalence among healthy Italian male sexual partners of women with cervical HPV infection. J Med Virol. 2008;80(7):1275–81.

[44] Nicolau SM, Camargo CG, Stávale JN, Castelo A, Dôres GB, Lörincz A, et al. Human papillomavirus DNA detection in male sexual partners of women with genital human papillomavirus infection. Urology. 2005;65(2):251–5.

[45] Sudenga SL, Ingles DJ, Pierce Campbell CM, Lin HY, Fulp WJ, Messina JL, et al. Genital human papillomavirus infection progression to external genital lesions: the HIM study. Eur Urol. 2016;69(1):166–73.

[46] Garland SM. Prevention strategies against human papillomavirus in males. Gynecol Oncol. 2010;117(2 Suppl):S20–5.

[47] Pirotta M, Stein AN, Conway EL, Harrison C, Britt H, Garland S. Genital warts incidence and healthcare resource utilisation in Australia. Sex Transm Infect. 2010;86(3):181–6.

[48] Sotlar K, Diemer D, Dethleffs A, Hack Y, Stubner A, Vollmer N, et al. Detection and typing of human papillomavirus by e6 nested multiplex PCR. J Clin Microbiol. 2004;42(7):3176–84.

[49] Wikström A, Hedblad MA, Johansson B, Kalantari M, Syrjänen S, Lindberg M, et al. The acetic acid test in evaluation of subclinical genital papillomavirus infection: a comparative study on penoscopy, histopathology, virology and scanning electron microscopy findings. Genitourin Med. 1992;68(2):90–9.

[50] Giraldo P, Gonçalves AK, Pereira SA, Barros-Mazon S, Gondo ML, Witkin SS. Human papillomavirus in the oral mucosa of women with genital human papillomavirus lesions. Eur J Obstet Gynecol Reprod Biol. 2006;126(1):104–6.

[51] Giraldo PC, Eleutério J, Cavalcante DI, Gonçalves AK, Romão JA, Eleutério RM. The role of high-risk HPV-DNA testing in the male sexual partners of women with HPV-induced lesions. Eur J Obstet Gynecol Reprod Biol. 2008;137(1):88–91.

[52] Kumar B, Gupta S. The acetowhite test in genital human papillomavirus infection in men: what does it add? J Eur Acad Dermatol Venereol. 2001;15(1):27–9.

[53] Backes DM, Bleeker MC, Meijer CJ, Hudgens MG, Agot K, Bailey RC, et al. Male circumcision is associated with a lower prevalence of human papillomavirus-associated penile lesions among Kenyan men. Int J Cancer. 2012;130(8):1888–97.

[54] Bleeker MC, Hogewoning CJ, Voorhorst FJ, van den Brule AJ, Berkhof J, Hesselink AT, et al. HPV-associated flat penile lesions in men of a non-STD hospital population: less frequent and smaller in size than in male sexual partners of women with CIN. Int J Cancer. 2005;113(1):36–41.

[55] Morales R, Parada R, Giuliano AR, Cruz A, Castellsagué X, Salmerón J, et al. HPV in female partners increases risk of incident HPV infection acquisition in heterosexual men in rural central Mexico. Cancer Epidemiol Biomarkers Prev. 2012;21(11):1956–65.

[56] Blomberg M, Friis S, Munk C, Bautz A, Kjaer SK. Genital warts and risk of cancer: a Danish study of nearly 50000 patients with genital warts. J Infect Dis. 2012;205(10):1544–53.

[57] Vandepapeliere P, Barrasso R, Meijer CJ, Walboomers JM, Wettendorff M, Stanberry LR, et al. Randomized controlled trial of an adjuvanted human papillomavirus (HPV) type 6 L2E7 vaccine: infection of external anogenital warts with multiple HPV types and failure of therapeutic vaccination. J Infect Dis. 2005;192(12):2099–107.

[58] Park IU, Introcaso C, Dunne EF. Human Papillomavirus and Genital Warts: a Review Of The Evidence for the 2015 Centers for Disease Control and Prevention Sexually Transmitted Diseases Treatment Guidelines. Clin Infect Dis. 2015;61(Suppl 8):S849–55.

[59] Kalra R, Singh SP, Savage SM, Finch GL, Sopori ML. Effects of cigarette smoke on immune response: chronic exposure to cigarette smoke impairs antigen-mediated

signaling in T cells and depletes IP3-sensitive Ca(2+) stores. J Pharmacol Exp Ther. 2000;293(1):166–71.

[60] Dunne EF, Nielson CM, Stone KM, Markowitz LE, Giuliano AR. Prevalence of HPV infection among men: a systematic review of the literature. J Infect Dis. 2006;194(8): 1044–57.

[61] Iribarren-Díaz M, Ocampo Hermida A, González-Carreró Fojón J, Alonso-Parada M, Rodríguez-Girondo M. [Practical considerations for high resolution anoscopy in patients infected with human immunodeficiency virus]. Enferm Infecc Microbiol Clin. 2014;32(10):676–80.

[62] Castellsagué X, Bosch FX, Muñoz N, Meijer CJ, Shah KV, de Sanjose S, et al. Male circumcision, penile human papillomavirus infection, and cervical cancer in female partners. N Engl J Med. 2002;346(15):1105–12.

[63] Nyitray AG, Lin HY, Fulp WJ, Chang M, Menezes L, Lu B, et al. The role of monogamy and duration of heterosexual relationships in human papillomavirus transmission. J Infect Dis. 2014;209(7):1007–15.

[64] Rombaldi RL, Serafini EP, Villa LL, Vanni AC, Baréa F, Frassini R, et al. Infection with human papillomaviruses of sexual partners of women having cervical intraepithelial neoplasia. Braz J Med Biol Res. 2006;39(2):177–87.

[65] Albero G, Castellsagué X, Lin HY, Fulp W, Villa LL, Lazcano-Ponce E, et al. Male circumcision and the incidence and clearance of genital human papillomavirus (HPV) infection in men: the HPV Infection in men (HIM) cohort study. BMC Infect Dis. 2014;14:75.

[66] Lu B, Wu Y, Nielson CM, Flores R, Abrahamsen M, Papenfuss M, et al. Factors associated with acquisition and clearance of human papillomavirus infection in a cohort of US men: a prospective study. J Infect Dis. 2009;199(3):362–71.

[67] Gray RH, Serwadda D, Kong X, Makumbi F, Kigozi G, Gravitt PE, et al. Male circumcision decreases acquisition and increases clearance of high-risk human papillomavirus in HIV-negative men: a randomized trial in Rakai, Uganda. J Infect Dis. 2010;201(10): 1455–62.

[68] Albero G, Villa LL, Lazcano-Ponce E, Fulp W, Papenfuss MR, Nyitray AG, et al. Male circumcision and prevalence of genital human papillomavirus infection in men: a multinational study. BMC Infect Dis. 2013;13:18.

[69] Petrosky E, Bocchini JA, Hariri S, Chesson H, Curtis CR, Saraiya M, et al. Use of 9-valent human papillomavirus (HPV) vaccine: updated HPV vaccination recommendations of the advisory committee on immunization practices. MMWR Morb Mortal Wkly Rep. 2015;64(11):300–4.

[70] Markowitz LE, Hariri S, Unger ER, Saraiya M, Datta SD, Dunne EF. Post-licensure monitoring of HPV vaccine in the United States. Vaccine. 2010;28(30):4731–7.

[71] Moreira ED, Giuliano AR, Palefsky J, Flores CA, Goldstone S, Ferris D, et al. Incidence, clearance and progression to disease of genital human papillomavirus infection in heterosexual men. J Infect Dis. 2014 Jul 15;210(2):192–9.

[72] Reiter PL, Gupta K, Brewer NT, Gilkey MB, Katz ML, Paskett ED, et al. Provider-verified HPV vaccine coverage among a national sample of Hispanic adolescent females. Cancer Epidemiol Biomarkers Prev. 2014;23(5):742–54.

[73] Nakagawa M, Greenfield W, Moerman-Herzog A, Coleman HN. Cross-reactivity, epitope spreading, and de novo immune stimulation are possible mechanisms of cross-protection of nonvaccine human papillomavirus (HPV) types in recipients of HPV Therapeutic Vaccines. Clin Vaccine Immunol. 2015;22(7):679–87.

[74] Bosch FX, Broker TR, Forman D, Moscicki AB, Gillison ML, Doorbar J, et al. Comprehensive control of human papillomavirus infections and related diseases. Vaccine. 2013;31(Suppl 8):I1–31.

10

HPV Infection and Prevention of HPV Infection in Men who have Sex with Men (MSM)

Corinna Sadlier, Orla Sheils and Colm Bergin

Abstract

The research landscape in relation to human papillomavirus (HPV) infection has evolved rapidly since the causal association between the virus and cervical cancer was made in the 1970s. Cervical screening programmes have resulted in a dramatic decrease in the incidence of cervical cancer. The first vaccine for HPV was licensed in 2006 with real-world data demonstrating high levels of vaccine efficacy.

In the setting of decreased rates of cervical cancer, the burden of HPV-associated disease in men (including genital warts, anal cancer, penile cancer and oropharyngeal cancer) has become more apparent. The incidence of anal cancer is increasing steadily. Men who have sex with men (MSM) in particular HIV-infected MSM are disproportionately affected. In contrast to the successes observed with cervical screening programmes, anal cancer screening tools have not demonstrated improvements in morbidity or mortality, and while many experts recommend screening high-risk groups for anal cancer, no consensus recommendations exist.

HPV vaccine has potential to decrease HPV-related malignancies including anal cancer. The majority of countries including Ireland offer HPV vaccine to females through national immunization programmes. However, only a minority of countries have extended the HPV vaccine recommendation to include males. The HPV vaccine is most effective prior to sexual debut; thus, immunisation programmes, including boys and girls, offer the greatest preventative opportunity. However, such programmes will not impact the high burden of HPV-associated disease currently observed in groups at high risk of HPV infection and HPV-associated disease such as men who have sex with men (MSM).

This chapter focuses on HPV infection and associated disease in MSM with particular focus on HIV-infected MSM. Host and viral factors influencing HPV infection and progression to disease are reviewed.

The potential for primary preventative strategies such as vaccination as well as secondary preventative strategies such as screening to impact on the burden of anal cancer in this cohort are reviewed.

Keywords: HPV, MSM, HIV, anal cancer, vaccine, screening

1. Introduction

Human papillomavirus (HPV) is the most common sexually transmitted infection (STI) worldwide. It is highly prevalent in the sexually active population and rapidly acquired after sexual debut [1]. The majority of HPV infections are subclinical and clear spontaneously; however, HPV can result in a wide variety of presentations ranging from benign genital dermatoses to disseminated invasive malignancy.

HPV is causally associated with genital warts, cervical cancer, vulvar cancer, anal cancer, penile cancer, and head and neck cancers [2]. HPV now accounts for approximately 5% of all cancers worldwide [3]. Over 150 types of HPV have been identified with over a dozen HPV types (16, 18, 31, 33, 35, 39, 45, 51, 52, 56, 58, 59, 68, 73, and 82) classified as highly oncogenic [4].

The incidence of cervical cancer has decreased dramatically since the introduction of cervical screening programmes [5]. In the same time period, the incidence of extra-cervical HPV-associated cancers, particularly oropharyngeal and anal cancers, have increased steadily [6].

Anal cancer is a relatively rare occurrence in the general population (1–2 cases per 100,000) [7]; however, certain risk groups including MSM (up to 40 cases per 100,000) and in particular HIV-infected MSM are disproportionately affected (up to 135 cases per 100,000) [8, 9]. The incidence of anal cancer in MSM is now greater than the incidence of cervical cancer pre-introduction of cervical screening programs [5, 10]. To date, screening programs for anal cancer have failed to demonstrate improvements in morbidity or mortality relating to anal cancer. Some experts advocate screening of at risk populations such as MSM for anal cancer [11, 12]. However, the utility of screening for prevention of anal cancer remains very much debated and no consensus recommendations for anal cancer screening exist.

Three HPV vaccines have been licensed. The bivalent HPV vaccine (HPV-2v) (Cervarix™, GlaxoSmithKline) protects against oncogenic HPV types 16 and 18. The quadrivalent HPV vaccine (HPV-4v) (Gardasil™, Merck and Co., Inc.) offers additional protection against HPV types 6 and 11, commonly associated with genital warts. The recently licensed nonavalent HPV vaccine (HPV-9v) (Gardasil 9™, Merck and Co., Inc.) provides protection against five additional oncogenic HPV types (31, 33, 45, 52, and 58).

National immunization programs delivering HPV vaccine to females have been established in the majority of developed countries. In recent years, there has been a move by countries including the United States, Canada, and Australia to recommend HPV-4v for boys also, given the broader benefits of the vaccine. The majority of European countries do not recommend

HPV vaccine for boys due to lack of cost-effectiveness data in the setting of high vaccine coverage in girls. Where high levels of HPV vaccine coverage have been achieved in females, heterosexual men have been observed to benefit from herd immunity; however, no protective effect has been observed in MSM, the highest group for HPV infection and associated disease [13].

HPV vaccine has been shown to be most effective prior to exposure to HPV [14]. Gender neutral immunization programmes providing vaccine for boys and girls will offer the greatest preventative potential; however, such programmes will not address the increased risk of HPV-associated disease in high-risk groups such as MSM. In addition, universal immunisation programmes are unlikely to be implemented in the short term given cost implication.

HPV vaccine has been demonstrated to be cost effective in MSM up to the age of 26 years over a range of assumptions [15]. Emerging evidence suggests that the vaccine may offer additional protective benefits in older MSM and that the vaccine may be cost effective in this group [16, 17].

The overarching aim of this chapter is to examine the burden of HPV infection and HPV-associated disease in MSM and HIV-infected MSM and to review potential preventative strategies.

Specifically this chapter examine the following:

1. Epidemiology of HPV infection and HPV-associated disease in MSM
2. Anal cancer screening in MSM
3. HPV vaccine for prevention of HPV infection and associated disease in MSM
4. Acceptability and feasibility of implementing targeted HPV vaccine programmes in MSM

2. HPV infection in MSM and HIV-positive MSM

HPV is the most common sexually transmitted infection worldwide. Lifetime risk of infection is estimated at 80% [18]. The vast majority of HPV infections are sub-clinical resolving spontaneously; however, a broad spectrum of presentations exist ranging from benign genital dermatoses to invasive malignancy. A complex interplay between host factors and viral factors impact on transmission and clearance as well as the clinical manifestation of HPV.

HPV infection in females has been the primary focus of research until recently given the causal link between HPV and cervical cancer. As the burden of extra-cervical HPV-associated malignancies has increased, and with the emergence of particular high-risk groups such as MSM, the research focus shifted.

While the natural history of HPV in females is well described, less is known about HPV infection in men. Numerous large longitudinal cohort studies have been undertaken in recent years to address this issue; however, eliciting the natural history of HPV infection is difficult.

Distinguishing between reinfection, reactivation of latent infection, incident infection, and clearance of infection is challenging in the setting of a multitude of host, viral, behavioral as well as sampling and analysis factors.

3. Prevalence of HPV infection in MSM

Prevalence of ano-genital HPV infection in men in the general population has been reported 1–84% [19, 20]. The wide range in prevalence observed is likely multifactorial relating to differences in study populations, sampling methods (including the anatomical sites of sampling), and analysis methods used.

The prevalence of anal HPV infection in MSM is higher than that observed in heterosexual men (47.2% versus 12.2%) [21]. The prevalence of high-risk (hr) or oncogenic anal HPV infection is documented at 26–73% in HIV negative MSM [10, 22, 23]. Prevalence of hr HPV has been shown to be significantly higher in HIV-infected MSM compared to HIV negative MSM with prevalence reported at up to 93% [24-26]. Receptive anal intercourse, number of sexual partners in the preceding six months and HIV infection have been identified as independent predictors of anal HPV infection [27, 28].

Prevalence of oropharyngeal and genital HPV infection has also been reported at significant rates (up to 45%) in MSM and HIV-infected MSM [29, 30].

Studies examining point prevalence of HPV infection provide important epidemiological insights. However, it is persistence of hr HPV infection that is the critical factor associated with development of malignancy.

4. Clearance of HPV infection

Clearance rates of hr HPV 16 anal infection have been reported at 12.2–18.7 per 1000 person months [31, 32]. Decreased clearance rates of hr HPV have been observed in HIV-infected compared with HIV-negative MSM, after adjusting for sexual behavior [28].

HIV infection has been identified as an independent predictor of HPV infection. Neither CD4 count nor nadir CD4 count has not been shown to influence clearance of HPV infection [10, 28, 33, 34]. This may partly explain high incidence of anal cancer observed in HIV-infected individuals despite immune reconstitution in the setting of highly active antiretroviral therapy (HAART).

5. Persistence of anal HPV infection

Persistence of hr HPV infection is the most important factor associated with anal cancer. MSM are frequently found to have multiple concurrent HPV infections in the anal canal. The most oncogenic hr HPV type 16 has been identified as the most likely HPV type to persist over time [35].

Given that prevalence of hr HPV is more common in HIV-infected MSM and rates of clearance are decreased, it is unsurprising that persistence of anal HPV in HIV-infected individuals is higher compared to HIV negative individuals [29, 36].

6. Incidence of HPV infection

Incidence of hr HPV type 16 in HIV-negative MSM ranged from 4.5 to 12.4 per 100 person-years. Incidence of hr HPV-16 in HIV-infected MSM is reported at 7.1 to 13.0 per 100 person years [28, 31, 32]. It remains unclear whether CD4 T cell count influences the incidence rate of anal hr HPV infection. One study reported increased hazards ratio in people with CD4 counts 200–499 cells/mm^3, compared to those with CD4 >500 cells/mm^3 [37]; however, this has not been a consistent finding [38].

7. Anal cancer

Anal squamous cell cancer (ASCC) accounts for 80% of all anal cancers. ASCC is a relatively rare occurrence in the general population with a reported incidence of 1–2 cases per 100,000 [8]; however, certain risk groups such as MSM and HIV-infected MSM are disproportionately affected. The incidence of anal cancer in MSM is reported at up to 40 cases per 100,000 [39] with up to 135 cases per 100,000 reported in HIV-infected MSM [8, 35].

The majority of AIDS defining malignancies have decreased since the advent of HAART; however, the incidence of anal cancer has increased dramatically [40]. The survival benefits associated with HAART have unmasked a cumulative risk of anal cancer which was not evident previously due to premature mortality relating to HIV infection.

HPV infection is causally associated with over 80% of anal cancers. HPV type 16 causes 66% of anal cancers while HPV type 18 is responsible for an additional 6% of cases [41]. Prevalence and persistence of the oncogenic HPV 16 are high in MSM and particularly HIV-positive MSM. So too is anal intraepithelial neoplasia (AIN), the precursor lesion for anal cancer. The natural history of progression from AIN to anal cancer differs from that of cervical intraepithelial neoplasia and remains poorly understood.

8. Similarities between anal cancer and cervical cancer

A number of similarities exist between ASCC and cervical cancer. Both cancers occur at the squamo-columnar junction epithelium. These transformation zones are characterised by high turnover epithelium that is thought to be particularly vulnerable to malignancy-inducing genetic alterations [42]. Both cancers are HPV associated. HPV is thought to promulgate changes to cells' DNA [43]. Immunosuppression is an important risk factor for both cancers with increased incidence observed in immunosuppressed patients such as transplant recipients and HIV-infected individuals [28, 44]. Both types of cancer also have widely divergent outcomes for early *vs* late presenting disease [45].

Similar to cervical cytology, cytological examination of anal cells can detect dysplastic cells. In contrast to the successes observed with cervical screening programmes, no effective screening modality has been demonstrated to impact on the morbidity and mortality associated with anal cancer.

9. Anal cancer and screening for anal cancer

Anal cancer frequently presents late (39% stage 3A or higher at diagnosis) with a lump, bleeding, incontinence from sphincter infiltration, fissure or fistula, and pain but also with nonspecific symptoms such as pruritus, discomfort, pelvic mass sensation, or change in bowel habit [46, 47].

Progression from normal epithelial mucosa to anal cancer transits through several precancerous stages, named anal intra-epithelial neoplasia (AIN) 1 to 3. AIN1 is considered low grade AIN (LGAIN); AIN 2 and 3 are considered high-grade AIN (HGAIN). AIN of any grade is common in MSM with rates of up to 50% reported in the literature [35].

Nearly a quarter of HGAIN lesions regress spontaneously within one year, while a minority of HGAIN (~1% per year) progresses to anal cancer [48].

Screening for anal cancer is a topic of much international debate. Some experts advocate for screening of high-risk populations such as MSM [49, 50]. However, no screening tool has been shown to impact morbidity or mortality of anal cancer.

Anal cytology is a poor predictor of HGAIN [51]. High resolution anoscopy (HRA) and biopsy of suspect lesions is considered the gold standard for detection of AIN in high-risk groups, although there are several important challenges including high cost, intra and inter-observer variability, and varying acceptability rates for HRA in patients [52]. In addition, the optimal treatment for HGAIN is yet to be established. Rate of recurrence of HGAIN after treatment is relatively high [50].

10. Head and neck cancer

Persistent infection with human papillomavirus (HPV) type 16 is also a major risk factor for the development of head and neck squamous cell carcinoma (HNSCC) and particularly development of oropharyngeal squamous cell carcinoma (OPSCC) [53]. HNSCCs include cancers of the oropharynx, oral cavity, and larynx. The incidence of HNSCC is increasing [54] and HNSCCs are now one of the 10 most common cancer seen worldwide [55].

HPV positive OPSCC has a unique clinical, histological, and molecular profile compared to HPV-negative OPSCC. Prognosis for HPV positive versus HPV negative OPSCC is significantly better independent of stage at diagnosis [56, 57]. HPV-negative OPSCC is associated with exposure to traditional carcinogens, such as tobacco and alcohol.

HIV-infected individuals are at increased risk of HPV infection and persistence of HPV infection. Similar to findings with other HPV-associated malignancies, prevalence of HNSCC is higher in HIV-infected individuals compared to the general population [58, 59]. The incidence of HNSCC is reported at 2–3 folds higher in HIV-infected individuals [60].

11. Penile cancer

Invasive penile cancer is rare. Over a third of penile cancer is associated with HPV, most commonly HPV type 16 and 18 [61]. The risk of penile cancer is up to four fold greater in HIV infected individuals compared to the general population [59].

12. HPV vaccine

Three vaccines have been licensed for the prevention of persistent HPV infection. All are subunit vaccines which use a recombinant form of the L1 major capsid protein of HPV as an antigen. L1 proteins self-assemble into noninfectious, nononcogenic units called virus-like particles (VLP).

The bivalent HPV vaccine HPV-2v (Cervarix™, GlaxoSmithKline) was approved by the FDA in 2009. The vaccine is approved for females 9 through 25 years of age. HPV2 is not approved for males. It protects against oncogenic HPV types 16 and 18 [62].

The quadrivalent HPV vaccine (HPV-4v) (Gardasil™, Merck and Co., Inc.) was approved by the FDA in June 2006. The vaccine is approved for females and males, 9 through 26 years of age. It offers additional protection against HPV types 6 and 11 commonly associated with genital warts as well as oncogenic HPV types 16 and 18 [63].

The nonavalent HPV vaccine (HPV-9v) (Gardasil 9™, Merck and Co., Inc.) was approved by the FDA in December 2014 and provides protection against 5 additional oncogenic HPV types (31, 33, 45, 52, and 58) [64].

HPV vaccines are highly immunogenic. More than 99% of recipients develop an antibody response to HPV types included in the respective vaccines one month after completing the three-dose series with comparable levels of antibody response following two doses [65]. However, there is no known serologic correlate of immunity and no known minimal titer has been determined to be protective.

HPV-4v has been demonstrated to be highly efficacious in preventing infection with HPV vaccine types related to external genital lesions, and anal intraepithelial neoplasia (AIN) in men [66]. The HPV-9v has been demonstrated to be highly efficacious in preventing infection with HPV vaccine types and disease related to the additional 5 types HPV-31, 33, 45, 52, and 58 in a susceptible population. Antibody response generated to HPV-6, 11, 16, and 18 were non-inferior to that generated by the HPV-4v vaccine, and thus the same indication as HPV-4v was applied [67]. No HPV vaccine has demonstrated protection beyond type covered in the vaccine.

The majority of developed countries have introduced national HPV immunization programmes for girls. A minority of countries including the US, Canada, and Australia now recommend provision of HPV vaccine for boys and girls.

While gender neutral vaccination programmes offer the best preventive opportunities, such programmes are unlikely to be implemented where levels of female vaccination coverage is high due to lack of cost-effectiveness evidence [68]. HPV vaccination of boys and male adolescents is not yet recommended in Ireland or in the majority of European countries that provide HPV vaccination for girls through national immunisation programs due to lack of cost effectiveness data.

High levels of female vaccination coverage have been shown to decrease genital warts in both females and unvaccinated heterosexual males through herd immunity; however, no protection has been observed in MSM. [13] Targeted vaccination of MSM has been shown to be cost-effective up to and beyond the age of 26 years [15, 16].

Despite the substantial clinical benefit of HPV vaccine in males, mathematical models suggest that HPV vaccination of males would exceed a cost-effectiveness threshold when vaccination coverage in females is high [68].

As yet no therapeutic benefit of the HPV vaccine has been demonstrated for the treatment of active disease present at the time of vaccination although early data suggests possible benefit of HPV vaccine in the setting of previous disease. This finding may represent an important opportunity for intervention in older high-risk patient groups such as HIV-infected MSM [69].

A single study has indicated that if the HPV vaccine proved efficacious in the HIV-positive population against vaccine sub-types, the potential reduction in anal cancer rates could be up to 61% [25].

In addition, data from female studies suggests that HPV vaccine of seropositive individuals who have cleared infection will provide increased protection against future infection [26].

In November 2014, the Joint Committee on Immunisation and Vaccination in the United Kingdom HPV sub-committee recommended implementation of a targeted programme of HPV vaccination for MSM >18 years to 40 years of age in GUM and HIV clinics if it could be delivered cost effectively [27].

13. Targeted HPV vaccine programmes

For HPV immunization programmes to have the desired effect, high levels of vaccine uptake are required. When considering feasibility of targeted HPV immunization programmes for MSM, HPV vaccine acceptability and factors influencing vaccine acceptability must be examined.

HPV vaccine acceptability in MSM is in Ireland is reported at 31–78%. Acceptability varied with stated vaccine cost and efficacy [70]. A meta-analysis of HPV vaccine acceptability in MSM including data from North America and Australia (where HPV vaccine is offered to boys and MSM up to the age of 26 years through national programmes) reported similar acceptability (47–74%) [71].

Factors identified as positively associated with HPV vaccine acceptability include knowledge of HPV infection and associated disease in MSM and no cost vaccine. Recommendation from a medical practitioner was also identified as being associated with HPV vaccine acceptability [72].

Evidence suggest that uptake of HPV vaccination in MSM would likely be high and would be expected to increase following implementation of health education programs outlining the risks of HPV-associated disease and efficacies of the HPV vaccine. Much of this education could be delivered synergistically using existing infrastructure alongside HIV prevention programmes.

14. Conclusion

The incidence of anal cancer is high in MSM, particularly HIV-infected MSM. Almost 80% of anal cancer is caused by persistent infection with hr HPV type 16 which is preventable through vaccination. While many experts advocate routine screening for anal cancer in high-risk groups such as MSM, it has not been demonstrated to impact on anal cancer related morbidity or mortality to date.

A growing body of evidence supports the potential of HPV vaccine to prevent development of HPV-associated disease in older MSM [69, 73]. Although no definite therapeutic benefit of HPV vaccine has been demonstrated for the treatment of active disease present at the time of vaccination, emerging data suggests a possible benefit of HPV vaccination in the setting of previous disease [16, 17].

Sexual health and HIV clinics would be well placed to facilitate targeted/catch-up HPV vaccination for the high-risk groups including HIV-infected and HIV negative MSM, particularly in the setting of similar effective models for hepatitis B vaccination[74, 75].

Further research is needed to assess potential for alternative screening modalities to impact the burden of anal cancer currently observed in MSM. Targeted HPV vaccine has potential to greatly reduce the burden of HPV-associated anal cancer in MSM and HIV-infected MSM in the future. Given the potential individual and population health benefits conferred, the HPV vaccine should not be withheld.

Author details

Corinna Sadlier[1,2*], Orla Sheils[3] and Colm Bergin[1,2]

*Address all correspondence to: sadliecm@tcd.ie

1 Department of Genitourinary Medicine and Infectious Diseases (GUIDE), St James's Hospital, Dublin, Ireland

2 Trinity College Dublin, Dublin, Ireland

3 Department of Histopathology, Trinity College Dublin, St James's Hospital, James's Street, Dublin, Ireland

References

[1] Einstein, M.H., et al., *Clinician's guide to human papillomavirus immunology: knowns and unknowns.* Lancet Infect Dis, 2009. 9(6): pp. 347–356.

[2] Giuliano, A.R., et al., *Epidemiology of human papillomavirus infection in men, cancers other than cervical and benign conditions.* Vaccine, 2008. 26 Suppl 10: pp. K17–K28.

[3] Forman, D., et al., *Global burden of human papillomavirus and related diseases.* Vaccine, 2012. 30 Suppl 5: p. F12–F23.

[4] Chen, Z., L.B. de Freitas, and R.D. Burk, *Evolution and classification of oncogenic human papillomavirus types and variants associated with cervical cancer.* Methods Mol Biol, 2015. 1249: pp. 3–26.

[5] Gustafsson, L., et al., *International incidence rates of invasive cervical cancer before cytological screening.* Int J Cancer, 1997. 71(2): pp. 159–165.

[6] Parkin, D.M. and F. Bray, *Chapter 2: The burden of HPV-related cancers.* Vaccine, 2006. 24 Suppl 3: p. S3/11-25.

[7] van der Zee, R.P., et al., *The increasing incidence of anal cancer: can it be explained by trends in risk groups?* Neth J Med, 2013. 71(8): pp. 401–411.

[8] Patel, P., et al., *Incidence of types of cancer among HIV-infected persons compared with the general population in the United States, 1992-2003.* Ann Intern Med, 2008. 148(10): pp. 728–736.

[9] D'Souza, G., et al., *Incidence and epidemiology of anal cancer in the multicenter AIDS cohort study.* J Acquir Immune Defic Syndr, 2008. 48(4): pp. 491–499.

[10] Machalek, D.A., et al., *Anal human papillomavirus infection and associated neoplastic lesions in men who have sex with men: a systematic review and meta-analysis.* Lancet Oncol, 2012. 13(5): pp. 487–500.

[11] Palefsky, J.M., *Anal cancer prevention in HIV-positive men and women.* Curr Opin Oncol, 2009. 21(5): pp. 433–438.

[12] Barroso, L.F., *Anal cancer screening.* Lancet Oncol, 2012. 13(7): pp. e278–279; author reply e280.

[13] Ali, H., et al., *Genital warts in young Australians five years into national human papillomavirus vaccination programme: national surveillance data.* Bmj, 2013. 346: p. f2032.

[14] Medeiros, L.R., et al., *Efficacy of human papillomavirus vaccines: a systematic quantitative review.* Int J Gynecol Cancer, 2009. 19(7): pp. 1166–1176.

[15] Kim, J.J., *Targeted human papillomavirus vaccination of men who have sex with men in the USA: a cost-effectiveness modelling analysis.* Lancet Infect Dis, 2010. 10(12): pp. 845–852.

[16] Deshmukh, A.A., et al., *Clinical effectiveness and cost-effectiveness of quadrivalent human papillomavirus vaccination in HIV-negative men who have sex with men to prevent recurrent high-grade anal intraepithelial neoplasia.* Vaccine, 2014. 32(51): pp. 6941–6947.

[17] Deshmukh, A.A., et al., *Long-Term Outcomes of Adding HPV Vaccine to the Anal Intraepithelial Neoplasia Treatment Regimen in HIV-Positive Men Who Have Sex With Men.* Clin Infect Dis, 2015. 61(10): pp. 1527–1535.

[18] Weaver, B.A., *Epidemiology and natural history of genital human papillomavirus infection.* J Am Osteopath Assoc, 2006. 106(3 Suppl 1): pp. S2–8.

[19] Dunne, E.F., et al., *Prevalence of HPV infection among men: A systematic review of the literature.* J Infect Dis, 2006. 194(8): pp. 1044–1057.

[20] Smith, J.S., et al., *Age-specific prevalence of human papillomavirus infection in males: a global review.* J Adolesc Health, 2011. 48(6): pp. 540–552.

[21] Nyitray, A.G., et al., *Age-specific prevalence of and risk factors for anal human papillomavirus (HPV) among men who have sex with women and men who have sex with men: the HPV in men (HIM) study.* J Infect Dis, 2011. 203(1): pp. 49–57.

[22] van der Snoek, E.M., et al., *Human papillomavirus infection in men who have sex with men participating in a Dutch gay-cohort study.* Sex Transm Dis, 2003. 30(8): pp. 639–644.

[23] Chin-Hong, P.V., et al., *Age-Specific prevalence of anal human papillomavirus infection in HIV-negative sexually active men who have sex with men: the EXPLORE study.* J Infect Dis, 2004. 190(12): pp. 2070–2076.

[24] Sadlier, C., et al., *Prevalence of human papillomavirus in men who have sex with men in the era of an effective vaccine; a call to act.* HIV Med, 2014. 15(8): pp. 499–504.

[25] Parisi, S.G., et al., *Anal and oral human papillomavirus (HPV) infection in HIV-infected subjects in northern Italy: a longitudinal cohort study among men who have sex with men.* BMC Infect Dis, 2011. 11: p. 150.

[26] Palefsky, J.M., et al., *Prevalence and risk factors for human papillomavirus infection of the anal canal in human immunodeficiency virus (HIV)-positive and HIV-negative homosexual men.* J Infect Dis, 1998. 177(2): pp. 361–367.

[27] Goldstone, S., et al., *Prevalence of and risk factors for human papillomavirus (HPV) infection among HIV-seronegative men who have sex with men.* J Infect Dis, 2011. 203(1): pp. 66–74.

[28] Mooij, S.H., et al., *The effect of HIV infection on anal and penile human papillomavirus incidence and clearance: a cohort study among MSM.* Aids, 2016. 30(1): pp. 121–132.

[29] Sadlier, C., et al., *Human papillomavirus (HPV) and the usefulness of the HPV vaccine for men who have sex with men.* J Infect Dis, 2014. 210(10): p. 1679.

[30] Beachler, D.C. and G. D'Souza, *Oral human papillomavirus infection and head and neck cancers in HIV-infected individuals.* Curr Opin Oncol, 2013. 25(5): pp. 503–510.

[31] de Pokomandy, A., et al., *Prevalence, clearance, and incidence of anal human papillomavirus infection in HIV-infected men: the HIPVIRG cohort study.* J Infect Dis, 2009. 199(7): pp. 965–973.

[32] Darwich, L., et al., *Prevalence, clearance, and incidence of human papillomavirus type-specific infection at the anal and penile site of HIV-infected men.* Sex Transm Dis, 2013. 40(8): pp. 611–618.

[33] Beachler, D.C., et al., *Natural history of anal vs oral HPV infection in HIV-infected men and women.* J Infect Dis, 2013. 208(2): pp. 330–339.

[34] del Amo, J., et al., *What drives the number of high-risk human papillomavirus types in the anal canal in HIV-positive men who have sex with men?* J Infect Dis, 2013. 207(8): pp. 1235–1241.

[35] Sahasrabuddhe, V.V., et al., *Human papillomavirus genotype attribution and estimation of preventable fraction of anal intraepithelial neoplasia cases among HIV-infected men who have sex with men.* J Infect Dis, 2013. 207(3): pp. 392–401.

[36] Geskus, R.B., et al., *Incidence and clearance of anal high-risk human papillomavirus in HIV-positive men who have sex with men: estimates and risk factors.* Aids, 2016. 30(1): pp. 37–44.

[37] Hernandez, A.L., et al., *Risk factors for anal human papillomavirus infection type 16 among HIV-positive men who have sex with men in San Francisco.* J Acquir Immune Defic Syndr, 2013. 63(4): pp. 532–539.

[38] Mbulawa, Z.Z., et al., *Impact of human immunodeficiency virus on the natural history of human papillomavirus genital infection in South African men and women.* J Infect Dis, 2012. 206(1): pp. 15–27.

[39] Jemal, A., et al., *Cancer statistics, 2003.* CA Cancer J Clin, 2003. 53(1): pp. 5–26.

[40] Brickman, C. and J.M. Palefsky, *Cancer in the HIV-infected host: epidemiology and pathogenesis in the antiretroviral era.* Curr HIV/AIDS Rep, 2015. 12(4): pp. 388–396.

[41] De Vuyst, H., et al., *Prevalence and type distribution of human papillomavirus in carcinoma and intraepithelial neoplasia of the vulva, vagina and anus: a meta-analysis.* Int J Cancer, 2009. 124(7): pp. 1626–1636.

[42] Schiffman, M., et al., *Human papillomavirus testing in the prevention of cervical cancer.* J Natl Cancer Inst, 2011. 103(5): pp. 368–383.

[43] Darragh, T.M., et al., *The Lower Anogenital Squamous Terminology Standardization Project for HPV-Associated Lesions: background and consensus recommendations from the College of American Pathologists and the American Society for Colposcopy and Cervical Pathology.* Arch Pathol Lab Med, 2012. 136(10): pp. 1266–1297.

[44] Berkhout, R.J., J.N. Bouwes Bavinck, and J. ter Schegget, *Persistence of human papillomavirus DNA in benign and (pre)malignant skin lesions from renal transplant recipients.* J Clin Microbiol, 2000. 38(6): pp. 2087–2096.

[45] Program, S.R., *SEER Stat Fact Sheets: Cervix Uteri Cancer.* Bethesda, MD: National Cancer Institute, 2015.

[46] Simpson, S. and R. Turner, *Four decades of anal cancer in Tasmania, Australia: what do the case data tell us?* Sex Health, 2012. 9(3): pp. 213–219.

[47] Simpson, J.A. and J.H. Scholefield, *Diagnosis and management of anal intraepithelial neoplasia and anal cancer.* Bmj, 2011. 343: p. d6818.

[48] Conley, L., et al., *Factors associated with prevalent abnormal anal cytology in a large cohort of HIV-infected adults in the United States.* J Infect Dis, 2010. 202(10): pp. 1567–1576.

[49] Abramowitz, L., et al., *Determinants of macroscopic anal cancer and pre-cancerous lesions in 1206 HIV-infected screened patients.* Colorectal Dis, 2016.

[50] Schofield, A.M., et al., *A prospective study of anal cancer screening in HIV positive and negative men who have sex with men; results of Analogy.* Aids, 2016.

[51] Botes, L.P., et al., *Anal cytological abnormalities are poor predictors of high-grade intraepithelial neoplasia amongst HIV-positive men who have sex with men.* Sex Health, 2013. 10(1): pp. 9–17.

[52] Hillman, R.J., et al., *Ability to detect high-grade squamous anal intraepithelial lesions at high resolution anoscopy improves over time.* Sex Health, 2016.

[53] Andersen, A.S., et al., *The interplay between HPV and host immunity in head and neck squamous cell carcinoma.* Int J Cancer, 2014. 134(12): pp. 2755–2763.

[54] Chaturvedi, A.K., et al., *Human papillomavirus and rising oropharyngeal cancer incidence in the United States.* J Clin Oncol, 2011. 29(32): pp. 4294–4301.

[55] Ferlay, J., et al., *Cancer incidence and mortality worldwide: sources, methods and major patterns in GLOBOCAN 2012.* Int J Cancer, 2015. 136(5): pp. E359–386.

[56] Fakhry, C., et al., *Improved survival of patients with human papillomavirus-positive head and neck squamous cell carcinoma in a prospective clinical trial.* J Natl Cancer Inst, 2008. 100(4): pp. 261–269.

[57] Ang, K.K., et al., *Human papillomavirus and survival of patients with oropharyngeal cancer.* N Engl J Med, 2010. 363(1): pp. 24–35.

[58] Picard, A., et al., *HPV prevalence in HIV patients with head and neck squamous cell carcinoma.* Aids, 2016.

[59] Grulich, A.E., et al., *Incidence of cancers in people with HIV/AIDS compared with immunosuppressed transplant recipients: a meta-analysis.* Lancet, 2007. 370(9581): pp. 59–67.

[60] Kreimer, A.R., et al., *Oral human papillomavirus infection in adults is associated with sexual behavior and HIV serostatus.* J Infect Dis, 2004. 189(4): pp. 686–698.

[61] Alemany, L., et al., *Role of Human Papillomavirus in Penile Carcinomas Worldwide.* Eur Urol, 2016.

[62] *FDA licensure of bivalent human papillomavirus vaccine (HPV2, Cervarix) for use in females and updated HPV vaccination recommendations from the Advisory Committee on Immunization Practices (ACIP).* MMWR Morb Mortal Wkly Rep, 2010. 59(20): pp. 626–629.

[63] *FDA licensure of quadrivalent human papillomavirus vaccine (HPV4, Gardasil) for use in males and guidance from the Advisory Committee on Immunization Practices (ACIP).* MMWR Morb Mortal Wkly Rep, 2010. 59(20): pp. 630–632.

[64] Petrosky, E., et al., *Use of 9-valent human papillomavirus (HPV) vaccine: updated HPV vaccination recommendations of the advisory committee on immunization practices.* MMWR Morb Mortal Wkly Rep, 2015. 64(11): pp. 300–304.

[65] Sankaranarayanan, R., et al., *Immunogenicity and HPV infection after one, two, and three doses of quadrivalent HPV vaccine in girls in India: a multicentre prospective cohort study.* Lancet Oncol, 2016. 17(1): pp. 67–77.

[66] Giuliano, A.R., et al., *Efficacy of quadrivalent HPV vaccine against HPV Infection and disease in males.* N Engl J Med, 2011. 364(5): pp. 401–411.

[67] Joura, E.A., et al., *A 9-valent HPV vaccine against infection and intraepithelial neoplasia in women.* N Engl J Med, 2015. 372(8): pp. 711–723.

[68] Kim, J.J. and S.J. Goldie, *Cost effectiveness analysis of including boys in a human papillomavirus vaccination programme in the United States.* Bmj, 2009. 339: p. b3884.

[69] Swedish, K.A. and S.E. Goldstone, *Prevention of anal condyloma with quadrivalent human papillomavirus vaccination of older men who have sex with men.* PLoS One, 2014. 9(4): p. e93393.

[70] Corinna Sadlier, A.L., Siobhan O'Dea, Sandra Delamere, Mick Qinlan, Susan Clarke, Orla Sheils (ORCID-0000-0002-4493-9496) & Colm Bergin *HPV vaccine acceptability in HIV-infected and HIV negative men who have sex with men (MSM) in Ireland.* Human Vaccines & Immunotherapeutics, 2016.

[71] Nadarzynski, T., et al., *Human papillomavirus and vaccine-related perceptions among men who have sex with men: a systematic review.* Sex Transm Infect, 2014. 90(7): pp. 515–523.

[72] Newman, P.A., et al., *HPV vaccine acceptability among men: a systematic review and meta-analysis.* Sex Transm Infect, 2013. 89(7): pp. 568–574.

[73] Swedish, K.A., S.H. Factor, and S.E. Goldstone, *Prevention of recurrent high-grade anal neoplasia with quadrivalent human papillomavirus vaccination of men who have sex with men: a nonconcurrent cohort study.* Clin Infect Dis, 2012. 54(7): pp. 891–898.

[74] King, E.M., *Human papillomavirus epidemiology in men who have sex with men: implications for a vaccine programme at sexual health clinics in the UK.* 2015, UCL (University College London).

[75] Rock, C., et al., *Impact of a new vaccine clinic on hepatitis B vaccine completion and immunological response rates in an HIV-positive cohort.* J Infect Public Health, 2013. 6(3): pp. 173–178.

Permissions

 Every chapter published in this book has been scrutinized by our experts. Their significance has been extensively debated. The topics covered herein carry significant findings which will fuel the growth of the discipline. They may even be implemented as practical applications or may be referred to as a beginning point for another development.

The contributors of this book come from diverse backgrounds, making this book a truly international effort. This book will bring forth new frontiers with its revolutionizing research information and detailed analysis of the nascent developments around the world.

We would like to thank all the contributing authors for lending their expertise to make the book truly unique. They have played a crucial role in the development of this book. Without their invaluable contributions this book wouldn't have been possible. They have made vital efforts to compile up to date information on the varied aspects of this subject to make this book a valuable addition to the collection of many professionals and students.

This book was conceptualized with the vision of imparting up-to-date information and advanced data in this field. To ensure the same, a matchless editorial board was set up. Every individual on the board went through rigorous rounds of assessment to prove their worth. After which they invested a large part of their time researching and compiling the most relevant data for our readers.

The editorial board has been involved in producing this book since its inception. They have spent rigorous hours researching and exploring the diverse topics which have resulted in the successful publishing of this book. They have passed on their knowledge of decades through this book. To expedite this challenging task, the publisher supported the team at every step. A small team of assistant editors was also appointed to further simplify the editing procedure and attain best results for the readers.

Apart from the editorial board, the designing team has also invested a significant amount of their time in understanding the subject and creating the most relevant covers. They scrutinized every image to scout for the most suitable representation of the subject and create an appropriate cover for the book.

The publishing team has been an ardent support to the editorial, designing and production team. Their endless efforts to recruit the best for this project, has resulted in the accomplishment of this book. They are a veteran in the field of academics and their pool of knowledge is as vast as their experience in printing. Their expertise and guidance has proved useful at every step. Their uncompromising quality standards have made this book an exceptional effort. Their encouragement from time to time has been an inspiration for everyone.

The publisher and the editorial board hope that this book will prove to be a valuable piece of knowledge for researchers, students, practitioners and scholars across the globe.

List of Contributors

J. Rajčáni, O. el Hassoun and M. Benčat
Pathology Ltd, Diagnostic Center, Alpha Medical Ltd, Záborského 2, 03601 Martin, Slovak Republic

M. Adamkov
Pathology Ltd, Diagnostic Center, Alpha Medical Ltd, Záborského 2, 03601 Martin, Slovak Republic
Department of Histology, Jessenius Medical Faculty, Comenius University, Martin, Slovak Republic

K. Kajo
Pathology Ltd, Diagnostic Laboratory, Alpha medical Ltd, Banská Bystrica, Slovak Republic
Department of Pathology, St. Elisabeth Cancer Institute, Bratislava, Slovak Republic

Noor Al-Antary
College of Medicine & Biomedical Research Centre, Qatar University, Doha, Qatar

Ala-Eddin Al Moustafa
College of Medicine & Biomedical Research Centre, Qatar University, Doha, Qatar
Oncology Department, McGill University, Montreal, Quebec, Canada
Syrian Research Cancer Centre of the Syrian Society against Cancer, Aleppo, Syria

Amber Yasmeen
Segal Cancer Centre, Lady Davis Institute for Medical Research, JGH, McGill University, Montreal, Quebec, Canada

Ruxandra Stanculescu
Obstetrics and Gynaecology Department, "Carol Davila" University of Medicine, "St. Pantelimon"Clinical Emergency Hospital Bucharest, Romania

Makbule Tambas
Department of Radiation Oncology, Okmeydani Training and Research Hospital, Istanbul, Turkey

Musa Altun
Department of Radiation Oncology, Istanbul Faculty of Medicine, Istanbul University, Istanbul, Turkey

Deniz Tural
Department of Medical Oncology, Bakirkoy Dr. Sadi Konuk Education and Research Hospital, Istanbul, Turkey

Laurence M. Vaughan, Brian R. Faherty, Erin C. Gutierrez, James M. Harris, William A. Nussbaumer and Ryan J. Schwab
Diagnostics Systems, BD Life Sciences, Sparks, MD, USA

Naveed Shahzad and Memoona Ramzan
School of Biological Sciences, University of the Punjab, Lahore, Pakistan

Muhammad Umer
National Institute for Biotechnology and Genetic Engineering, Faisalabad, Pakistan

Bilal Aslam
Department of Microbiology, Government College University Faisalabad, Pakistan

Slawomir A. Dutkiewicz and Anna Rezner
Department of Prevention and Epidemiology of Neoplasms, Medical School and Faculty of Health Sciences, Institute of Public Health, Jan Kochanowski University, Kielce, Poland

Witold Rezner
Neoplasm Pathology Department, The Holycross Cancer Centre in Kielce, Kielce, Poland

Jack Chalasinski
Atlantic University School of Medicine, Gros Islet Highway, Rodney Bay, Saint Lucia, West Indies

Elena López-Díez
Department of Urology, University Hospital of Vigo, Vigo, Spain

Sonia Pérez
Department of Microbiology, University Hospital of Vigo, Vigo, Spain

Amparo Iñarrea
Department of Obstetrics and Gynecology, University Hospital of Vigo, Vigo, Spain

Corinna Sadlier and Colm Bergin
Department of Genitourinary Medicine and Infectious Diseases (GUIDE), St James's Hospital, Dublin, Ireland
Trinity College Dublin, Dublin, Ireland

Orla Sheils
Department of Histopathology, Trinity College Dublin, St James's Hospital, James's Street, Dublin, Ireland

Index

www.ingramcontent.com/pod-product-compliance
Lightning Source LLC
LaVergne TN
LVHW060520210926
848485LV00005B/1111